Master Educator

Student Course Book

Part I—Basic Teaching Skills for Career Education Instructors

Part II—Basic Teaching Skills for Career Education in the Beauty and Wellness Disciplines

Part III—Professional Development for Career Education Instructors

Letha Barnes

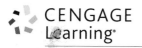

CENGAGE Learning

Australia • Brazil • Japan • Korea • Mexico • Singapore • Spain • United Kingdom • United States

CENGAGE
Learning®

Master Educator Student Course Book, Third Edition
Letha Barnes

Vice President, Milady & Learning Solutions Strategy, Professional: Dawn Gerrain

Director of Content & Business Development, Milady: Sandra Bruce

Associate Acquisitions Editor: Philip I. Mandl

Product Manager: Maria Moffre-Barnes

Editorial Assistant: Elizabeth A. Edwards

Director, Marketing & Training: Gerard McAvey

Associate Marketing Manager: Matthew McGuire

Senior Production Director: Wendy Troeger

Production Manager: Sherondra Thedford

Senior Content Project Manager: Nina Tucciarelli

Senior Art Director: Benj Gleeksman

For product information and technology assistance, contact us at
Cengage Learning Customer & Sales Support, 1-800-354-9706
For permission to use material from this text or product,
submit all requests online at **www.cengage.com/permissions**
Further permissions questions can be emailed to
permissionrequest@cengage.com

Library of Congress Control Number: 2012956270

ISBN-13: 978-1-133-69369-7

ISBN-10: 1-133-69369-5

Milady
Executive Woods
5 Maxwell Drive
Clifton Park, NY 12065
USA

Cengage Learning is a leading provider of customized learning solutions with office locations around the globe, including Singapore, the United Kingdom, Australia, Mexico, Brazil, and Japan. Locate your local office at **www.cengage.com/global**

Cengage Learning products are represented in Canada by Nelson Education, Ltd.

To learn more about Milady, visit **milady.cengage.com**

Purchase any of our products at your local college store or at our preferred online store **www.cengagebrain.com**

Notice to the Reader

Printed in the United States of America
2 3 4 5 6 7 17 16 15 14

This book is dedicated to my mother and best friend, "Pickle" Trapp, a talented and skilled educator and school owner who provided the foundation of my passion for improving career education. She was an inspiration to me and thousands of students throughout her career. Thank you, Mom, for your love, support, and dedication to career education. I miss you.

—Letha

About the Author

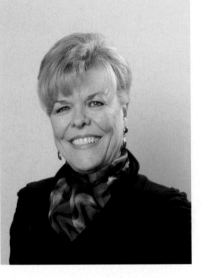

LETHA BARNES is a third-generation educator and school owner. In her more than 40 years in career education, she has earned many accomplishments.

She served the State of New Mexico for 10 years as the school representative on the Board of Barbers and Cosmetologists, holding the position of vice chairman or chairman during the entire tenure. She is a former president of the American Association of Cosmetology Schools (AACS), during which time she spearheaded the effort, with the assistance of a great team of professionals, to re-establish the educational branch of the association, which is known today as Cosmetology Educators of America. She was designated the AACS Person of the Year in 1995. She is the recipient of the AACS Special Recognition Award for her Contribution to Cosmetology Education and the AACS Award of Distinction for Lifetime Contribution to Cosmetology Education. Her schools were recognized in 1998 as runners-up for the American Salon Big Apple Award. She was also the recipient of the Dygve-Kretzmer 1999 Community Service Award. In addition, she was the 2001 recipient of the coveted N. F. Cimaglia Award.

As an approved provider of continuing education and former Director of the Career Institute, Ms. Barnes has presented continuing-education programs to tens of thousands of educators, professionals, and students throughout the United States and Canada. She has been a speaker at many regional, national, and international events, including Hairworld '96, Great Clips for Hair National Conventions, AACS Mid-Year Conferences, AACS annual conventions, the National Interstate Council of State Boards annual conferences, and numerous Cosmetology Educators of America conventions. She is well known for her highly energetic presentations and her passion for education. She has testified before the New Mexico State Senate and a U.S. Congressional Subcommittee on behalf of career education. She served as a school-owner commissioner, an academic commissioner, and first vice chairman for the National Accrediting Commission of Cosmetology Arts and Science (NACCAS) and she taught the NACCAS Accreditation Workshops for over 10 years.

In addition to this textbook, Ms. Barnes has authored numerous other works for Cengage Learning, including course management guides for cosmetology, fundamentals of esthetics, advanced esthetics, nail technology, and instructor training, as well as several editions of the Instructor Support Slides for those same disciplines. She has also developed and authored four editions of the *Essential Companion Study Guide* that accompanies the *Standard: Cosmetology* core textbook.

Foreword

by Bill Church

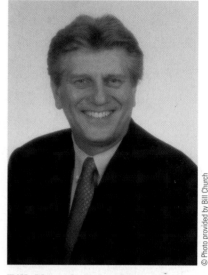

When asked by Letha Barnes to write a foreword for the third edition of the *Master Educator* textbook, several thoughts entered my mind. My first thought was that of Letha herself and how she has transformed career education by developing and impacting educators throughout the United States and beyond. Second, I was flattered at being asked to contribute in a small way to that endeavor. Third, and perhaps most important, I believe that the *Master Educator* textbook and its accompanying training modules impact instructors and students in ways that can hardly be measured.

Let me give you an example. I have taught for 30 years, both part time and full time at the public school and university levels. When I was first introduced to the Master Educator program and asked to teach a module for the Career Institute, I was completely "blown away" by the quality of material I saw. In both undergraduate and graduate school, I attended all of the university education courses required for my major. After reviewing all of the material contained in the *Master Educator*, I have come to this conclusion: once an instructor completes a program of study using the *Master Educator* textbook and/or attends all the accompanying modules offered by the Career Institute, he or she will have been exposed to more information than one who was trained at the university level. The material that Letha has developed for this book is that good.

Let's look for a moment at what that means to career education. Too often, new instructors are hired on a Friday, given a textbook to review over the weekend, and asked to begin teaching on Monday or Tuesday—a monumental task at best! If it were within my power, completing the Master Educator program would be a requirement for all instructors before they entered a classroom. Since such a requirement is not always practical, ongoing training, as early as possible, for both new and veteran instructors, is necessary. Better-trained instructors translate to better-trained students. Better-trained students translate to more professional employees. More professional employees translate to better incomes and more respect throughout any profession. The Master Educator program does all that and more. It was an inspiration for me when instructors in my Career Institute classrooms looked at me at the end of our session and said, "Thank you for empowering me with this information. Where has it been all my life?" Or, "This is the kind of material I have been looking for since I began teaching."

Read this book. Use this book. It will empower both you and your students, and ultimately make a difference in your graduates' career success. There is nothing I have seen for instructors that even comes close to the quality of information contained in this book.

Thank you, Letha Barnes, for your part in changing the face of career education. Keep up the good work!

Bill Church, BA., MA

Bill Church, BA., MA
Owner, Regency Beauty Institute, Cleveland Ohio
Past president, American Association of Cosmetology Schools (AACS)
Past chairman, National Accrediting Commission of Career Arts and Sciences (NACCAS)
2008 recipient of the N. F. Cimaglia Award

Foreword

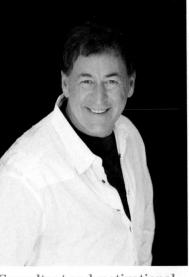

Consultant and motivational speaker
Director of Motivation for *Hair Color & Design Magazine*
Author of *Success Dynamics*
Inductee of North American Hairstyling Awards Hall of Leaders

by Geno Stampora

I can still remember the first day I entered the beauty academy to see if it was right for me. I ran into an instructor before seeing the registrar. She shared with me the importance of what a beauty professional provides the public. She even shared with me some of the history of beauty professionals. It was after our brief visit that I had made my decision, even before sitting down to discuss how it all works. I can still remember the feeling of opening my kit for the first time and having my instructor explain what was inside and how I would use these tools to forge a great future in beauty.

It was difficult for me. I always had the personality and the love of people on my side, but to learn the technical stuff was a challenge. I was fortunate to have instructors that took the time to understand me and my learning style. My respect for them is great and it grew as I progressed through my career. Then the feeling of standing in front of my first class and seeing the same excitement that I had in the faces of those future professionals was priceless.

A great educator does whatever it takes to discover and share with every different student just what they need to make it. They are selfless, giving, educated, and talented in breaking through and communicating what is necessary to every student they come in contact with. They know that for many students this relationship will never be forgotten.

Letha Barnes is the essence and substance of beauty. She is all the things above and more. This new and special tool, the *Master Educator,* is years of knowledge and experience compiled into a book written by a Master.

When well-studied, read, and reread, this textbook will provide you with much of what you need to create success for you and for all of the students whose lives you have the privilege to touch.

I have always said that the future of beauty is the four walls of an academy that has our students inside. That is where it starts. I thank Cengage Learning and Letha Barnes for providing the great tools of success, beginning with this book. The future of beauty is in your hands. Be a Master at what you do. Hold high the knowledge and skills needed to make our students the best they can be.

Geno Stampora

Preface

The purpose of the *Master Educator* is to offer teaching methodology, learning philosophy, and professional development for aspiring career educators. It is intended to be adopted by schools offering instructor training as a core program in the overall curriculum. The material is applicable to educators within any discipline of career education. It is designed to work effectively in an instructor-led classroom environment but can also be used in a mentor/self-study environment, allowing learners to move at their own pace, which encourages independent study. Part I is designed to address all the core information required to pass a basic instructor-licensing examination if one is required in your career discipline. Part II contains three additional chapters that are specific to disciplines within the Beauty and Wellness industry. Part III takes the basic instructor a step further and deals with subject matter more relevant to a seasoned educator or one who wants to pursue professional development. The entire textbook supports the Career Institute's Master Educator Certification program, which offers one-day training modules in educator development. For more information, please go to www.milady.cengage.com/careerinst.

Why This Text Was Developed

Education within career education has undergone a drastic series of changes in the past decade, and it continues to change, just as the businesses within the variety of career fields have experienced significant changes. Career education now demands new approaches in teaching and new directions for learning. The *Master Educator* is a core textbook that addresses these new approaches and directions.

Before the first edition of this textbook, there was an outcry for quality material that would prepare educators for the marketplace. As a third-generation educator, I have been blessed with a passion for career education and compassion for my students. I recognize those same characteristics in other educators throughout the United States. Many have told me how they would have given anything to have quality educational materials to help prepare them for their roles as educators. Others have told me that even though they have been teaching for a while and they are blessed with the passion, they did not feel they had the training or the tools to facilitate the best possible education for their students prior to the publication of the first edition of the *Master Educator*. It has been with those educators and the future educators of America in mind that this project evolved and has been revised. Initially, schools and educators throughout the United States were surveyed to determine what qualities and characteristics were sought in educators as well as the major educator challenges that schools face on a regular basis. Every possible attempt was made to address all of the issues identified in those surveys. Anyone who is a career practitioner in any discipline and wishes to become a provider of education to others within their field will benefit from studying this material. It has been tested and proven in classrooms within many disciplines.

Organization of Material

Written in a clear, easy-to-read style, the textbook is user-friendly and will serve as a resource that learners and educators can draw on to develop their own plans of action in the classroom. The book is divided into three parts to address training for career education instructors. The first part accommodates the needs of the most basic instructor training programs, such as those states that require 600 hours or less. Part two contains three additional chapters specific to the beauty and wellness career fields. The third volume is added to meet the needs of more comprehensive programs as well as the needs of those already licensed instructors who wish to further their professional development.

Part I contains the following chapters: The Career Education Instructor; The Teaching Plan and Learning Environment; Teaching Study and Testing Skills, Basic Learning Styles and Principles; Basic Methods of Teaching and Learning; Communicating Confidently; Effective Presentations; Effective Classroom Management and Supervision; Achieving Learner Results; Program Review, Development, and Lesson Planning; Educational Aids and Technology in the Classroom; Assessing Progress and Advising Students. Part II contains the following chapters: Making the Student Salon an Adventure; Career and Employment Preparation, and The Art of Retaining Students. Part III deals with more advanced subject matter as well as career development topics, with the following chapters: Educator Relationships; Learning Is a Laughing Matter; Teaching Success Strategies for a Winning Career; Teams at Work; and Evaluating Professional Performance.

Each chapter contains stated objectives, review questions, and a marginal glossary of key terms.

How to Use This Material

The text provides integration of theory and applied methods for master educators teaching any discipline, including those training to become an educator. The hope is to create a comprehensive, conceptual, and practical framework for generating learning outcomes for every learner type. The future of vocational careers depends in large part on the quality of education provided in career education schools throughout the world. In recent years, every area of education has been challenged to adjust to increasing diversity among students, changing social conditions, and significant personal "baggage" carried by today's students. For training to be effective, educators must be able to meet and overcome these challenges. As a master educator, you become a "facilitator" of growth, insight, change, and improvement. Your students will discover that answers come from within. Education in any field cannot rise above the quality and ability of its teachers.

This book can be used by educators to teach their students to become educators. In addition, it is designed to be used for independent study by those wishing to become educators. Each learner should review the objectives listed at the beginning of each chapter, read the chapter thoroughly, complete the review questions found at the end of each chapter, and observe the accompanying videos. The comprehensive *Instructor Resource* provides detailed lesson plans with supplementary educational materials to make the information even more meaningful. It will be up to the educator within the course of study to use those materials to make learning even more effective for those enrolled in a teacher-training program.

In your quest for excellence as a master educator, you must be a role model for your students. Your own behavior, attitude, and image will set the example for your students. Your personal planning, your adherence to the rules of learning that you set forth, your enthusiasm, and your interest in your students and their goals will make an everlasting impression on your students. You must move from a *teacher-centered* method of education to a *student-centered* environment. This textbook is designed to help you make that transition and unleash the learning potential of the adults whom you train.

By completing this course of study using the *Master Educator*, you will learn valuable qualities needed in an educator. You will discover and gain knowledge of educational methods that assist in learner attention and retention.

Features

The textbook and accompanying ancillaries have several distinctive features:

Text book

- Pedagogical use of color accelerates learning through illustrated material.
- Measurable performance objectives needed for success are spelled out at the beginning of each chapter.
- Forms, charts, and illustrations are used for clarification.
- The Critical Concept feature opens each chapter.
- The Master Educator board feature found at the beginning of each chapter lists key performance measures of master educators.
- It's Worth Remembering feature includes quotable information relevant to the topic.
- The Consider and Connect feature contains key points relevant to the topic.
- Insights that reflect the philosophies of several highly successful educators.
- A glossary that contains key terms and definitions for use in creating flash cards.
- The Wrapping It Up feature contains a brief summary of the important points contained in the chapter.
- The In Retrospect feature contains review questions included in each chapter.

Instructor Resource on CD

- Detailed lesson plans for each chapter of the text and more.
- Learning-reinforcement ideas and activities for each lesson.
- Multiple-choice tests for each chapter.
- Computerized test bank.
- Instructor support slides with instructor notes.

Master Educator CourseMate

- Content follows the Master Educator core text.
- Content-rich, web-based learning aid that presents information in a new and different way.
- 24×7 access
- Provides tools and content that allow for more effective management of time, progress checks, exam preparation, and organization of notes.
- Designed for integration of additional technology into programs that accommodate the ever-changing learning styles.
- Student Features include: Chapter Learning Objectives, Study Sheets, Online Chapter Quizzes, Webinars, Discussion Topics, Web Links and Activities.

Acknowledgments

I would like to thank the many schools and educators who participated in the industry-wide surveys that provided essential feedback for the preparation of this text and the reviewers who read the revision proposal and offered valuable input as to how to implement changes to make the book even better.

I would also like to acknowledge two other very special people who found the time to write a foreword for this work. My special thanks to Bill Church, fellow educator, friend, and colleague. As a cosmetology school owner, former director and past president for the American Association of Cosmetology Schools, and school owner commissioner for the National Accrediting Commission of Cosmetology Arts and Sciences, Bill continues to make a great difference in our industry. Thanks, Bill, for your kind words.

In addition, I would like to thank my friend, Geno Stampora, whose accomplishments and awards in this industry are too numerous to list but include being a leading-edge consultant and motivational speaker; being an owner, operator, and manager of salons, schools, and a distributorship; having served as a coach, image consultant, and salon educator; authoring *Success Dynamics*; serving as Director of Motivation for *Hair Color & Design* magazine; and so much more. Thank you, Geno, for your support of this book and our industry.

I would also like to express my heartfelt gratitude to Steve and Brandon Martin, owners of Avenue Five Institute in Austin, Texas. They and their staff and students opened the doors of their beautiful facility and extended their gracious hospitality to our team during the photo shoot that provided the majority of the photos for this book.

After many months and many, many hours of work on this project, I must give a heart-felt and sincere thanks to my very special friend and husband, Tom Barnes. He remains my partner in business and in life. Without his support, his willingness to manage our other business endeavors, and his dedication to my cause, this book would not have been possible. Like the song says, he is my hero; he is everything that I wish and hope to be. I have had many opportunities to fly higher than eagles only because of his wind beneath my wings. He continues to take me even higher. Thank you, Tom. I love you.

My fervent hope is that this effort, which has sincerely been a labor of love, will be a blessing and benefit to many, many educators for years to come. I dedicate this book to *you, the educators,* who are the very foundation of every career field and the hope of our future. If this book has touched you in any way, I would appreciate hearing from you. I look forward to receiving both your positive comments and your constructive criticisms. It is only through sincere feedback from other professionals that we can make the next revision of this text even better. You can reach me by e-mail at letha@thebarnes.net. I look forward to hearing from you and will do my very best to respond to any comments received.

Letha Barnes, author, educator, president of Training, Education and Management, Inc.

Contents

Chapter 3   Teaching Study and Testing Skills

Chapter 4   Basic Learning Styles and Principles

Chapter 5   Basic Methods of Teaching and Learning

Chapter 8   Effective Classroom Management and Supervision

Chapter 9   Achieving Learner Results

Chapter 10   Program Development and Lesson Planning

Chapter 11   Educational Aids and Technology in the Classroom

Chapter 12   Assessing Progress and Advising Students

Part II Basic Teaching Skills for Career Education in the Beauty and Wellness Disciplines

Part II includes content specific to most beauty and wellness disciplines required by most regulatory oversight agencies and national testing agencies for licensure as an instructor.

Chapter 13 Making the Student Salon an Adventure

Chapter 14 Career and Employment Preparation

Chapter 15   The Art of Retaining Students

Part III   Professional Development for Career Education Instructors

Part III covers more advanced material that is not considered critical for basic licensure. This volume is recommended for states requiring more than 600 clock hours for basic licensure and for licensed instructors who want to improve their performance as educators.

Chapter 16   Educator Relationships

Chapter 19 Teams at Work

Chapter 20 Evaluating Professional Performance

Master Educator

PART 1

Basic Teaching Skills for Career Education Instructors

1 The Career Education Instructor

Objectives (Desired Performance Goals):

After reading and studying this chapter, you should be able to:

● List the qualities and characteristics desired in a master educator.

● List the key concepts in time management and event control.

● Practice the strategies for building self-confidence.

● Adopt steps for independent action and self-control.

● Implement the actions for self-motivation.

● Develop enthusiasm.

● Practice the steps to develop a winning personality and a positive attitude.

! CRITICAL CONCEPT

Master educators unfailingly practice and model all the qualities and characteristics required for success.

Qualities and Characteristics of a Master Educator

TEACHING REQUIRES DYNAMIC, conscious effort on the part of the educator, whose basic function is to facilitate learning among students. Teaching is an intellectual experience that demands the ability to invent, adapt, and create new techniques and procedures to meet the changing demands of learners. In order to be effective in the role of educator, certain qualities, characteristics, traits, skills, and practices are essential. Because educators are also human (contrary to what their students may think on occasion), no two educators will be exactly alike. However, they will have learned that possessing certain qualities aids their success as an educator, whether they are teaching in the classroom, in the laboratory, or in specially developed classes for a varied audience.

The profile of a master educator will vary depending upon individual strengths, weaknesses, abilities, and attitudes. It may even change from one group of students to another. Qualities of a great educator cannot be reduced to a single list, but rather create a collage in which the various roles and characteristics of educators are combined to achieve the ultimate goal of success with learners.

Roles of a Master Educator

During your career as a master educator, you will find yourself filling the role of motivator, coach, mentor, friend, disciplinarian, peace-maker, negotiator, arbitrator, nurturer, and entertainer. In other words, you will find that to fill the role satisfactorily you must be a well-rounded individual. The classroom is a businesslike environment wherein learning occurs and knowledge is born. It is also, however, a place where adults interact on a continuous basis through verbal and nonverbal communication. The educator who is knowledgeable in a variety of subject areas will be a more interesting role model and educator to students. Take the time to ensure that you have interests outside the classroom and that you can converse confidently about people, places, and events. This life balance will serve you well both as an individual and as an educator.

Research was conducted across the United States regarding the qualities, characteristics, and personality types that managers and directors look for in the educators they hire as well as the qualities students look for in their teachers, as discussed in the following sections.

Loyalty to the Institution and Its Mission

This is one of the most frequently cited characteristics that managers and directors require in their educators. Employers expect loyalty in their employees. You become much more valuable to your organization if you practice unswerving faithfulness and allegiance to your institution and its purpose. Why is loyalty so important? The predominant goal or purpose of the institution cannot possibly be accomplished if every member of the team within the institution is not working faithfully to accomplish that mission. Employers need to feel confident that you have, at all times, the

+ MASTER EDUCATOR

1. Wakes up singing and enters each classroom with vigor and enthusiasm.
2. Is confident and projects professionalism at all times.
3. Models all the professional behaviors expected of students.

Figure 1–1   Practice unswerving faithfulness and allegiance to your institution.

best interest of the institution and its students in mind (Figure 1–1). If your purpose is consistent with that of the institution, your actions and performance can do no permanent harm to the school, even if you make mistakes. If, on the other hand, you are not faithful to your institution and harbor ill feelings for your supervisors or for the school itself, a great deal of irreparable harm can be done, especially to the students.

As an educator, you will have ample opportunities to bring about positive change within your organization by working *with* management rather than complaining or working *against* management. As you develop as an educator, you may also wish to adopt a personal mission statement or philosophy to live by. Following is an example of one educator's mission statement. *"I am committed to ensuring the success of my graduates in their chosen field while providing an energetic environment that facilitates the confidence and skills necessary for them to attain success. I am dedicated to helping students unlock their creativity and imaginations, improve themselves, and ultimately achieve professional success while observing loyalty before all else except honor and integrity."*

Welcome Advice from Colleagues

You've heard it said that "two heads are better than one." This aptly applies to educators. There will always be more than one method of doing a task or facilitating learning. Your fellow educators may have had great success with delivering specific material that could be very beneficial to you. Their success can only be useful to you if you are willing to listen to them and apply those techniques or principles that may work for you as well. In other words, be receptive to competent counsel from colleagues and be guided by that counsel as long as it does not compromise or impair the dignity and responsibility of your position as an educator. Remain open to the knowledge of all those around you, especially your own students. You will gain a wealth of information from your learners if you keep an open mind and listen attentively. You may have heard the saying that our minds are like parachutes—they work better when they are open!

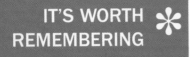

Constant Pursuit of Knowledge

Educators must possess a high level of expertise and knowledge in the various disciplines they teach. Educators will be judged by their knowledge of the subject matter. Students will ultimately admire and look up to those educators who are experts in their chosen fields. Educators must also be well grounded in the theory as well as any applicable practical applications of the disciplines they teach. In doing so, they will earn and maintain the respect of their students while at the same time imparting information that will allow the students to improve their own skills, knowledge, attitudes, appreciations, and habits.

Education is a continuing process for your students and for you. Changes and improvements in techniques and technology take place daily. It is in the best interest of the educator and the students to stay constantly alert and maintain competency in the changing trends.

Your career development does not end with the basic technical and theoretical knowledge needed within the disciplines you teach. You must also continue to develop your abilities and expertise as an educator. Continuing education in teaching methods and other related topics may be required for institutional reaccreditation or credential renewal by state regulatory agencies, if applicable. Employer surveys are very clear that they are looking for educators who participate in professional development classes on an ongoing basis. For some disciplines, regulatory agencies may require from 8 to 36 hours of continuing education per year. Employers are disappointed to discover that many educators never do more than the absolute minimum.

To be a master in any profession, it takes more than minimum participation. A good rule of thumb for effective professional development as an educator is to obtain at least 40 contact hours per year. Master educators recognize this as a personal responsibility related to the position. The most successful individuals in any field are those who invest in themselves. They do not expect the institution or employer to arrange for and provide for all their continuing education. Master educators seek learning opportunities because they understand that learning is the basis for all thinking. They will be active members in professional organizations. They will read industry publications on a regular basis. They will pursue continuing knowledge of their career field and maintain practical and current methods of teaching as well as cooperate with professional organizations and individuals engaged in activities that enhance the development of their profession.

Effective Time Management and Organized Work Methods

Time is one of the most valuable resources of life, and every human being has exactly the same amount of it. Your supervisor, your children, your students, your neighbors, highly successful CEOs, and you have the same 365 days per year, the same 24 hours per day, and the same 60 minutes per hour. Why is it that some educators achieve greatness in the classroom and have time left over for a balanced, harmonious life outside the institution, while others seem to be buried under an endless sea of papers, projects, assignments, and details? How you organize and use your time determines how much you get done at school, how much time you spend with your family,

CONSIDER AND CONNECT

Your commitment to personal career development is another quality greatly desired by employers. Obtaining a credential to teach does not conclude your learning as an educator; it merely signifies its beginning.

IT'S WORTH REMEMBERING

Enthusiastic teachers who are devoted to student success will know the triumph of high achievement and will enjoy the victory of seeing their students excel and succeed.

and whether you have a sense of moving forward or regressing. How you use your time will determine whether you feel you are managing your life or it is managing you!

time a continuum that is measured in terms of events that succeed one another from past through present to the future.

According to *Webster's Dictionary*, **time** is a continuum that is measured in terms of events that succeed one another from past through present to the future. Therefore, the basic elements of time are *events*. The key to managing your time effectively is mastering "event control." It is not a mysterious gift or talent you are born with—it is a skill that can be learned and practiced. While you will probably never have enough time to do everything you want to do, you certainly can become more systematic in your approach to managing it. It will be helpful to identify some important key concepts in time management and event control (Figure 1–2).

You really can learn to make things less complicated and even to make them more fun. It begins by identifying a level of performance or achievement that you can reach, both at home and on the job. Then, when you do more than you have actually scheduled or expected, you feel like a hero instead of criticizing yourself for falling short of your own expectations. The **Time Utilization Log** in Table 1–1 will help you get better acquainted with yourself, which is the first step in changing your ways and using your time more efficiently. For one day, record your time on the log following the instructions provided. Review the log carefully and ask yourself these key questions.

Time Utilization Log a document used to help you track how you spend your time, which is the first step in changing your ways and using your time more efficiently.

When answering these questions, keep in mind that there are some common time wasters that may affect your performance as an effective

IT'S WORTH REMEMBERING

The more you have to do, the more time you will have to do it in. Everyone has the same 24 hours in a day so make the most of it. If you take care of the minutes, the hours are likely to be more productive.

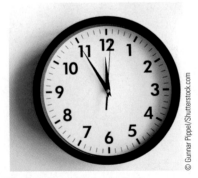

Figure 1–2   Schedule important tasks during peak productivity hours.

TOP TEN QUESTIONS FOR EFFECTIVE TIME ANALYSIS

1. Did I accomplish what I hoped to?

2. Did I spend the appropriate amount of time on the most important tasks?

3. Which tasks or projects took my time but contributed nothing to important goals?

4. Were there activities I could have delegated to someone else?

5. Did I spend valuable time on unimportant work?

6. At what point during the day did the longest period of uninterrupted time occur?

7. How many times was I actually interrupted?

8. How many of those interruptions were actually necessary?

9. How much time was spent on time wasters?

10. What could I do differently next time?

Table 1–1

TIME UTILIZATION LOG

TIME	PLANNED WORK	INTERRUPTION	UNPLANNED	SUBJECT/ACTIVITY	PRIORITY				TIME-SAVING IDEAS
					A	B	C	OTHER	

INSTRUCTIONS. TIME: Record every activity as it occurs. **TYPE:** Check whether the activity was planned, unplanned, or an interruption. **SUBJECT:** Provide a brief description of the activity. **PRIORITY:** Check the appropriate column with A—most important, B—average importance, C—low importance. **TIME-SAVING IDEAS:** Record any ideas that might improve or correct time lost owing to the activity. Review the log carefully and evaluate what was accomplished compared with what you hoped to accomplish. Determine which activities could have been delegated or eliminated. Identify your most productive, uninterrupted time during the day. This will aid in future planning.

educator. When analyzing your log, identify any of the applicable time wasters and determine whether they are caused internally or externally.

Interruptions: These may be the hardest to control. It is essential that you learn to say "no." You can also ask people to talk with you later. Limit your personal calls or visitors, which impose on your productivity at work.

Waiting: This can be infuriating for anyone. A certain degree of it is inevitable each day, but you can work to minimize it. If your dentist, your students, or your friends are late, explain the value of everyone's time. Consider going to the bank at a different hour to avoid lines or do your banking online. When waiting is absolutely necessary, put the time to good use by reading an industry periodical, planning your next class presentation, writing a list of things you need to do, or using your cellular device to catch up on important correspondence.

Procrastination: Delaying starting a project or task is often caused by the desire for perfection. Don't set standards so high for any project that they cannot be accomplished. Otherwise, your fear of failure will prevail and you will probably never even begin the task. Warning signs for **procrastination** are: "I'm going to start this job and I'm not going to stop until it's finished," and "I'll do it as soon as I (enter your favorite excuse)." This can be overcome by starting with the easiest part of the project. Write an outline, obtain important background information, and make necessary contacts. It is not recommended to begin with the most important part of the task because you may become frustrated at your lack of progress toward completion. Beginning with the simpler elements allows you to enjoy the feeling of accomplishment sooner and allows you to celebrate your accomplishment. Giving yourself small rewards as you cross certain thresholds toward completion will encourage you to continue your work.

We've all heard the expression, "mind your p's and q's." In developing a plan for the most effective use of your time, it will be helpful to consider the p's and q's of event control (see Table 1–2).

We change our lives by changing our attitudes and perceptions. We become what we think about ourselves. Practice will not necessarily make something perfect, but it will make it permanent. Therefore, we must correctly practice what we do. Certainly, by practicing event control and time management, we are better able to maintain efficiency and consistency in the performance of the administrative tasks of teaching.

procrastination to put off doing something until a future time; to postpone or delay needlessly.

IT'S WORTH REMEMBERING ✳

You can either control the events in your day or sit back and let the events of your day control you.

☑ **Authority, Order, and Self-Confidence**

authority an individual cited or appealed to as an expert; the power to influence or command thought, opinion, or behavior.

With respect to your role as an educator, **authority** is defined as:

1. an individual cited or appealed to as an expert and
2. the power to influence or command thought, opinion, or behavior.

Neither definition indicates the need for an educator to be a drill sergeant. The definitions do, however, imply that an educator holds a great a deal of responsibility. If you impose and use authority fairly and consistently, it will gain you the respect and loyalty of your learners. It will allow you the privilege of influencing or commanding the thoughts, opinions, and behaviors of your learners. It is important for young educators to fully

Table 1–2

THE P'S AND Q'S OF EVENT CONTROL

P'S	Q'S
PLAN: Predetermine a course of events for long-range, short-range, and immediate goals and activities. Master educators know they must have a realistic, workable plan for today, this week, this month in order for their classes to have direction and momentum. Remember that lack of planning on your part should not cause a state of emergency for someone else.	**QUESTIONS:** A master educator will ask, "What is the most important use of my time right now? Why is this important to me?"
PRIORITIZE: Make a list of tasks that need to be accomplished and give a value (A, B, or C) to each task. Determine the order or sequence in which the tasks need to be completed.	**QUALITY:** If you are really good in one particular area and you spend the entire day working on that, the day will have been well spent. Strive to bring quality into all your work. Time will be saved from not having to do unnecessary corrections.
PEAK TIME: Energy, creativity, and productivity come in peaks and valleys. A master educator will determine when peak time occurs and schedule the most important tasks during that time and the less important activities when energy levels are low.	**QUANTITY:** Master educators will make sure their efforts really count. Don't spend time on lots of small things in an effort to appear to have accomplished a lot unless those small things are contributing to the greater goal. Don't do a lot of "busy work" just to gain a feeling of satisfaction.
PROCRASTINATION: A master educator will not put off until tomorrow what can be accomplished today. It is not uncommon to want to put off those tasks that are difficult or unpleasant. Avoidance of such projects can be overcome by chipping away one small task at a time and giving yourself small rewards for the accomplishment.	**QUIRKS:** Learn what works for you. You may communicate best when wearing a certain color. You may reflect on important issues best during the middle of the night. Whatever your style, if it is effective, keep doing it.
PRACTICE: Event control and time management take behavior modification and practice. Developing the habit of daily event control takes effort at first, but soon becomes second nature.	**QUIET TIME:** A master educator will schedule some quiet, personal time daily that can be used to reflect on life's events and to relax. This is a perfect time to dream, think, plan, and organize. During this time, don't do any work, make phone calls, or schedule appointments. This small investment in yourself will result in big payoffs.
PERFECTION: A master educator understands that perfection only exists in our imagination. Since perfection can never be accomplished, striving for it will only result in frustration and fear of failure. Learn to be realistic in your goals for quality.	**QUIT:** Master educators know when to quit any task or project. They also know when to quit for the day. Never spend three or four hours on a project that is really only worth one hour of your valuable time. Recognize when you are no longer being productive due to fatigue or burn-out. Take a break, relax, breathe deeply, and get refueled for the rest of the project or day.

grasp the awesome responsibility they have in the role of teaching. A high degree of maturity is required to manage all the different roles required of an educator.

For an educator to achieve recognition as an authority, he or she must first have self-esteem and self-confidence. To hold someone in high esteem, according to *Merriam Webster's Dictionary*, is to hold him in high regard and prize accordingly. Therefore, **self-esteem** is the deep-down feeling you have in your own soul about your own value or self-worth. Self-confidence, on the other hand, is confidence in oneself and in one's own powers and abilities. An educator who lacks confidence will not believe that he has the ability to do the kinds of things that other educators have done and, oftentimes, won't even try. Master educators, however, have unshakeable confidence in their

self-esteem pride in oneself; the deep-down feeling you have in your own soul about your own value or self-worth.

ability to achieve anything they really want to accomplish. They have no fear of failure whatsoever. Not all of us are blessed with that belief in self. If you should fall into the latter category, there are some steps you can take to build confidence in yourself.

Engage in systematic, purposeful action, consistent with your values, to move in the direction of goals. Stretch your abilities to the maximum and you will feel positive and more confident about yourself. You can achieve or have whatever you dream of if you have the self-confidence to go for it.

For an educator to influence the classroom, self-confidence and a climate for serious learning is required. Learning will occur if the environment is student-centered and fun. However, the outcomes expected must be serious. You must be able to define what is expected of your students and never allow the quality of their work to be compromised.

Your recognition as an authority in your chosen field will not happen automatically or overnight. It has already been established that you must be a subject-matter expert in every subject you teach in order to gain the respect of your students. That is the first step from which you will acquire and accumulate your authority. Once your authority has been established, you will be able to effortlessly maintain order in your classes. As an authority, you have the power to influence your students and the ability to command thoughts and behavior in them that will ultimately result in aspiration (Figure 1–3).

Having authority in the classroom requires that you establish a formal distance between yourself and your learners. You can be friendly with your students. You can be supportive and nurturing with your students, but you will face many unnecessary hurdles in the educational process if you fraternize or socialize with your students as a friend outside the institution. Such relationships will result in a challenge to your authority and, more than likely, disrupt the order that you have strived to develop in your classroom. Conversely, maintaining order ensures that your classes have direction and momentum. It implies that your classes are comfortably disciplined and peaceful. Clearly, to establish authority and order in your classroom, you must set an example for your students and fairly and equitably enforce the standards of conduct expected of them. You must strive to achieve the highest standards of excellence at all times and you must respect your students,

CONSIDER AND CONNECT

An educator's goal is to achieve a level of authority that will encourage a strong desire in learners to achieve something great within their career field. Once they have developed that aspiration, the job of an educator becomes much simpler.

IT'S WORTH REMEMBERING

Master educators learn to embrace and master change and growth but never compromise their core values and principles.

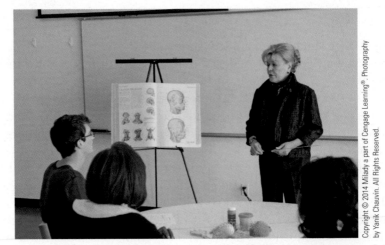

Figure 1–3   To gain learner respect use authority in the classroom fairly.

TOP TEN SELF-CONFIDENCE BUILDERS

- **Like and accept yourself unconditionally.** Consider yourself a valuable and worthwhile human being. Respect yourself, consider yourself a good person, and believe in yourself, and you will be confident in your ability to say and do the right thing at the right time.

- **Be clear about your own values.** The more you understand what you believe in and stand for, the more you will like yourself. Ultimately, you will gain a deep-down sense of self-assurance and calmness.

- **Be true to yourself.** Live your life in accordance with your highest aspirations and the highest values you have established for yourself.

- **Never compromise your integrity.** Be courageous and accept yourself for who you really are (not as who you might be or as who someone else wants you to be). After taking everything into consideration, know that you are a pretty good person.

- **Enjoy your uniqueness.** You have your own skills, talents, and abilities that make you extraordinary. Become aware that you are unique, and incorporate that awareness into your personality and your attitude toward your career.

- **Practice self-control.** You will feel confident to say and do the things that are consistent with your values when you are in control of yourself and your life. Obtaining control can be accomplished by setting clear goals or objectives, establishing a sense of direction based on what you hope to achieve in life.

- **Work step by step toward desired goals.** When you achieve predetermined goals, you feel strong and capable and in control. You feel like the winner you are. Your self-confidence soars and your willingness to take on even greater challenges grows. The more you achieve, the more you feel you are capable of achieving.

- **Become an expert.** Self-efficacy is the ability to perform effectively in your chosen area. Whenever you teach well, your self-esteem and self-respect will skyrocket. You will experience a sense of personal pride and obtain the self-confidence to take on even greater challenges.

- **Make a commitment to excellence.** When you resolve to pay any price, make any sacrifice, invest any amount of time and money to be the best that you can be, you will become a master educator. At that point, you will elevate yourself above the average educator who drifts from job to job, class to class and accepts mediocrity as the adequate standard.

- **Avoid the enemies of human happiness.** Fears and doubts undermine our self-esteem and self-confidence and cause us to think in negative terms about ourselves. When referring to the story of the human race, Abraham Maslow said that it is the story of men and women "selling themselves short." Don't magnify your difficulties and minimize your opportunities.

Take action to overcome the doubt, worry, and fear.

coworkers, and fellow educators if you are to be respected yourself. Such leadership skills will earn your recognition as an authority and ensure that your classes are conducted in an orderly manner.

Professionalism: Ethics and Character

Educators who are of high moral excellence and firmness and who hold dear a set of moral principles or values that are above reproach are in great demand in the workforce. **Ethics** are the moral principles by

ethics the moral principles by which we live and work.

IT'S WORTH REMEMBERING ✳

The performance of your students is a portrait of your work. Are you willing to autograph the portrait?

which we live and work. It is important to emphasize the relationship between effectiveness in teaching and ethical conduct. The potential for abuse of students and the abuse of the school and management is constant. Great educators recognize the potential harm that can be brought upon both the students and the school through irresponsible, unethical behavior. They will exercise extreme care to avoid breaches of good ethics that would bring dishonor upon themselves or their institution. Master educators are aware of the ethical standards of their profession, and they model and teach those standards in their everyday interactions with students. They will work for honesty and truth in fulfilling the requirements of their position. They will supervise and instruct without prejudice and avoid unethical practices at all times. They will avoid criticism of others and never gossip, keeping confidentiality where appropriate.

Dependability and Flexibility

It has been said that all it takes to be considered in the top 20% of your profession is to (Figure 1–4):

- show up
- be on time
- be ready to work

It seems to be true, because research indicates that dependability and flexibility are two of the most important characteristics sought when hiring new educators. When institutions enroll students in various programs, they are making a commitment to provide quality education to those students. This cannot be accomplished if the educators are not present to facilitate that educational process. In 1995, baseball legend Cal Ripken, Jr., broke Lou Gehrig's record of playing in 2,130 consecutive baseball games. He received

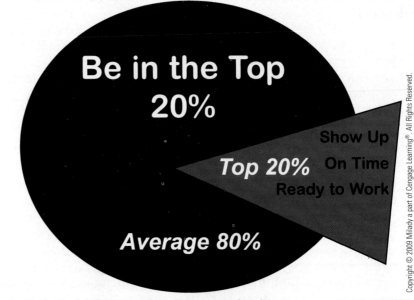

Figure 1–4   Be in the top 20% of your profession.

much praise and many accolades, which he brushed off, instead praising America's real working heroes. One of the individuals he referred to was a woman by the name of Mildred Parsons, who at the time was 82 years of age and had not missed a day of work as secretary for the Federal Bureau of Investigation in 56 years. Can you imagine the consistency and security that the students in our nation's schools would feel if their educators were that dedicated and dependable?

In addition to dependability, employers are actively seeking educators who are flexible. They are looking for educators who readily adapt to new, different, or changing requirements. Many educators are extremely resistant to change in any form. If you think about it, though, when you change, you take action, you affect the future. Change is inevitable as we proceed in the new millennium. Without change and growth, educators will go the way of the dinosaur. As a master educator, your ability to perform effectively in this world of ongoing, never-ending change really is a true measure of how well-developed a person you are. One of the most common challenges faced by school managers and directors is having seasoned educators who use teacher-centered, rather than student-centered, education and present lessons the same way they did many years ago. Such educators are unwilling to update their teaching methods and materials and move into learner-centered education.

Employers are also looking for educators who are willing to adapt to any role that may be assigned on any given day. They want educators who are willing to step in and take whatever actions are necessary to achieve the mission and objectives of the institution. They state that a common challenge to providing quality education derives from educators who are unwilling to "go the extra mile" and who avoid certain tasks because "it is not my job." A master educator will always be willing to give that little extra that can make a significant difference.

By giving a full day of work for a full day of pay, committing to punctuality and preparedness, and practicing the habit of giving everything your best *and then some*, you will demonstrate your dependability and be in great demand.

> ### IT'S WORTH REMEMBERING ✳
>
> If you learn to become a *change master* rather than a *change resister*, the results you can achieve will be unlimited.

Cooperation and Teamwork

It is no wonder that the ability to cooperate is a characteristic employers seek in their educators. All institutions of higher education hope their students will attain uncommon results. **Teamwork** creates synergy, which has been described as what happens when one plus one equals three. Whether you are completing the everyday tasks of running a school or getting together with other staff members to solve a problem or to create a great new improvement plan for the institution, teamwork benefits everyone involved.

> **teamwork** a cooperative effort by a group of individuals working together to achieve a common goal.

Teamwork does not exist in all schools. If one educator believes that his assigned students are his only students and doesn't pay any attention to students in other classes, there is no school team. If an educator believes he is assigned to teach only one class or subject and remains unwilling to cross-train or to take over other areas when needed, the team is deficient. Many independent educators work in the same facility, but often they are not working together toward the common goals or mission of the institution. When this occurs, the students and the clients sense the tension.

For a dynamic team to exist in any institution there has to be a spirit of cooperation and communication among all members of the organization. Successful cooperation is a two-way street. If you are not willing to give an inch, it is unlikely that you can expect others to cooperate with you. Developing cooperative relationships with your coworkers is essential to your success as an educator. When you place other people's interests higher than your own, cooperation will flourish. A successful school team doesn't mean looking "at" each other, but looking in the same direction, toward the same goals, together. Table 1–3 lists some of the stumbling blocks to building a dynamic school team and some positive steps for creating successful cooperation within the institution.

Interest in Other People

A dynamic educator actively cultivates an interest in other people, personnel, educators, and students. This will bring joy into the educator's own life and into the institution. The eternal law of cause and effect will begin to work. When you show interest in others, they will ultimately show interest in you. A dynamic team needs to share a spirit of passion and focus on the same goal. When you're part of a dynamic school team:

- You will get help from your coworkers at times when you're overwhelmed and you will return the favor when they need your help.
- You will be able to refer your students requesting assistance to another educator when you are not feeling well or when you are swamped with administrative responsibilities.
- You will be able to share knowledge with other educators and learn from them.

Table 1–3

DYNAMIC TEAM BUILDING: STUMBLING BLOCKS AND STAIR STEPS

STUMBLING BLOCKS TO DYNAMIC TEAM BUILDING	STAIR STEPS TO DYNAMIC TEAM BUILDING
Selfishness	Empathy
Dishonesty	Honesty and Integrity
Unreliability	Reliability
Hostility	Goodwill, Positive Attitude
Suspicion and Interference	Trust and Openness
Laziness	Willingness and Energy
Untidiness	Neatness and Order
Controversy	Adaptability
Trouble Making	Cheerfulness
Poor Communications	Open, Clear Communications
Rudeness	Courtesy

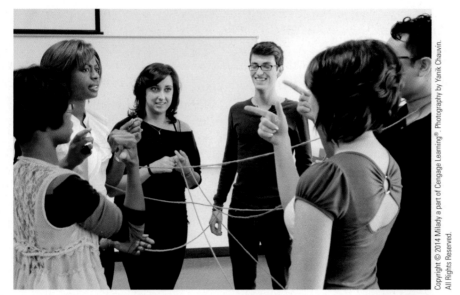

Figure 1–5 **Teamwork creates a spirit of cooperation and communication among all members.**

- You will work to project a unified, professional image for the institution.
- You will work in an atmosphere of colleagues helping other colleagues rather than competitors working in disharmony.
- You, your fellow educators, the students, and the institution will enjoy greater success. Everyone wins.

Expectations of goodwill are contagious. Put the interests of others ahead of your own and practice the positive self-expectancy that they will do the same thing. If you pledge your commitment to counsel and assist fellow educators in the performance of their duties and strive for teamwork and cooperation, you will almost always achieve it. An Ethiopian proverb says that when spider webs unite, they can tie up a lion! Imagine what can be accomplished with that same effort of unity within your school (Figure 1–5).

Initiative and Ability to Work Independently

In today's higher education environment involving adult learners, a master educator needs to exercise **initiative** in starting and following through on assigned work. He must learn to work independently with little close supervision. He must learn to initiate actions required to solve problems whenever possible without intervention from supervisory or management personnel. The master educator must maintain steady performance under varying work pressures. Educators who have adopted and developed these particular skills will become much more valuable to their employers. Employers are looking for educators who are "self-starters." They need individuals who are in harmony with the institution's mission and who know that providing quality education to its students is the first and foremost priority. Schools need educators who will take whatever steps are necessary to ensure that objective is met.

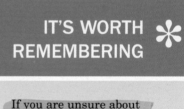

IT'S WORTH REMEMBERING

If you are unsure about your future, take control of it, manage it, and create it.

initiative the power, ability, or instinct to begin and/or follow through with a plan or task.

STEPS TO INDEPENDENT ACTION

- **Study your position description.** What is expected of you in your educator role within the institution? What are the specific job duties for which you are responsible? Study and learn this information and be prepared to fulfill those requirements on a daily basis.

- **Read and study the school's operating procedures.** Become knowledgeable of the institution's written operating procedures, which address the various functions and departments within the institution. This will allow you to know the actions or procedures that should be followed for those situations that occur only occasionally.

- **Read and study rules established by oversight agencies.** Become knowledgeable of the state statutes and regulations governing the operation of your institution. Make yourself aware of the policies, standards, and criteria established by the institution's accrediting agency. This information will allow you to make independent, but informed, decisions when the situation calls for it.

- **Be willing to take risks.** Know that if you wait until everything is "perfect," you will never do or accomplish anything. If your goals and objectives are on target and you know that your actions are performed with the best interest of the institution and your students in mind, then dive in. There will be times when what you did was the wrong thing to do, but you will take comfort in knowing it was not because of the wrong reason. Most employers will appreciate and respect your willingness to take action.

- **Follow the steps for building self-confidence.** When your level of self-confidence rises, you will be able to take action without worrying that the action is the right thing to do. You will *know* it is the right thing to do.

There are certain steps you can take to ensure you have initiative and can work independently without a great deal of close supervision, as noted in the accompanying box.

Remember, the less supervision or "maintenance" you require, the more valuable you are to your employer.

Patience and Self-Control

As a master educator, you will face countless challenges posed by your students on a daily basis. Your students will easily recognize and appreciate your honesty and straightforwardness when dealing with those challenges. You will only be able to lead your students if you can control your own

IT'S WORTH REMEMBERING ✳

The educator who is sincere, patient, and in control can turn challenges into opportunities.

emotions. Your students will quickly lose respect for you if you lack poise and frequently display fits of temper and unprofessional behavior. Preparation and proper planning will go a long way toward accomplishing self-control. When faced with a situation that would otherwise cause your blood to boil, follow these important steps:

1. Pause and breathe. Take a deep breath and count silently to 10. This gives you the opportunity to get in control and evaluate the situation.
2. Consider the circumstances. What actions or events caused you to want to react in an uncontrolled manner? What has caused your student to behave in this manner? Are there factors unknown to you that could have caused the student's behavior?
3. Evaluate the options. What actions are available to resolve the situation? Choose the most effective approach—if possible, one in which everyone "wins" or benefits.
4. Behave professionally. Identify and display the professional behavior you want your students to observe in you; behavior you won't regret or be embarrassed about later.
5. Listen to the student. Hear what the student has to say. You will learn what unknown circumstances led to the volatile situation.
6. Apply the best approach. In a controlled manner and with an even, moderate voice, follow the best approach to resolve the situation.

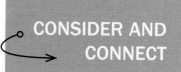

CONSIDER AND CONNECT

Remember, you never have to apologize for something that was not said or done. Maintaining patience and self-control will aid you significantly in facilitating a safe and effective learning environment.

TOP TEN STEPS TO A PROFESSIONAL IMAGE

1. Shower or bathe daily.

2. Use appropriate deodorants or antiperspirants.

3. Follow proper oral hygiene by brushing and flossing teeth daily and using mouthwash.

4. Wear freshly laundered, properly pressed clothing that is in good repair.

5. Wear shoes that are clean and in good condition.

6. Maintain clean, healthy, and appropriately styled hair.

7. Maintain well-manicured hands and nails.

8. Wear appropriate makeup if female; maintain clean-shaven face or neatly trimmed facial hair if male.

9. Wear appropriate jewelry and keep it to a minimum.

10. Practice proper posture and deportment.

By following these steps, you will maintain the respect you have earned from your students. You will convey professionalism that cannot be questioned or criticized. You will display poise and self-control, which will increase your self-confidence. Thinking clearly and acting in this manner is an excellent way to prevent irreparable harm from an emotional storm.

☑ Professional Image

Portraying a professional image to your students is essential. Educators must pay particular attention to their own wardrobe while also observing the boundaries and guidelines established by the institution. A master educator will practice impeccable grooming and never consider arriving for work without all aspects of personal appearance being properly addressed (Figure 1–6).

Stand in front of the mirror each morning before departing for work and ask yourself whether or not you would hire the person standing before you. If you fail to follow steps 1 through 10 daily, you send a message to your coworkers and students that you don't care enough about them or yourself to project a positive, professional image. Even those students whose appearance and image leave something to be desired may be inspired to improve when you set the perfect example for them. In fact, consider following one school's example: Install a full-length mirror on or near the door entering

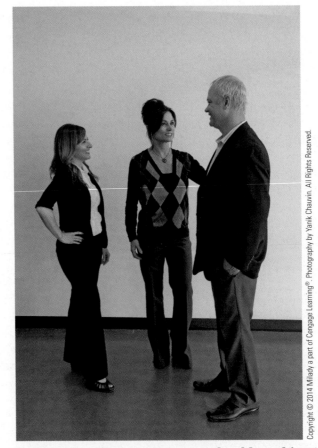

Figure 1–6   All elements of your appearance should combine to make a memorable and pleasing impression on others.

the classroom with a full-sized, red "stop" sign above it. Mount the question, "Would you hire this person?" just above the mirror and below the stop sign. Your example and this exercise will go a long way in stressing the importance of portraying a professional image at all times to your students. A master educator will make certain that everything about his or her appearance—from clothing to grooming, from scent to smile—combine to make a memorable and pleasing impression on others.

Courtesy, Compassion, and Consistency

Other qualities essential to success as an educator are courtesy, **compassion**, and consistency. Good manners and old-fashioned politeness are basic to being effective as an educator. Being on time to work, starting class on time, and keeping appointments as scheduled with your students all amount to simple, common courtesy. By being courteous, you can command the same behavior from your students. In addition to courtesy, having compassion for your students suggests you hold a sympathetic consciousness of your students' distress and have a desire to help alleviate that distress. Compassionate educators will be able to put themselves in the learner's place and understand what has caused certain behaviors and actions on their part. When you have compassion for your students, you will want to know all you can about them: their background and family history, their culture and beliefs, their interests and goals. Your compassion for your students will make your approval of them even more enjoyable, and it will make your correction of their performance more palatable to them. All humans, including students, need to feel needed, appreciated, and important. Compassion will convey approval at every opportunity without showing favoritism in any manner.

Your compassion will help ensure that rules and standards are applied fairly and equitably. It is poor practice to firmly enforce a rule today and ignore it tomorrow. This sends a message to your students that you are not sufficiently interested in them, and they won't know what to expect from you. Consistency can be likened to justice: Justice ensures fairness and righteousness. The master educator will look for the best in all students and treat them fairly, courteously, and compassionately.

compassion the deep feeling of sharing or feeling the pain or suffering of another; sympathy.

Desire and Motivation

As we build fragments into the collage that profiles a master educator, two key ingredients must be added: strong personal desire and self-motivation. Desire is the ingredient that makes the difference between an average educator and a *master educator*. It has been referred to as the "great equalizer" because it is the factor that allows individuals of average knowledge or ability to compete successfully with those who have far more ability.

Desire creates what Abraham Maslow has defined as **unconscious incompetence**. His theory states that "we don't know that we don't know." Perhaps it can best be related to the bumble bee. According to twentieth-century folklore, the laws of aerodynamics prove that the bumblebee is incapable of flight. It does not have the capacity in terms of wing size or beats per second to achieve flight with the degree of wing loading necessary.

unconscious incompetence Abraham Maslow's theory states that unconscious incompetence means that "we don't know that we don't know."

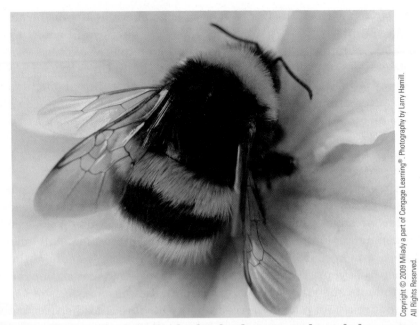

Figure 1–7   Desire allows individuals of only average knowledge or ability to compete successfully.

Therefore, the assumption is that it is impossible for the small creature to fly. Perhaps the bumble bee has unconscious incompetence. It does not know that it cannot fly and, of course, it does not read. It does, however, fly!

Something desired is something longed for or hoped for; it is something craved or coveted. It therefore becomes the foundation for all self-motivation. *Merriam Webster's Dictionary* defines a motive as a need or desire that causes a person to take action. So, everyone is motivated, educators and students alike. The amount of success you achieve as an educator will greatly depend upon the degree of your self-motivation and the direction that motivation takes (Figure 1–7).

You may have heard that as an educator, you will have the responsibility of motivating your students. This theory would imply that motivation is an external factor. The fact is that motivation is internal. On an external level, however, you can create circumstances or situations by which your students can be motivated. For example, you could publicly criticize and humiliate a student during a class, causing him to get up and stalk out of the classroom. Would you have really motivated the student to leave the class, or did your behavior cause in your student the internal motive of anger or frustration, which ultimately resulted in his action? A number of external motivators can be used in the classroom, such as exciting presentations, pep talks, student success rallies, group projects and activities, incentives, motivational guest speakers, and more. The bottom line is that most of those external motivators will have very little effect until your students make the personal decision to want to change their lives for the better. They have to be ready to internalize and accept your messages. So, the most important aspect of motivation lies in the fact that it is an internal decision influenced by external situations or circumstances.

Your responsibility as a master educator will be to awaken in students the personal desire to take the actions necessary to attain their own goals

CONSIDER AND CONNECT

A dream becomes reality when it is pursued with a plan and a timeline.

for success. It is not likely that you will be able to awaken such a desire in your students if it has not been awakened in you. We all have the power within us to become motivated, but some of us are afraid to risk going after our own dreams. Motivation can be compared to the motor of an automobile. It is the driving force behind everything an individual will accomplish, whether positive or negative, intentional or unintentional. Motivation is your inner drive that will keep you moving toward your goals in spite of mistakes, setbacks, or discouragement. For human beings, there are some fundamental physical and mental motivators basic to life, such as hunger, thirst, love, money, pleasure, faith, and survival. The two most powerful emotions that influence our behavior are desire and fear. Fear can cause anxiety, stress, and hostility, which defeat plans and goals, whereas desire will excite and energize; *desire* will encourage enthusiasm for excellence.

For motivation to be effective and active, it must focus on a specific need, goal, or aim. It can be likened to steam that, if released into the air, evaporates and disappears. If it is contained in a small room, inhabitants of the room would feel hot and uncomfortable. However, if that same steam is harnessed to an engine, it can propel a thousand-ton ship. It is important that your motivation doesn't simply evaporate into inertia or become trapped inside, causing you to feel frustrated or agitated. By attaching your motivation to a desired goal, your accomplishments will become limitless.

If you feel that you lack strong personal motivation, there are some actions you can employ to help you stay positively self-motivated, as discussed next.

Do Things That You Enjoy Doing. There are many people in today's society who are unhappy because they are working in areas they don't enjoy. As a master educator, you will experience and enjoy many rewards as you watch your students grow and hear them say, "Aha!"

Associate with Positive, Motivated, Successful People. Your environment affects, to some degree, who you are. If you associate with negative thinkers, it will be far too easy for you to acquire some of their behavior. If, on the other hand, you associate regularly with high achievers who set a positive example, you are likely to adopt some of the same positive behaviors.

Identify Motivating Activities and Situations. Hobbies can be personally uplifting. Upbeat music is another example of how you can set the mood for positive thinking and get reenergized. It can help to improve your attitude and prepare mentally and physically for tasks that lie ahead.

Improve Your Physical Fitness. As you become more healthy and fit, your energy level will soar. Physical activity, whether it is routine exercise, playing tennis, swimming, yoga, taking nature walks, or running, helps keep you both healthy and positive (Figure 1–8).

Listen to Motivational Tapes and Read Inspirational Publications. Many great thinkers and authors have great ideas to share with you both in books and on tapes. It has been said that you will be the same five years from now except for the people you meet and the books you read. Spend some time browsing the self-improvement section at the local bookstore.

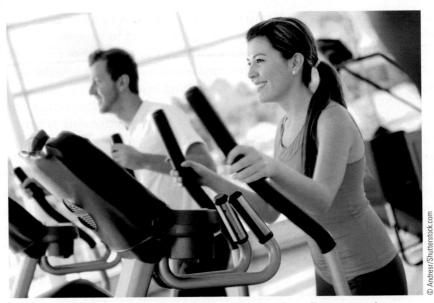

Figure 1–8   Your mind as well as your body needs a fitness regimen.

Purchase books that address specific needs, desires, or concerns in your life and read them actively. Underline or highlight key ideas and then take action by applying the principles you learn to your life.

Eliminate "I Can't" from Your Vocabulary. Saying you can't do something is merely another way of saying you won't even try. In reality, you "can do" almost anything you set your mind to and are willing to work to achieve.

Change "I wish" to "I will." Concentrate on how you can accomplish the things you desire and then take action. Don't focus on things you wish you could do "if only" someone or something didn't prevent it.

Identify Major Life Goals or Desires. Again, desire is the fuel for motivation. You cannot work toward achieving a goal until you have identified it. Your desires cannot be achieved instantly. You must reaffirm your goals daily and have an action plan to attain them.

☑ Enthusiasm and Energy

It is impossible to finish any task or to achieve even the smallest goal if enthusiasm is lost. The term *enthusiasm* is derived from the Greek word "enthous," which means *inspired*. Today it is defined as strong warmth or feeling, keen interest, or fervor. It is the inner fire that, combined with desire, can set you apart from those who have far superior abilities. Enthusiasm does not depend upon how you have been raised, or on your individual talent, or even on your intelligence. It is a winning spirit that comes from within. The medical profession now agrees that fatigue, in large part, is of mental origin rather than a result of any physical ailment. Today's society is plagued with feelings of boredom, frustration, anxiety, worry, and resentment, all of which can eclipse enthusiasm in a moment. It is important to understand that *energy* and *enthusiasm* are two essential halves of a very important whole. To have energy, you must be enthusiastic; to be enthusiastic, you must have energy. When the two

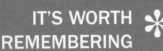

IT'S WORTH REMEMBERING

Many great accomplishments in education have resulted when unique ideas are shared with enthusiasm.

work hand in hand, a high degree of energetic enthusiasm can be maintained throughout the day.

Motivational experts concur that enthusiasm can be developed. Following are some behaviors and activities that can help even the most sluggish educator become enthusiastic.

Wake Up Singing. That's right. Sing in the shower; sing in the car on the way to work (ignore the strange looks you get from other travelers). Singing indicates that you are happy, and when you are happy, you generate happiness for those around you, even your students.

Smile, Smile, Smile. There is no such thing as an "unattractive smile." Smiling actually relieves facial tension and produces a subtle chemical change in your body. Smiling makes your endorphins start pumping, and soon you're feeling more enthusiastic. Your students will appreciate the boost they receive from your smiles because they are contagious . . . what a great emotion to spread!

Be a "First-Timer." As an educator, you must perform many routine tasks each day. You must prepare lesson plans, tests, handouts, and learning activities. You must prepare your classroom and organize your presentations. Try to remember to approach each task as if you were performing it for the very first time. Handle each assignment with a fresh mind. Even though you may have taught the subject a hundred times, you owe it to your students to make your class as fresh and interesting as if you were presenting it for the first time ever.

Apply the "Pretend Principle." This behavior piggybacks on being a "first-timer." When your work as an educator requires you to perform routine and boring tasks, pretend they are interesting and exciting. Make a game of it. Attempt to do the task perfectly, perhaps even faster than you normally do it. Set quotas or time limits; discover new and creative ways in which the work can be performed. Pretend you are having fun doing a menial task and, before you know it, you will actually be enjoying it. Adopting this principle will leave you with a great deal more energy and enthusiasm at the end of the day to apply to your personal life as well.

Practice Proper Posture. By standing up straight with your chest out, stomach in, and shoulders back, you will actually feel uplifted mentally and physically. Body language can literally distinguish winners from losers. Let your posture identify you as an enthusiastic and successful educator.

Have Personal Pep Rallies. Your mind as well as your body needs a fitness regimen. In addition to your regular physical fitness routine, coach your mind to be positive. Positive self-talk is a great way to get oneself mentally prepared for a challenging day of teaching.

Attach Yourself to a Purpose. This will generate a great new surge of power. We can be compared to tickets of admission containing a line that reads, "Invalid if detached." It is the same with people. We lose our value and importance when we become detached from commanding aims and purposes. Keep focused on your goals. The enthusiasm you use to tackle your responsibilities as an educator grows in direct proportion to the clarity of your purpose.

Seize the Spirit of Adventure. Nothing can squelch enthusiasm more than a rigid, inflexible, routine, and boring lifestyle. Be willing to try new foods and attempt things you've never tried before. Take a few risks. View each new challenge as an opportunity and an adventure (Figure 1–9).

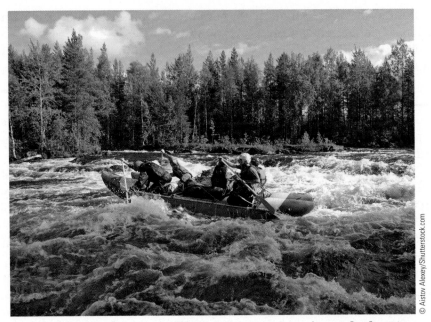

Figure 1–9   View each new challenge as an opportunity and adventure.

Take a different route to work each day. Bring some variety into your life. Robert Frost is a perfect example of this principle. Before he became famous as a poet, Mr. Frost had dropped out of school a number of times. He was considered nonteachable. He took odd jobs that never lasted. His grandfather, who felt that becoming a poet was demeaning, gave Robert a farm in New Hampshire with the directive to work the farm to feed his family. He and his wife raised six children there in poverty and lost two of them to death. Frost clung to his vision and purpose of becoming a poet. At the age of 40, he and his wife left the farm and moved to England, where he pursued his dream of writing poetry. History has proven that it was the turning point in his life. In 1916, when reflecting upon his life, he wrote *The Road Not Taken,* which said, in part:

> *Two roads diverged in a wood, and I—*
> *I took the one less traveled by,*
> *And that has made all the difference.*

Expand Your Mind through Learning. Stretching and expanding the mind through learning is a rich and inexhaustible source of enthusiasm. Continue to read, write, and learn with insatiable curiosity. Ceaseless intellectual activity is a common characteristic among many great world leaders who remained active until very late in life. As you learn, new interests will be awakened, igniting sparks of enthusiasm in your life.

Think Enthusiasm. Wake up each morning saying that you are enthusiastic. As you progress through the day, tell yourself that you are enthusiastic. As you face each new challenge with your students, do it with enthusiasm. It has been said that you will become what you think. If you want to be energetically enthused, you must think and act with enthusiasm!

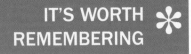

IT'S WORTH REMEMBERING

When we stretch our mind with new ideas, dreams, and concepts, it will never return to its original limitations.

Your personality as a master educator will become brighter, warmer, and more alive if you are enthusiastic. Pursue a dominant purpose in your teaching career, create the spirit of adventure in your classrooms, and never stop learning.

Imagination and Pleasure

Educators who are in great demand in the workforce are resourceful; they have creative ability and active minds. You may be thinking right now that you are not creative. However, creativity is not something mysterious that only a few educators possess. All of us are born with creativity. If you do not believe that, give a four-year-old a simple object such as a stick and watch what happens (Figure 1–10). Over the course of a morning, the stick will become many things: a baton, a cane, a sword, a horse, or even an orchestra conductor's wand. It's the child's imagination, his ability to form a mental image of something not present, that allows him to create and enjoy all the toys his imagination and creativity allow.

Master educators believe that they have the resourcefulness to facilitate learning for their students. They are confident that knowledge will be transferred to their learners. Developing a vivid and clear imagination as an educator in the educational process will not only help learners expand their own imaginations but also will help them grasp the shared information. When students can form a mental image of something not present or something

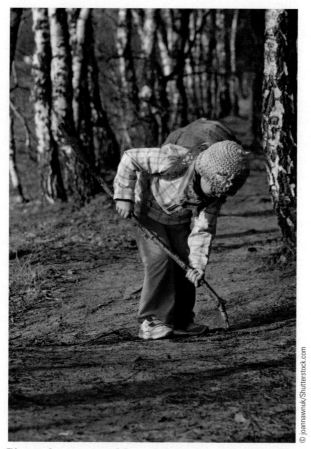

Figure 1–10   Give a four-year-old a stick and watch what happens.

they have not yet done, it makes actually doing it for the first time much easier. As an educator, you must be able to see students as successful career professionals in order to be able to instill that same vision in them.

A creative imagination will help facilitate the presentation of various course topics. It will aid you in making sure that new ideas are used for delivery, that new activities for student participation are implemented, and that new projects or assignments are used to reinforce learning and increase retention of the material presented. By introducing new ideas and activities into classes daily, you will bring surprise and excitement into the educational process. This is a sure way to ensure that students return to class the following day. If our students take one day of class at a time, they will ultimately graduate and be prepared to enter the workforce as professionals.

It is an established fact that stress and anxiety obstruct the learning process. Start to see your adult learners as babies in big bodies. They like to play and explore and, in doing so, combine fun with learning. Human nature dictates that humor and laughter help people to bond. As a master educator, your connection to your learners is important to their participation in the learning process. If your students like and enjoy your classroom style, they are more likely to learn from you. Don't misunderstand—learning is a very serious matter; the outcomes of learning must never be compromised. The process, however, can be fun! It's a fact that when the process is fun, the outcomes are generally positive. Later on in this text, we will discuss in detail the various skills, techniques, and ideas that can make learning more fun and more effective.

IT'S WORTH REMEMBERING ✳

Learning happens more quickly and lasts much longer if you are having fun in the process.

Effective Communications and Generational Skills

The national survey of post-secondary career school managers and directors indicated that educators must be able to master the art of communication with their coworkers and students, who vary greatly in age, background, culture, beliefs, and attitudes. In fact, Chapter 6 of this textbook has been dedicated to developing the ability to communicate confidently. An educator is unique in that he is called upon to speak before groups of learners *every day*. It is not so with other professions. Courtroom attorneys address juries occasionally; doctors speak with individual patients, not groups, on a daily basis; clergy speak a few times a week to their congregations. As a master educator, however, you are responsible for your own material (unlike clergy) and must present that material to a diverse audience of learners on a daily basis. Those learners include underachievers, high achievers, students with little or no personal discipline, students with little respect for the rules, students with dysfunctional families, and students who are aggressive.

Winning Personality and Positive Attitude

As an educator, you will never be 100 percent efficient—no matter how thoroughly you know the subject matter or how completely you master the techniques of teaching—unless you have developed a personality that fosters both learning *and* genuine human relationships. In addition to knowing yourself and your own attitudes, you must also know how others,

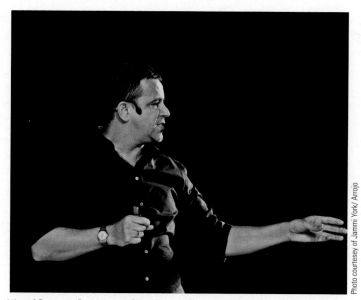

Photo courtesey of Jammi York/ Arrojo

Figure 1–11   Always have enthusiasm for your subject matter.

specifically your students, perceive you. This can be accomplished through feedback from students and coworkers and through self-evaluation. A master educator must also sincerely enjoy working with students. Finally, and possibly most importantly, as a master educator, you must convey a sincere positive attitude toward your subject matter.

If you do not have a *passion* for your career field and *compassion* for your students, you should pursue another career avenue. Without enthusiasm for your subject matter and your students, you can hardly hope to motivate your students or help them achieve their career goals (Figure 1–11).

If you feel your personality is lacking some positive qualities, there are a number of steps you can take to develop a pleasant, enjoyable, gracious, and amiable personality, as discussed next.

Maintain an Open Mind. Seek out different ideas, cultures, and creeds that may be different from your own. A healthy curiosity promotes interesting questions and unlimited learning (Figure 1–12). Others will always appreciate the opportunity to explain their backgrounds and experiences. Even if you are not comfortable with the speaking role in conversation, you can still become an interested listener and learner.

Build a Bank of Poise. Learn to smile and shrug off awkward moments. A smile will go a long way toward turning what could be a very awkward situation into an insignificant matter. You put those around you at ease when you show that you don't take yourself too seriously. This can be especially important and effective when dealing with students. They need to know you are human.

Make the Best of What You Have. Accept the fact that no one has everything, including you. Count your blessings and realize that you have the time and energy to contribute to your students' self-satisfaction and success, sometimes with nothing more than a kind, encouraging word or two. You may sometimes feel that life is less than fair, but never forget that self-pity is an acid that eats holes in contentment.

IT'S WORTH REMEMBERING ✳

The attitudes we make our own and project daily impact our dreams and affect our future.

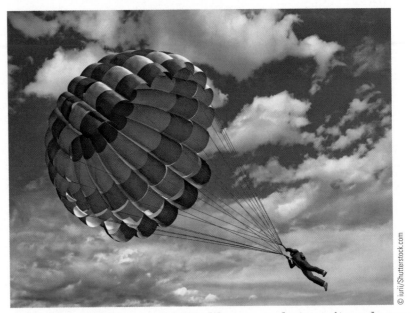

Figure 1–12 **Remember, your mind is like a parachute . . . it works much better when it is open!**

Do Not Hold Grudges. A life can be wasted by spending time keeping bitter moments alive. A well-known country song popular in the late 1990s said it best: "We bury the hatchet but leave the handle sticking out." That behavior can be deadly when applied to students. Even though your anger or hurt may be justified, dwelling on such feelings will only make you—and them—more unhappy. When you are hurt, hostile, or nursing a grudge, you pass on those negative feelings to your coworkers and students. They will naturally find any way possible to avoid your negativity.

Do Not Live in Fear. What is going to happen tomorrow, next week, or next year will happen whether you're worried about it or not. Learn to live life one day at a time, even one hour at a time, if necessary. This can be very helpful in achieving a calm, cheerful attitude—and remember, cheerfulness is contagious. What a great emotion to spread!

Focus on the Future Rather Than the Past. Let go of past mistakes and try to discover what you can learn and do to correct them in the future. Make a personal resolve to do better. Have confidence in your ability to improve instead of sulking about what cannot be undone.

Avoid Sarcasm at Someone Else's Expense. It really only sends the message that you are dissatisfied with yourself or lack self-confidence. An ego can never be built at the expense of others without losing friends in the process.

Practice Sharing Pleasing Remarks. This is also known as practicing random acts of kindness. Use your voice and your mind to practice delivering only kind and pleasant remarks to both those you know and to strangers. Such behavior will go a long way toward making you feel much better about yourself. Others will find you more pleasing to be around as well. Before you know it, you will be in demand, as a teacher, as a guest, and as a friend (Figure 1–13)!

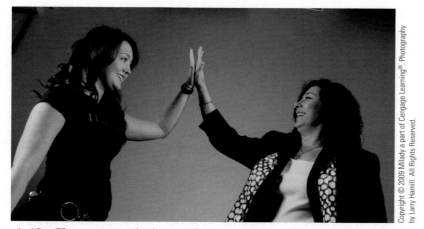

Figure 1–13   Show appreciation and recognition of student performance.

Do Not Be Critical. You have all heard the expression that people who live in glass houses should not throw stones. For example, have you ever approached an intersection while driving and the driver coming from the other direction suddenly turned left in front of you without signaling? If so, you probably entertained some not-so-positive thoughts about the other driver then a few blocks down the road, you found yourself displaying the exact same behavior—turning without a proper signal. Somehow, nature has a way of balancing our actions and criticisms. Thinking about similar situations you have experienced should help keep you from being so quick to criticize others.

Do Not Insist on Having the Last Word. This can be especially difficult for an educator. However, even if you may be right most of the time, sometimes things are better left unsaid. Remember, it is never necessary to apologize for things you *have not* said or done.

By following these simple steps, you will find that others are drawn to you and will look forward to conversation and interaction because you are kind and considerate.

General Instructor Responsibilities

There is no doubt that a positive mental attitude is indispensable to success and achievement. You can build and maintain a positive attitude by focusing on doing what appears immediately in front of you. This automatically leads to the next step until you ultimately reach your goal. Your personal desire should be to develop an attitude that is so strong that no matter what happens, you are able to remain positive and optimistic. After all, what good is an attitude that is only positive when things are going well? This relates back to your self-confidence and your faith that no matter how distressing situations may seem in the here and now, they will work out positively in the long run. It has been determined that successful people are really no different from anyone else, with the exception of one special characteristic: They choose to work toward achieving their goals rather than thinking and worrying about the challenges and difficulties that face them daily.

> ## IT'S WORTH ❋ REMEMBERING
>
> We can choose to be negative (take the "red pill" every day) or we can choose to be positive (take the "green pill" every day). Either way, we are making choices that determine how we build our futures.

Respected neuropsychologist Dr. Karl Pribram has found that the "law of attraction" is prevalent in today's society. He concludes that any visual image, especially one that is visualized in complete detail, sets up an energetic force field that attracts into your life the ideas, things, people, and circumstances that are consistent with your visual image. Think about that: If your image is positive, it will eventually bring about positive, desired outcomes. If it is negative, you achieve the same results. This relates to the theory that we are, in fact, in control of our own attitudes.

It is has been said that a healthy self-esteem and positive self-talk are the spiritual seeds of happiness and success. It is up to us as individuals to get those seeds to sprout. Nothing is more nourishing for those seeds than a positive attitude. Conversely, any chance for happiness or success can be squelched by negativity. If that sounds like exaggeration or hype, consider the discovery in the second half of the twentieth century that a positive mental attitude is one of the single most important traits toward achieving health and happiness. Medical researchers discovered endorphins, the natural, internal opiates secreted and used by the brain that screen out unpleasant stimuli and reduce the experience of pain. In a study related to this discovery, actors were connected to electrodes and blood catheters that measured the rate at which the body produced endorphins. The actors were then asked to act out various scenes that portrayed a wide range of emotions. When the actors portrayed characters who were joyful, confident, and full of love, the rate of endorphin production in the body soared. Conversely, when they portrayed characters who were depressed or angry or devastated and without hope, the endorphin production dropped significantly. These scientific studies and experiments have shown that endorphins engender feelings of optimism, satisfaction, and safety. What's more, the studies prove that you are in control of your own attitudes. If actors can pretend to be positive and enthusiastic, and actually become positive and enthusiastic due to the increased rate of endorphin production, there is no justification for feelings of negativity ever again . . . unless, of course, you just want to indulge in a "pity party."

Remember that negativity can spread like flames in a forest fire. Negative attitudes can literally destroy a school, harm interpersonal relationships, and cease the growth of creativity among students. Negative people are usually frustrated, lonely, and profoundly unhappy. They are often driven to external means to cure their depression. They hope to find the answer in drugs, alcohol, tranquilizers, food binges, shopping sprees, gambling, or promiscuity. In order to save themselves, they must learn that they have the ability to control their own thoughts and can therefore change for the better.

Viktor Frankl wrote, when reflecting on his experiences in Nazi concentration camps, that the last great freedom of man is the freedom to choose his own attitude under any given set of circumstances. We cannot control what happens to us in some cases, but we can control our attitude toward what happens to us. As a master educator, you will be responsible for your own actions and attitudes. Educators who are happy, satisfied with themselves, and successful in attaining their goals are self-made, and their positive attitudes helped them get there! Remember, it is nearly impossible for even the most difficult student to remain argumentative, neutral, or

IT'S WORTH REMEMBERING ✳

The greatest thing about the discovery of how endorphins function is that it is now known that we no longer have to lose control. We can pretend, imagine, and play-act certain emotions, feelings, and attitudes and, ultimately, we can determine our own behavior. This is much better than "reacting," without control, to others' behavior and actions.

indifferent in the presence of a positive educator. You will radiate energy, good humor, and motivation. Students will become infected by your endearing and positive outlook. Your attitude is definitely a choice you make, and a positive attitude is indispensable to your success!

Wrapping It Up ✓

Educators are unique in that they are required to prepare and present information to a group of learners from diverse backgrounds on a daily basis. In doing so, they must interact effectively with coworkers, clients, and students. The profile of a master educator will vary based upon individual strengths, weaknesses, abilities, and attitudes. Our national survey of school managers and directors, however, established that a number of attitudes and behaviors are required of educators to ensure success in the institution. First and foremost, they are looking for *loyalty* to the institution and its mission. They also seek educators who *welcome advice and counsel from their colleagues*. At the top of the list was the *constant pursuit of knowledge* and professional development within the beauty industry and as an educator. They expect their educators to *organize* their work in advance and *manage their time* effectively. Educators who are *self-confident authorities* in their given field and maintain order and tranquility in their classrooms are also in demand.

Employers are, of course, always seeking educators of high moral excellence who hold dear a set of *moral principles* and *ethics* that are above reproach. They have stated that it is essential for their educators to maintain *dependable*, regular attendance as well as a *willingness to adapt* to the inevitable changes that occur daily in the industry. The dynamics of *teamwork* and *cooperation* among all personnel are also essential ingredients in the profile of a master educator. Schools are also looking for educators who exercise *initiative* in starting and following through on assigned work; they need educators who *work independently* with little close supervision. In addition, they recognize that educators must be able to convey *patience* and master *self-control* in light of today's educational environment. As educational institutions, schools also consider a *professional image* to be essential for educators. How can educators possibly serve as role models for students if they do not project a positive, professional image as an example? Schools have determined that many of the other qualities and characteristics required of a master educator can be more easily accomplished if the educator is *courteous*, *compassionate*, and *consistent* when dealing with learners.

Based on the many years of experience held by the schools surveyed, it was established that to be a master educator, you must have strong *personal desire* and *motivation*. With desire and motivation, a certain amount of *energy* and *enthusiasm* comes naturally. These are also key ingredients necessary for success as a master educator. Schools are looking for educators who have developed their *imagination* and *creative ability* and who share that creativity in the classroom. They state that *effective communications skills* are needed to reach the variety of generations and backgrounds in today's learners. Finally, all survey respondents agreed that the master educator will possess a *winning personality* and a *positive attitude* on a daily basis.

IT'S WORTH REMEMBERING ✳

As a master educator you will have countless opportunities to strike a match to the inner spirit and potential of your students. What a powerful responsibility!

IT'S WORTH REMEMBERING ✳

If you give just a little, you will get just a little. If you give yourself fully to building your character and your career through excellent actions and performance, you will build a future that impacts many lives over many years.

By developing all these qualities and characteristics, the master educator is better equipped to fill the demanding roles required of the position: motivator, coach, mentor, friend, disciplinarian, peace-maker, negotiator, arbitrator, nurturer, and entertainer!

In Retrospect

1. List the qualities and characteristics desired in a master educator.

2. What are the key concepts in time management and event control?

3. List at least five strategies for building self-confidence.

4. What are at least three steps you can take for taking initiative and practicing self-control?

5. List at least five actions for self-motivation.

6. What can an educator do to develop his or her personal enthusiasm?

7. What steps can be taken to develop a winning personality and a positive attitude?

2

The Teaching Plan and Learning Environment

Desired Performance Goals:

After reading and studying this chapter, you should be able to:

- List the benefits of effective organization and teacher preparation.

- List the characteristics that are common among adult learners.

- State the goals of classroom arrangement and organization.

- Perform the administrative tasks required of the educator and explain what they include.

! CRITICAL CONCEPT

Master educators know things that begin well are more likely to end well. Thus, they plan carefully for the learning experience to begin well.

The Teaching Plan

THE EDUCATOR'S ABILITY to lead and inspire students to a sincere desire for learning is critical in the educational process. That ability must also be accompanied by the educator's regular performance of routine duties and effective management of the classroom. It should be the goal of every educator to create a positive learning environment that will provide a pathway to career success for students. The educator of the twenty-first century is better known as a facilitator of learning than as a teacher. To **facilitate** means to make easier or to bring about. Learning can clearly be made *easier*, if the classroom environment is well organized, pleasant, and conducive to education. That can be accomplished with careful planning and consideration of several key issues.

facilitate
make easier, aid, assist.

Teacher Organization and Preparation

The ease and efficiency of each class or course greatly depends on the organization and preparation time the instructor invests. Classroom organization includes knowing your subject matter and the most recent developments in your chosen field that will impact what you teach. The teacher who is planning ahead will learn how many students will be in the class and then plan activities to learn about them and what brought them to this particular educational program. In addition, the instructor will identify the materials and equipment necessary to properly facilitate learning of the subjects covered in the course. The classroom where instruction will take place will be carefully assessed, and options available for offering a varied environment during instruction will be considered.

+ MASTER EDUCATOR

1. Prepares and organizes prior to the actual start of class.
2. Maintains current knowledge relevant to the field of study.
3. Develops organized work habits to ensure that administrative tasks such as record keeping and reports are completed accurately and timely.
4. Ensure classrooms are safe while also providing a motivating and comfortable environment for learning.

CONSIDER AND CONNECT

The more time an educator spends in preparation, the more time will be available for engaging students in active learning.

Proper organization and preparation help educators to:

- understand their group of students
- properly allot and designate class time
- allow for appropriate office time to fulfill administrative responsibilities
- properly set up effective records management
- plan daily activities throughout the course
- be current in their chosen educational field
- maximize the budget allowed for the course of instruction
- organize needed educational aids and course resources
- develop handouts in a professional manner
- review course materials and supplemental resources to refresh knowledge
- create an environment that is welcoming and safe
- create appropriate checklists for the classroom or laboratory as applicable
- establish the appropriate tone, expectations, and motivational environment for the class

Setting the appropriate tone for the first day of class is critical to creating a dynamic learning environment. It also plays a part in facilitating appropriate closure to the course. If the teacher is organized, the typical class will run smoothly. Student records will be properly maintained and current (Figure 2–1). Students will know how they are progressing through the course. They will receive relevant and timely feedback from the instructor and reach the end of the course in a satisfactory manner.

General Organization

We have more data available to us now than ever before. Organized educators will take full advantage of that information and plan a system that works for them (Figure 2–2 a and b). That may be a hard-copy system with paper documents properly filed in an organized filing cabinet or it may be an electronic system where files and folders are organized on a hard drive. The most important thing that you should remember as an instructor is that you need to organize your materials in a system that works for you. Failure to do so will likely mean that you do not use all the information and data available to you. Following are some suggestions to aid in organizing for your course.

- Copy the material, either electronically or in print. Place information in a folder, either on your hard drive or in a paper folder.
- Properly file the material. It is suggested that you create a large folder for each unit of study and then insert separate files for each of the topics to be covered. For example, you might have a folder titled "Business" and then have several files within, such as Financial Statements, Retail Sales, Marketing, Advertising, Policies and Procedures, and so on.
- File trade journals and articles by date. If you subscribe to popular trade magazines, consider purchasing sturdy magazine files at the local office supply store. A simpler and less expensive method is simply to file them in chronological order in a bookcase. If the spines do not contain the date of publication, insert tabs containing that important information.
- Arrange reference or resource books and texts on a book case. Label the books by subject area.
- Schedule office time if it is shared with another educator or adjunct faculty member.
- Create a support system among faculty. This can be achieved through regular staff meetings, which promote effective communication among faculty members. It will also help them to stay abreast of institutional news, events, and policies.

Knowing Students and Organizing Student Information

It will be to your advantage to learn as much about your students as possible. Doing so promotes understanding of your students as individuals, promotes beneficial discussions with students, enables student internal motivation, and facilitates instruction specifically directed toward student interests and goals. Students who believe you have taken a personal interest in their success will enjoy the educational experience more, have

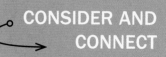

CONSIDER AND CONNECT

Educators who are prepared maximize student learning and minimize behavioral issues.

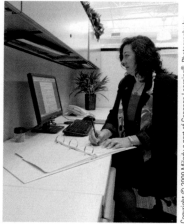

Figure 2–1   A prepared educator will organize and properly maintain student records.

IT'S WORTH REMEMBERING

A good plan may end up as only a good intention unless it is effectively put into action.

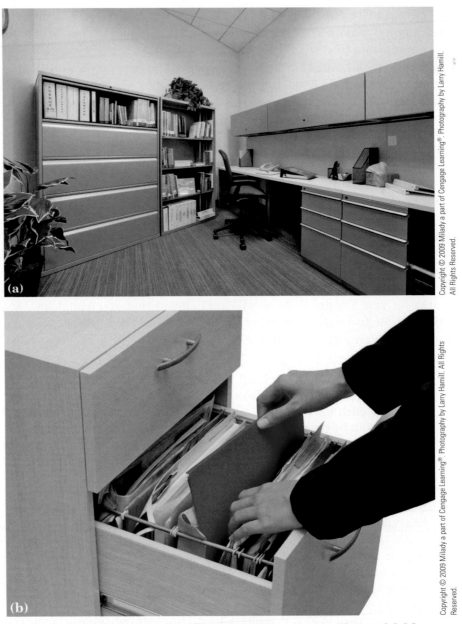

Figure 2–2 (a, b)   Successful educators will organize files and folders in a system that works best for them.

Confidential Student Profile a document containing personal student information and other relevant information, including copies of successful projects, thoughts on what motivates the student, goals and interests of the student, and any learning obstacles that affect the student.

better attendance, and study harder. They will likely encourage their fellow classmates to do the same.

Your school will have already established certain procedures for maintaining student information. It is imperative that you become completely familiar with those systems and procedures and follow them implicitly. Some additional ideas for gathering and using student information follow.

- **Create a Confidential Student Profile.** An example of a student profile questionnaire is shown in (Figure 2–3). Include initial opening-activity results, copies of successful projects, thoughts on what motivates the student, goals and interests of the students, and any learning obstacles that affect the student. Always follow school policies as well

Student name: _____

Educational background: _____

Prior work experience: _____

_____

Why you chose this field of study: _____

_____

List any obstacles that might impact your progress through the course of study: ___

_____

_____

What are your one-year, three-year, and five-year career goals? _____

_____

_____

_____

Birth location: _____

Number, age, and gender of siblings: _____

Hobbies/personal interests: _____

Favorite color: _____ Favorite restaurant: _____

Favorite vacation: _____

Favorite flower: _____ Favorite fragrance: _____

Favorite book: _____ Favorite movie: _____

Favorite music/song: _____ Favorite TV show: _____

List something unique about you that very few people know about: _____

Figure 2–3   Sample student profile questionnaire.

as those established by the Family Educational Rights and Privacy Act and any other regulatory oversight agency with respect to student files and information.

- **Create a Record of Student Progress.** This may include student attendance, absences, completion of learning objectives, attitude, class participation, professionalism, and withdrawal dates. This record may be written or electronic as defined by your school. Numerous published products allow students to complete work by means of a student CD-ROM or an online program. Many of these types of products allow instructors to either import grade information or access student progress via the computer.

- **Document Student Contacts.** This does not have to be a time-consuming or overwhelming task. Simply complete the documentation immediately and file it appropriately. You may choose to use an electronic system, a hand-written system, or a combination of both. A spiral notebook is a simple way to document phone conversations. Always remember to note the date, time, student name, and details of the conversation. A similar system can be used for personal meetings or conversations. Since we now live in the Internet age, e-mail is a routine method for communicating. Be sure to set up a system of saving e-mails in an electronic file cabinet. You should consider keeping a list of student names with their e-mails.

Managing the Atmosphere

The classroom is the domain of the educator. It is the place where you will spend a significant part of your life. You should take pride in its appearance and take whatever measures are necessary to create a safe haven and place where educators and learners alike can enjoy being there (Figure 2–4). You must ensure that the physical condition of the classroom is comfortable, safe, well-ventilated, and organized and has proper lighting. A cluttered, disorganized, or poorly arranged classroom will have a negative impact on the learning process. You should make certain that you know how to safely operate all tools and equipment used in the classroom. You will see that all such materials are properly stored upon completion of their use. You will ensure that all implements or tools are properly cleaned and stored at the end of the class or day as applicable. You will insist that waste materials are properly contained and removed regularly as well.

The educator's desk and/or work area should set an example of good housekeeping for the students. It should be organized and free of dust, debris, or food and any noneducational items. This will set the pace for the general housekeeping required in the classroom. Bulletin boards should be updated regularly. Books and shelves should be dusted routinely. Boards should be cleaned daily. A master educator will set such an example for order and cleanliness that students will easily be inspired to model that behavior. It is also important that the educator make routine inspections of the facilities and the equipment for which she is responsible and prepare written reports to ensure that needed repairs can be performed when necessary.

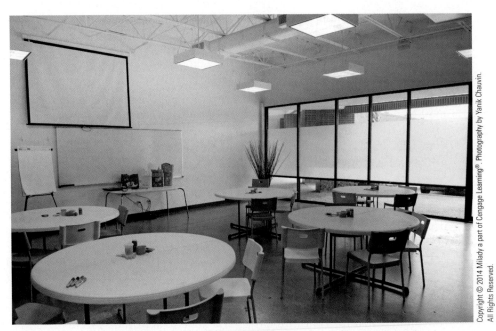

Figure 2–4   Educators should create a safe haven and comfortable, well-organized classroom.

Consider the Environment

The primary objective of every educator should be to create an environment that facilitates optimal instruction and learning. This includes classroom characteristics—from how the classroom is arranged to library resources and equipment—and includes the interpersonal environment as well. A large part of your preparation will be to assess your classroom environment and make the necessary adjustments to achieve optimum results. You will want to consider the following:

- Student demographics and adult learner characteristics. Who makes up your class? How can their backgrounds and characteristics be used to positively impact the environment?
- The physical classroom. Is the lighting sufficient? Does the ventilation meet the needs of the class? Will students be comfortable? Can they learn here?
- The seating arrangements. Will students be able to have eye contact with each other? Will students be able to communicate effectively with each other? How much control will the educator be able to maintain?

Adult Learner Characteristics

Before an educator begins any educational program, it is important to have a firm understanding of who the learners will be. It is important to know why they are being trained, what experience they bring with them to the classroom, and, perhaps most important, what anxieties and expectations they have. By understanding your learners, you will be taking the first step toward becoming a master educator. Researchers and psychologists have identified a number of characteristics common among adult learners, as discussed next.

Goal Orientation. Adult learners tend to be more goal-oriented than younger learners. Relevance is important to them—they need to be able to apply what they've learned right away. They recognize the need for their learning to make a difference in their careers—they want more than theory; they want information they can grasp and put into practical use.

Past Educational Experience. Adult learners have already experienced a wide array of training beginning at home, in school, and then perhaps in various jobs prior to pursuing career education. Some of those experiences may have been positive while others may have been not so positive. If your adult learners did not do well in school, for example, they may tend to be apprehensive or defensive when placed in an adult learning environment.

Ingrained Habits. Adult learners may come to your classrooms with behavior patterns that may be contrary to what you will be presenting. Adult learners may be less flexible or more difficult to persuade than other learners. They may feel threatened when told that former behaviors must change. The master educator will take advantage of the learners' past experiences and behaviors and, whenever possible, use them to improve procedures or techniques.

Established Opinions. Adult learners often arrive with established opinions about what is being taught. Those opinions may not always be productive or appropriate but should be recognized as important. Adults need to be told that their ideas and opinions have value and weight, and that they are significant, if they are to be actively involved in the learning process.

Relationship with Prior Knowledge. Adult learners tend to make connections with information or knowledge they already have. The master educator will continually relate new information to familiar situations or procedures. This gives the adult learners familiar ground on which to stand while you are also asking them to stretch or expand into unfamiliar territory. This makes the training process less threatening, more accessible, and more comfortable. In addition, the practicality and usefulness of the new information becomes more relevant.

Involvement Is Needed. Adult learners are not willing to simply sit in a classroom and receive information passively. They need to participate in the learning process and know that their participation is having a positive effect on the learning process. Master educators will limit lecture to absolutely essential information and then involve the learners by having them use that information. Educators should ask questions, ask for learners' opinions, challenge learners to think, and incite reaction on the part of the learners as to what is taking place in the classroom. If students have an active role in the learning process, they will have a personal stake in making that process successful.

☑ Student Demographics

Clearly, there has never been a time in history where the student body in any classroom was more diverse. Student demographics will have a significant impact on how you present information and interact with the class as well as how students will interact with each other (Figure 2–5). It makes sense, then, that instructors need to learn as much as they can about all

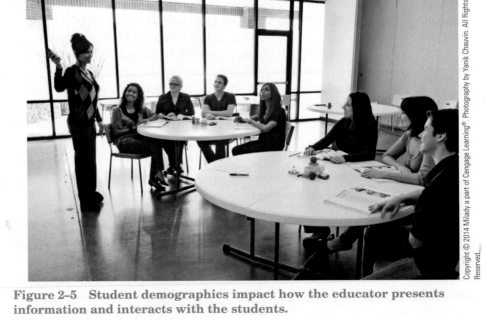

Figure 2–5   Student demographics impact how the educator presents information and interacts with the students.

their students individually and collectively. You may want to consider the following elements.

Age. It is likely that you will have students ranging in age from 18 to 60. That means they will bring different backgrounds, education, experiences, opinions, and expectations to your classroom. You will need to model respect for each age range in order to expect the same respect from your students. Invite perspectives from all age ranges. Recognize differences that result from age; likewise, recognize similarities. By facilitating learning that involves students from varied age groups working together, you will be better preparing your graduates for the workforce.

Gender. It will be important for you to understand the differences between male and female learners and maximize the strengths that each brings to the classroom. Research shows that male students tend to keep speaking when interrupted until their point is adequately made, whereas female students are less likely to reenter class discussion after being interrupted. The instructor should monitor who is contributing to discussion and the interactions between students. Group dynamics should also be noted, including identification of the leaders and the listeners.

Ethnicity. The ethnic background of a student may influence how the student perceives and learns information as well as how she engages in interpersonal relationships. Instructors should make every effort to understand and honor cultural and ethnic differences and avoid stereotyping students at all costs. Remember that recognizing and sharing cultural perspectives adds depth and richness to the learning experience.

Unique Interests. All adult learners have developed and experienced a wide range of hobbies and special interests. Relating as much of the education as possible to what students already know will increase learner interest and retention.

Making It Happen

You can take a number of approaches to get to know your students better and gain a deeper understanding of the student body as a whole. One idea is to simply ask the student to write a personal profile on the first day of school. Explain that you are requesting the information to make your instruction more applicable to individual interests. Ask them to write a brief description of their educational and cultural background, past work experiences, special interests, and why they have chosen their particular field of study. In lieu of a written profile, have a brainstorming session where students simply share the information verbally.

As a dedicated educator, it is important for you to be aware of learners' attitudes, past experiences, habits, and opinions. In doing so, you will be able to understand their perspectives and be able to help them discover how useful a change in behavior can be. Involve them actively in the learning process and those behavior changes will occur more quickly.

The Physical Environment

Both your teaching and student learning will be influenced by the physical environment of your class. You will need to consider room size, acoustics, lighting, ventilation, windows, audiovisual aids, and seating. For example, lighting needs will vary based on the learning activity. It is important to know how to operate the lights properly to deliver smooth and professional presentations. If your windows are treated with blinds, check ahead of time to see how they affect shadows or reflections on the board or screen. Determine where the controls are for heating and cooling and plan ahead for the increased temperature that will occur when the classroom is full of students. Identify where the vents are and how adjustment can affect the room temperature. Prepared educators will also make note of the audiovisual equipment and supplies needed to meet the objectives of the course. They will practice operating the equipment and know where replacements supplies such as bulbs for projectors are stored. A determination must be made regarding sufficient electrical outlets for needed equipment and whether heavy-duty extension cords or surge protectors will be needed. In addition, depending on the size of the classroom and student body, the acoustics must also be considered. Educators will need to determine whether a microphone is needed and whether there is potential for distracting noise and what to do about it.

The Motivating Classroom

The manner in which the educator arranges the classroom and learning space is an integral part of classroom management. The room should be organized to:

- allow varied instructional activities to occur simultaneously;
- suit the needs of the educator and learners;
- properly store all supplies and equipment;
- ensure there are no auditory or visual distractions for learners;
- ensure the educator has a clear view of all learners at all times;
- ensure that frequently needed materials and supplies are readily accessible to the educator and the learners; and
- create excitement and facilitate internal motivation for learners.

The room design can communicate to learners that participation in the lesson is expected and encouraged. Classroom arrangement includes everything from the educator's presence in the room to the arrangement of the seats to the use of the walls and bulletin boards. A master educator will have fully prepared the lesson prior to class, arrive early for class and greet students as they enter, preassign seats or lab stations if appropriate based upon class objectives, have learning activities designed to motivate students, and will use color and visuals in the classroom to promote learning. Many content-related and motivational posters are available that can be positioned around the classroom to inspire learning and motivate students. (For more information on this topic, please refer to Chapter 11, "Educational Aids and Technology in the Classroom.") Bulletin boards can be used to enhance learning, increase content retention, and notify students of important information such as assignments, procedures, and so forth. Having students create motivational bulletin boards in teams is a great way for students to discover important information about a given subject.

The use of color in the educational facility can also have a major impact on learning. Educators may find that using color to attract attention and reinforce learning is a useful technique. Some colors seem to be automatically soothing, while others can be irritating or distracting. For example, some researchers have determined that pale yellow and almond are the best colors for not causing irritation. Pale pink and light rose colors have been determined to be very soothing and have been used in jails and behavior-disorder classrooms for young children. Green gives a sense of security and seems to inspire creativity and would be appropriate for a lab or clinic where creativity is greatly needed. Blue is relaxing and causes the brain to secrete tranquilizing hormones. It has been identified as the color of academics and it is a good color for general classrooms. Because it is a soothing color, computer screens are often light blue. Color and brain research indicate that orange seems to agitate learners, and bright yellow excites the brain and the body. Research also shows that data conveyed in natural colors as compared to black and white are retained at a much higher rate.

The seating arrangement helps determine educator control, sight lines with and among learners, and overall student participation. Several different arrangements that can be effective for teaching are depicted in this chapter. In each diagram, the large X represents the position of the facilitator or educator.

U-shaped Arrangement. The **U-shaped arrangement** is effective for small classes up to about 15 people. It is effective for lecture, demonstration, and discussion. This arrangement can accommodate use of a flip chart or multipurpose board/chalkboard near the educator. This shape gives the educator or facilitator high control over the classroom, but its drawbacks include less eye contact among learners and less participation of the learners (Figure 2–6a).

Circle Arrangement. The **circle arrangement** is also effective for small classes up to about 15 people. It is suitable for conducting lectures, discussion, role-playing, and completing case studies. It would not be effective for use with projected visual aids, because it would be difficult for everyone in the circle to see a screen from a suitable angle. This arrangement provides the educator with high control of the group, opportunity for excellent eye contact among learners, and the promotion of good participation within the class (Figure 2–6b).

Boardroom Arrangement. The **boardroom arrangement** is suitable for roundtable-type discussions. It is also known as the solid or hollow rectangle arrangement. This arrangement is suitable for situations such as meetings of staff or consultations with an advisory committee. It is not an arrangement used often in a career education classroom. This arrangement allows only medium control by the educator and limits eye contact and participation among learners (Figure 2–6c).

Semicircle Arrangement. The **semicircle arrangement** can be highly effective for small classes up to about 10 learners. This might be a good option for small phase I or beginner classes where the educator wants to form a close bond with all students and ensure good interaction among students. It can be used for informal discussion, allowing the facilitator or educator to be seated. It also allows for effective use of visual aids that can be seen by all. It provides the educator with a high degree of control, excellent eye contact with and among the learners, and a high degree of participation by the learners (Figure 2–6d).

Classroom-Style Arrangement. The **classroom-style arrangement** may be the most commonly used in traditional classrooms but is clearly not

U-shaped arrangement an arrangement for small classes up to about 15; effective for lecture, demonstration, and discussion; facilitator has high control.

circle arrangement an arrangement for small classes up to about 15; effective for lectures, discussion, role-playing, and completing case studies; facilitator has high control.

boardroom arrangement an arrangement suitable for roundtable-type discussions or meetings; not often used in career education classroom; facilitator has medium control.

semicircle arrangement an arrangement effective for small classes up to about 10 learners; effective for informal discussion; facilitator has high degree of control.

classroom-style arrangement an arrangement commonly used in traditional education; can be used for lecture, demonstration, discussion, or panel discussions; facilitator has high control; provides poor opportunity for participation and interaction.

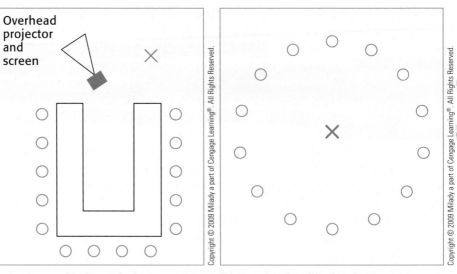

Figure 2–6a   U-shaped classroom arrangement.

Figure 2–6b   Circle classroom arrangement.

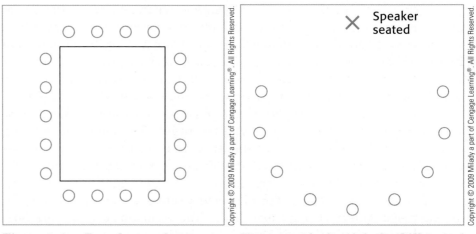

Figure 2–6c   Boardroom classroom arrangement.

Figure 2–6d   Semicircle classroom arrangement.

chevron-style arrangement an arrangement also known as the V-shape; can be used for lecture, demonstration, discussion, role-playing, and case studies; suitable for small and large groups; facilitator has medium control.

theater-style arrangement an arrangement suitable for lecture, slide use, and video projection; can be used for small or very large groups; facilitator has high control; provides for poor opportunity for participation and interaction.

the most effective. It can be used for lecture, demonstration, discussion, or panel discussions. It provides the educator with a high degree of control of the classroom. However, it provides poor opportunity for eye contact and interaction among the learners present. It can be used for both small and large groups (Figure 2–6e).

Chevron-Style Arrangement. The **chevron-style arrangement** is also known as the V-shape. It only allows the educator to have medium control of the classroom, but it allows for good eye contact among many learners and encourages effective learner participation. It can be used for lecture, demonstration, discussion, role-playing, and case studies. It is suitable for both small and large classes and is often used for classes and seminars presented in hotels or convention centers (Figure 2–6f).

Theater-Style Arrangement. **Theater-style arrangement** is less likely to be used in schools that teach in career education institutions. Generally, in theater-style arrangement, there is no desktop available for use by the learners. The arrangement is suitable for lecture, slide use, and video projection.

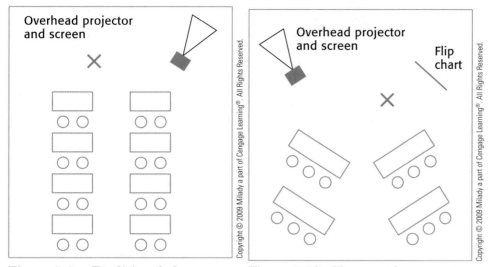

Figure 2–6e   Traditional classroom arrangement.

Figure 2–6f   Chevron classroom arrangement.

It can be used for small classes or groups up to several hundred. It gives the educator or facilitator a medium degree of control of the room, provides for very poor eye contact among the learners, and discourages participation of the learners (Figure 2–6g).

Amphitheater Arrangement. The **amphitheater arrangement** is not as common in small career education institutions. However, it is highly effective for lecture, demonstration, slide or video projection, and role-playing. The educator has a high degree of control over the classroom. However, only medium eye contact will occur among those present, as well as a lesser degree of participation or interaction among the learners (Figure 2–6h).

Half-round or Crescent Arrangement. The **half-round or crescent arrangement** has also been referred to as *cabaret*. This is by far the most popular style for learner-centered education. It can be used for lecture, demonstration, discussion, slide or video projection, role-playing, group projects, and activities. In this setting, communication can take place within groups, between groups, and with the instructor. It provides for a high degree of eye contact and participation among the learners, which results in the educator having a slightly lower degree of control over the classroom. However, as we move away from teacher-centered education and focus on learner-centered, discovery-driven education, this classroom arrangement is highly effective and encouraged in adult education (Figure 2–6i).

Master educators will learn to adapt the arrangement of their classroom to the style most appropriate for the method of instruction delivery and the objectives of the lesson. Changing the arrangement of the classroom periodically creates interest and reduces the monotony the students might feel if it never changes.

The Practical Classroom

If your assigned course of study includes practical skills, you will need to visit the facility to ensure that the environment is also conducive to active learning. A number of elements should be considered when evaluating and preparing your lab space.

amphitheater arrangement an arrangement that is highly effective for lecture, demonstration, slide or video projection, and role-playing; facilitator has high degree of control; provides poor opportunity for participation and interaction.

half-round or crescent arrangement an arrangement also called cabaret; most popular for learner-centered education; used for lecture, demonstration, discussion, slide or video projection, role-playing, group projects and activities; facilitator has lower degree of control, but this arrangement provides for high degree of eye contact, participation, and interaction.

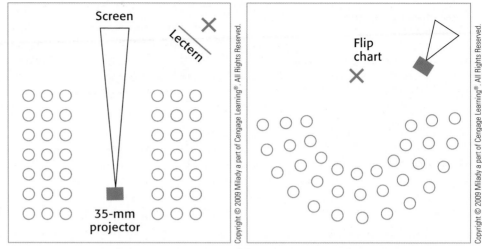

Figure 2–6g   Theater-style classroom arrangement.

Figure 2–6h   Amphitheater classroom arrangement.

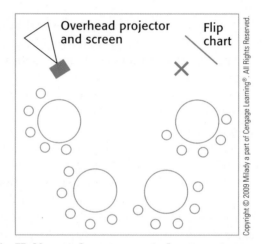

Figure 2–6i   Half-round or crescent classroom arrangement.

Special Needs Accessibility. Under the Americans with Disabilities Act (ADA) of 1990, students with a documented disability are entitled to receive special accommodations. Such accommodations are designed to provide the student with equal access to educational facilities. For a more detailed discussion of the ADA and teaching students with disabilities, please see Chapter 9, "Achieving Learner Results." When preparing for class and assessing lab facilities, consider what accommodations can be made for students with special needs. You will work with individual students to assess their needs and determine how best to meet them.

Number of Learning Stations. To ensure the optimal learning experience, there should be a sufficient number of learning stations that are appropriately equipped for the largest class size assigned to the lab.

Equipment. Determine that all lab equipment is working properly; an ill-equipped lab will prevent students from attaining learning outcomes. Make sure you know who to contact regarding maintenance and repairs. More important, ensure you know how to properly operate all equipment and can demonstrate the operation effectively for your students.

Supplies. As you familiarize yourself with the class schedule, you will be able to list the required supplies for each lab activity and create a schedule for obtaining them. Your planning regarding lab supplies will include the proper storage of supplies in accordance with any applicable storage and disposal guidelines set forth by regulatory agencies such as the Occupational Safety and Health Administration (OSHA).

Policies and Procedures. Your school will have established policies regarding the operation of labs. Review those policies carefully and determine if you need to supplement them. Further, make sure that the policies are clearly communicated to all students. Explain them, provide them to students, post them, and enforce them. Policies might include hours of operation, required staff supervision, consumption of food or beverages, equipment check-out procedures, and equipment or supply replacement procedures.

Learning Facilities Checklist

The checklist in Table 2–1 has been adapted from Delmar Cengage Learning's Faculty Development Program, Module 2, Teacher Preparation.

Table 2–1

LEARNING FACILITIES CHECKLIST

ELEMENT	STATUS	COMMENTS
Room Size and Arrangement		
—Room size appropriate	_____	
—Seating appropriate for class activities	_____	
—Seating variations possible	_____	
Acoustics		
—Speaking conditions evaluated	_____	
—Microphones tested	_____	
—Microphone operation is understood	_____	
—Noise distractions identified and adjustments made	_____	
Lighting and Blinds		
—Switches located	_____	
—Electrical system located	_____	
—Blinds assessed for shadows and reflections	_____	
Ventilation		
—Controls located	_____	
—Vents located	_____	
—Adjustment methods understood	_____	

continued

ELEMENT	STATUS	COMMENTS
Audiovisual		
—Equipment needs identified	_____	
—Check-out procedures known	_____	
—Equipment is in working order	_____	
—Replacement procedures understood	_____	
—Trial run completed	_____	
—Supplies (markers, erasers, flip charts, etc.) available	_____	
—Marker colors appropriate	_____	
—Electrical outlets located and sufficient	_____	
—Extension cords and surge protectors obtained if needed	_____	
Lab Stations		
—Configuration is optimal for learning needs	_____	
—Student-to-station ratio is optimal and meets accreditation standards	_____	
—Policies in place for station assignment	_____	
—Equipment is in working order	_____	
—Repair procedures known	_____	
—Trial run completed	_____	
—Equipment operation understood	_____	
Lab Supplies		
—Resources are identified	_____	
—Reorder needs and time frames identified	_____	
—Supply budget known	_____	
—Allocation of supplies identified, documented, and made known to students	_____	
—OSHA regulations followed	_____	
Policies and Procedures		
—Institutional and instructor policies and procedures identified and documented	_____	
—Policies provided to students	_____	
—Students have acknowledged policies	_____	
Special Needs Students		
—Special needs identified	_____	
—Accommodations reviewed	_____	
—Adaptations made	_____	
Other		
—Additional considerations may be added in this space	_____	

Teaching Materials

Well-organized, focused, and clear educational materials and resources will serve students effectively in their learning experience. A few elements for consideration when reviewing textbooks follow.

Relevance. Does the textbook cover the relevant topics? Does it meet the objectives of the course of study? Are supplemental resources available to support the content?

Student Level. What is the educational background of the student body? Is the textbook reading level appropriate? Is it too fundamental or too comprehensive?

Timeliness. Evaluate the textbook in relation to the rate of change in the applicable field of study. Consider the publication date. Will supplemental information be needed to ensure an effective course of study?

Credibility. The credibility of the publisher and the professional experience of the authors are significant in textbook evaluation. Consider authors' credentials, background, and experience relevant to the field of study.

Organization and Layout. The table of contents and preface should be thoroughly reviewed as well as the glossary, appendices, and index. Ask: Are the major learning objectives of your course covered? Does the organization assist students in locating and studying important content? Is quality paper used that prevents "bleed through" from color and graphics on the opposite side? Is the font clean and easy to read? Are there wide margins with white space used appropriately? Too much clutter is visually distracting and frustrating for learners. Wider margins and dividing the page into columns or portions provide for more effective visual organization, and information can be read and digested more easily (Figure 2–7).

For a more detailed discussion of educational materials and aids, refer to Chapter 11.

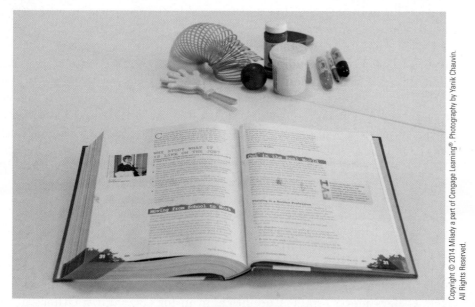

Figure 2–7   An example of an effectively designed textbook page.

Textbook Evaluation Checklist

The form in Table 2–2, adapted from Delmar Cengage Learning's Faculty Development Program, may be used to compare your choices of at least two textbooks for a particular class. In each of the categories provided, record your impressions of each book that you review. Completing the comparison in this manner allows you to do a side-by-side comparison of the applicable elements of each textbook.

Table 2–2

TEXTBOOK EVALUATION CHECKLIST			
Title of Text:			
Relevance of Text:			
Student Level of Text:			
Timeliness of Content:			
Credibility of Publisher and Authors:			
Organization and Layout:			

Administrative Responsibilities

Educators are responsible for a certain amount of record keeping and reports pertinent to managing a classroom. Such administrative requirements are set forth by the institution, by the state regulatory agency, and by the accrediting body. In order to comply with such requirements, educators must first become knowledgeable of all the rules and regulations governing their schools. Educators will maintain accurate records of student attendance, grades, and progress reports. Educators must document academic advising of students (a topic thoroughly covered in Chapter 12, "Assessing Progress and Advising Students"). Educators must develop and maintain daily lesson plans. Educators are often responsible for inventory and requisitions, at least within their area of responsibility. Educators may have to prepare monthly hours reports, as well as process student registrations, graduations, and withdrawals (Figure 2–8).

Other administrative tasks required of educators may be conducting surveys of students, attending advisory council meetings, writing reports about the facilities and equipment, giving feedback for the completion of institutional self-studies prepared for accrediting agencies, and more. Educators may also be requested to provide written reports on continuing education programs or seminars they have attended. Completion of such records and reports is a viable part of achieving the mission of the institution. Educators must be accurate and current if they are to be effective. The master educator will take the responsibility of record keeping seriously and schedule time to ensure that it is done in a quality manner.

Attendance

A number of methods can be used to track student attendance. Most clock-hour schools use some form of electronic or computerized time clock. Others merely have students sign in for class daily. Others use a

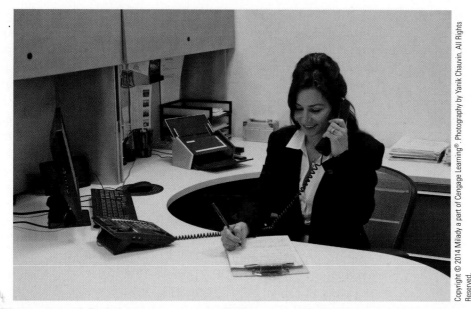

Figure 2–8   Administrative responsibilities may include inventory, record keeping, report writing, conducting surveys, and much more.

combination of both. Educators will need to monitor the procedures at their institution and make certain that students are following them diligently. If students are clocking in manually on a time clock, the educator may be charged with the responsibility of totaling hours at the end of the day. The educator may also have the authority to adjust those hours based on certain circumstances, such as rounding hours to the nearest quarter hour, giving credit for missed time through the approval of excused absences, recognizing time the student spent training through a scheduled lunch period if the school's policy and regulatory agencies allow it, and so forth. It is vital that all educators know all regulatory requirements regarding attendance and follow them explicitly. In addition, many students receive federal financial assistance to subsidize the cost of their career education. The U.S. Department of Education sets forth specific regulations governing student hours and financial aid disbursement. Attendance records for financial aid recipients are subject to an annual audit and periodic program reviews by the Department of Education. Therefore, all personnel, including educators, must take care to ensure that attendance records are accurate for every student enrolled.

Grade Records

The academic progress of students through a course of study is just as critical as their attendance progress. States, institutions, and federal agencies set forth satisfactory academic progress requirements for students in many areas. Oftentimes, students must meet certain grade averages and complete a prescribed number of skills in each learning category in order to graduate and be eligible for the state licensing examination. As with attendance, students must also meet certain grade requirements to be eligible to receive federal financial aid. Therefore, educators must grade students according to the institution's published grading criteria and record those grades appropriately. Chapter 12, "Assessing Progress and Advising Students," provides in-depth discussion of the foundations and purposes of grading as well as different grading procedures and styles.

The master educator understands that the administrative tasks that support the educational process are critical to the achievement of the institution's mission and objectives. Both quality education and careful administration of the institution's operations are integral elements necessary if students are to get the most from their educational experience.

Welcoming New Students

Dynamic educators recognize that the first day of class for new students sets the stage and mood for the remainder of the course of study. The "You never get a second chance to make a positive first impression" definitely applies to the first day of school. Developing a sound orientation program is one of the best ways to prevent future withdrawals from the program. Some key goals for the first day of school include setting the tone, establishing rapport, reviewing the standards, establishing expectations, introducing the course, clarifying course goals, answering questions, and teaching. Each of these areas will be discussed in detail in Chapter 10, "Program Review, Development, and Lesson Planning."

Wrapping It Up

We have established the importance of preparation and organization by the educator prior to the actual start of the class. Educators must maintain current knowledge relative to the field of study. It is necessary to develop organized work habits to ensure that administrative tasks such as record keeping and reports are completed accurately and in a timely manner. Classrooms must be safe while also providing a motivating and comfortable environment for learning. Course information requires organization to ensure that instructors have the required resources available when they are needed. Preparation and ongoing performance require organization to save time, work efficiently, and ensure greater opportunities for success.

In Retrospect

1. List the benefits and results of effective organization and teacher preparation.

2. List the characteristics that are common among adult learners.

3. List are the ultimate goals of classroom arrangement and organization.

4. List several administrative tasks required of an educator.

Objectives (Desired Performance Goals):

After reading and studying this chapter, you should be able to:

- List and explain reading skills.

- List note-taking and highlighting skills.

- Explain 15 strategies for effective studying.

- Avoid five failure habits.

- Identify key elements in developing a study group.

- Explain the importance of training students in test-wise strategies.

! CRITICAL CONCEPT

Master educators know that character is shaped by learning, so they help shape a student's character by acting as a learning catalyst.

MASTER EDUCATOR

1. Teaches study and test-wise strategies at the beginning of every program.
2. Enables students to learn success behaviors at the beginning of every program.
3. Works cooperatively with learners to reduce barriers to learning.

Learning Is Lifelong

LEARNING how to learn should be the first lesson every individual is taught. It is a lesson that may be even more important than what we learn.

It is essential that we teach our students the best possible learning skills. It doesn't matter whether our students are 17 or 70; we need to inspire in them the same openness to learning they experienced when they were three or four years old. As an educator, you will be giving them a gift that they will take with them through the rest of their lives. What they learn may become outdated, but the skill of how to learn will allow them to continue to master new information and skills for many years to come.

Developing Reading and Study Skills

A major barrier to learning is a student's inability to read and study effectively. As in any other educational endeavor, it is helpful to have a support system for the study process. Consider developing a handout for the parents or significant others in your students' lives that lists some of the things they can do to enhance the study environment, as described in the accompanying box.

IT'S WORTH REMEMBERING

We are never too old to learn. If we stop learning, we stop growing.

STUDY SUPPORT SYSTEM SAVVY

1. **Space Setup.** Create an area that is free of distraction, properly lit, and contains all the necessary supplies such as highlighters, colored markers for note taking and mind mapping, pencils, erasers, paper, dictionary, and so on.
2. **Establish a Routine.** Agree with the student on an organized and scheduled approach to study. Research shows that students with an organized study routine experience greater success.
3. **Eliminate Distractions.** Today's learners have been raised on MTV and may be able to concentrate with music on, but you should agree that study time is not the time for television. Turn off text messaging and cell phones during study time. An online computer, however, can be an added benefit.
4. **Establish Priorities.** The old saying that work comes before play applies here. Homework and study time must be the priority when in school. Help the student understand that fun and frolic may follow study time.
5. **Communicate with the Educators.** Support members may find it beneficial to find out what the student is learning and why. This allows you to place more emphasis and importance on what is expected of the student.
6. **Motivate and Encourage.** Students can be inspired to take their studying seriously by those they respect, but take care not to overdo it or nag.
7. **Get Involved.** Pay attention to learners' efforts, but don't do their work for them. For example, you can proofread papers, drill them on vocabulary, observe their technical skills, and provide feedback.

8. **Be a Role Model.** If their course of study requires them to do a lot of reading, it would be beneficial to observe you reading a lot as well.

9. **Provide Positive Reinforcement.** Give learners sincere praise when they do a good job or make a good grade.

10. **Be a Realist.** It's important to provide a positive support system, but students need to recognize that in the "real world," things are not always fair. They need to learn to *build a bridge and get over it*.

Reading Skills

Master educators will lay a solid groundwork of improved study skills upon which learners can build their career training experience. One of the first areas you may want to emphasize is their reading skills, as these should be developed even before study skills. Module 7 of Cengage Delmar Learning's Faculty Development Program, "Teaching Adults How to Learn," suggests a few strategies that your students may find beneficial. They are adapted here.

Time Allotment. Encourage students to allow ample time to read and comprehend material prior to testing. More difficult material requires more reading and comprehension time. Suggest that students break reading time into manageable segments and plot the reading on a timeline.

Skim First. Suggest that students should preview the material and identify concepts and topics they understand. They should pay attention to ways the material is organized, review chapter summaries, and note main ideas and headings. They should conduct additional research as needed.

Have References Handy. A good dictionary and access to the Internet are helpful. Students should refer to the school's library of resource information as necessary.

Employ Concept Connectors. Students should relate what they are reading to what they have previously learned in life and in school. They should examine what they are learning from the material and periodically review their progress and understanding.

Reread. Material may need to be reread until understanding is clear. Sometimes material has to be read in chunks; other times it will become clearer when the student reads all the way through the entire segment.

Evaluate. Teach students to assess what they know, what they have read, and what they need to review.

Underlining and Highlighting

Most students find that underling and highlighting text when reading and studying is an effective strategy. However, if 90 percent of the text is highlighted, the purpose has been defeated. It is beneficial to provide a few key strategies to students for this important step in learning. The following strategies have been found to be effective.

Create a System. As with note taking, students should be assisted in developing a system for organizing what they highlight and underline. Students should use different colors of highlighters for different concepts. For

I. Main Point
  A. Sub-point
    1. Subsub-point
    2. Subsub-point
  B. Sub-point

II. Main Point
  A. Sub-point
    1. Subsub-point
    2. Subsub-point
  B. Sub-point
    1. Subsub-point
    2. Subsub-point
  C. Sub-point
    1. Subsub-point
    2. Subsub-point

III. Main Point
  A. Sub-point
    1. Subsub-point
    2. Subsub-point
  B. Sub-point
    1. Subsub-point
    2. Subsub-point
  C. Sub-point
    1. Subsub-point
    2. Subsub-point
      a. Subsubsub-point
      b. Subsubsub-point

Figure 3–1   Traditional outlining may be preferred by highly analytical learners.

example, if teaching business skills, you might have students highlight the section on business ownership in yellow, the section on drafting a business plan in pink, and the section on marketing and advertising in aqua. Students will recognize and remember the content more readily based on the color used. In addition, if the content uses or reflects a specific symbol, the student should also use the same symbol in the notes.

Focus on Key Words or Phrases. Encourage selective highlighting based on important concepts, ideas, or facts.

Check for Meaning. Students should be advised to review their underlining and highlighting to ensure it all makes sense. If the highlighting is confusing or overdone, it will not be helpful. The student will then need to create a separate note-taking document or mind map to help clarify the information.

Note-Taking Skills

Another area you should emphasize early on is strong note-taking skills. Students use a variety of note-taking methods to capture the major points of a lesson. For the highly analytical learner, the standard outlining using Roman numerals may work (Figure 3–1). For the majority of our learners, however, less conventional methods, such as mind mapping, may be more appropriate (Figure 3–2). The method is not as important as the notes being well organized and understandable to the student. The following techniques for note-taking skills are adapted from Virginia Polytechnic Institute and State University, Division of Student Affairs.

- **Think about What You Are Hearing.** Remind students to actively think about how the information relates to other concepts they have learned in life or in class. Teach them to use reminder words or symbols that will be meaningful when they come back to the notes later.
- **Devise a Shorthand Method.** Recommend that students use standard paper (8.5" × 11") that allows them ample space to organize their notes more effectively. They can also write more legibly if they have sufficient space.

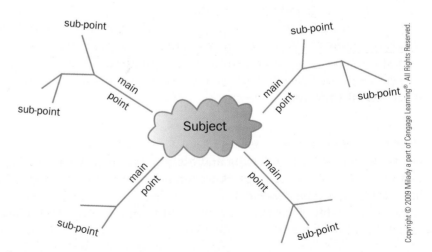

Figure 3–2   The majority of learners prefer less conventional methods for note taking, such as mind mapping.

- **Designate and Recognize Cues.** Let students know that if they see material written on the board or on an overhead slide, it will likely be on a test. Your voice emphasis may also be another cue for key information.
- **Clarify.** Encourage immediate questions if something is unclear. If students are unable to ask questions immediately, have students write them down on a Post-it and place them in an "Ask it Basket" or ask them later.
- **Reminder Notes for Discussion.** If the note-taking session is not part of a discussion, ask students to make a reminder note or symbol that will allow them to return to key points later during the scheduled discussion time.
- **Record Main Points.** Suggest that students write key or main points as major headings and leave space to fill in details later. Coach them to listen for main points.
- **Fill in the Blanks.** Suggest that students go back immediately following the presentation and fill in the details of each main point. They can use their textbook or other reference materials as a resource.
- **Use an Organizational System.** A system allows the student to separate notes into main points, details, questions, and follow-up points.
- **Make Separate Reference Pages.** Some information is best recorded in its own separate space outside the notes. A diagram on the board, for example, may be more easily understood if it stands alone and does not fall in the body of the notes.

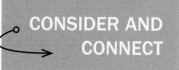

CONSIDER AND CONNECT

Educators should recommend that students use colored tabs to notate important information in the text or handouts for easy reference at a later time.

When to Study

As suggested earlier in the tips for the student's support system, the student should create a routine time of day for studying. Some experts believe that doing the same thing at the same time every day is the most effective way to successfully accomplish any task. Certain students, however, get easily bored with routine. The main thing to remember is that no matter what time of day students choose to study, they should keep the following factors in mind:

- **Study during Peak Performance.** This is the time of day that the student performs best. The peak performance period will vary from student to student. You've heard people say that they are just not a morning person. If that is the case, studying in the afternoon might be more effective. Students should select a time when they can concentrate and focus. That is the formula for efficient and effective studying.
- **Consider Sleep Habits.** As human beings, we must recognize that habits are a powerful influence over our lives and behavior. Therefore, if a student habitually gets up at 7:00 a.m. and goes to bed at 11:00 p.m., it is doubtful that getting up earlier or staying up later will facilitate an effective study period.
- **Take Advantage of the Circumstances.** The student's goal should be to study at optimum time and under optimum circumstances. However, while being at their best is a valid goal, it is not always possible. Therefore, if some unplanned time, such as waiting at the dentist's office, makes itself available, it could be used for studying.

- **Relate Time to Task.** Students must consider the complexity of the learning objective when assigning time to do it. For example, a student would not want to try to complete a 50-page reading assignment a half hour before the class or test.
- **Maximize Prime Time.** Students should tackle the most challenging assignments during peak time and schedule less important study tasks when the energy and motivation level may be lower.

Fifteen Effective Study Habits for Students

Take Charge. Be responsible for your own learning. Taking charge allows you to make decisions about your priorities, time, and resources.

Define Personal Values. Once you have established your own personal values and principles, center yourself around them. Don't let friends or family dictate to you what is important.

Set and Prioritize Goals. You must decide what is important to you in your career education. Then you must prioritize those goals in a logical and sequential manner. Then you must focus and not let anyone or anything distract you from attaining those goals.

Show Up! Don't miss class, even when you don't feel like attending or your car died or you stayed out too late last night. Go to class!

Get Correct Assignments. Make sure you get the assignments in the educator's exact words. Don't forget to include the due date.

Establish a Schedule. Construct a general, long-term schedule first. It will include the obligations you are required to meet weekly, such as job, school, organizations, family commitments, church, and so forth. Then make a list of the major events and amount of work to be accomplished in each subject in the current week. Finally, make a short-term, one-day schedule. This will include what specifically is to be accomplished, and when, each day. Follow the schedule to the best of your ability, but don't beat yourself up over varying from it. Simply regroup and try again. However, try to make your study time habitual on a daily basis whenever you can.

Pick the Place. Have a regular place set aside for you to study and do nothing but study. It should be quiet and free of distractions such as TV, radio, or other people. Make sure the area has good lighting and ventilation, a comfortable chair (but not too comfortable), and a desk or table large enough to spread out your books and papers. Adopt the routine of studying in this special place. Before long your attitude, attention, and behavior will automatically turn to studying when you go there (Figure 3–3).

Adopt a Mascot. Select one particular item or social symbol that you can relate to the act of studying. It can be a favorite T-shirt or cap or even a figurine or stuffed animal. Just before you begin to study, put on the cap or set the symbol on the desk. This small ceremony will aid in your concentration. First, going through this brief ritual helps get your mind set for studying. Second, it signals others that you are working and they shouldn't disturb you.

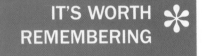

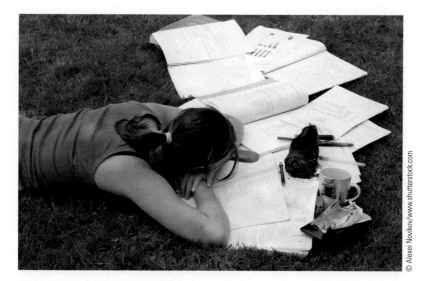

Figure 3–3   Why is this environment unsuitable for effective studying?

Stand Up and Look Away. It is inevitable that your mind will wander from time to time. Rather than staring at the book or getting up and leaving the room, simply stand up and look away from your books. Continue to daydream for a while if you must, but the physical act of standing up will usually bring your thinking back to the task at hand.

Don't Plan a Diversion. Make sure not to start a lengthy project or go back to any former unfinished tasks just before your scheduled study time. Try to be habitual with the time you begin studying and be careful not to get too distracted just prior to beginning studying. This will improve your concentration.

Divide the Work into "Mini" Assignments. Set a time when you expect to have the first "mini" assignment completed. You will feel a sense of accomplishment as you complete each one, and that will make continued study easier.

Keep a Reminder Pad. Oftentimes our minds wander to other things that need to be done, distracting us from our studies. Keep a pad and pencil nearby, and when you think of other things needing your attention, write them down and return to your studies. The list will be there later when you can turn your attention to the items listed.

Tackle the Difficult. Whenever possible, begin with the hard or boring part of the studying first. Save the fun stuff for dessert! Having gotten the less interesting or difficult material behind you, it may be easier to complete the lesson or assignment.

Expect Respect from Others. Notify others of when you will be studying. Don't answer the phone or door during your study time if at all possible. Explain that this is your study time and you will be ready to play, talk, party, go to the movies, or whatever when you have put in your scheduled study time (Figure 3–4). Hang a "do not disturb" sign on the door if you need to. Your future may be at stake (Figure 3–5)!

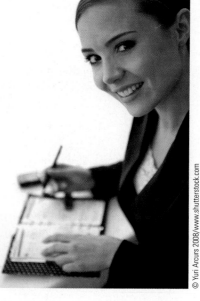

Figure 3–4   Keep a notepad handy to jot down things that may otherwise distract you from study.

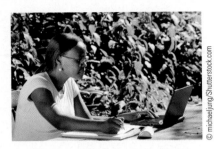

Figure 3–5   Take the necessary steps to eliminate distractions while studying.

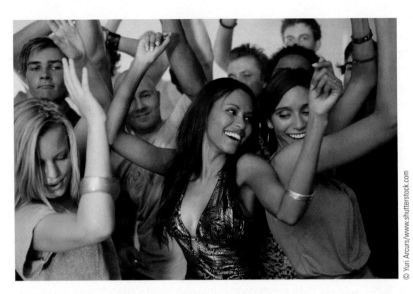

Figure 3–6   Reward successful study sessions with a favorite activity.

CONSIDER AND CONNECT

Teach students that when they study, they should study, and when they worry, they should worry, but they should never attempt to do both simultaneously.

failure behaviors
any behavior that prevents a student from completing course requirements, achieving educational objectives, and preventing the student from attaining success.

Reward Yourself. When you have completed your scheduled study session, reward yourself with a favorite activity. Listen to your favorite music, go out with friends, do whatever you enjoy the most. You deserve it. You are on your way to success (Figure 3–6).

Master educators help students learn to relax before they even begin to study. Your students may suffer from learned "book anxiety," which causes them to relate books or assignments to something unpleasant. The key to breaking this book-anxiety problem is to learn how to relax. When students are physically, deeply, and completely relaxed, it is very difficult for them to feel any type of anxiety. Students should learn to associate their textbooks or study materials with relaxation, not tension.

☑ Forget the Five Failure Behaviors

Master educators will recognize that fears sometimes grow so strong in learners that they can actually keep learners from even thinking about how to challenge fear. Learners can take action in the face of their study-related fears and avoid barriers to learning by also avoiding **failure behaviors**. Share the following failure behaviors and beliefs with your students so that they can identify them as they arise:

- **Skipping School.** Don't feel pressured to go to every class. After all, the educator probably won't even notice you are gone. Somebody can always tell you what went on in class, right? So don't sweat it, get to class when you can.
- **Skipping Homework.** Assignments are okay, but don't get too carried away. When you feel like doing homework, then do it. But you should never let studying or homework rule your life!
- **Skipping Mental Presence.** Bring your body to class but leave your brains at home. Just think of all the things you can accomplish during

class. You can think about your upcoming date or your son's soccer game or even catch up on a little lost sleep. No one will notice and you will accomplish what you wanted to.

- **Skipping Relationships.** Don't bother getting to know other students or establishing a relationship with your educators. They probably have less going for them than you do, right? No need for anyone to be asking nosy questions about dumb things like your future!

- **Skipping Town.** If you're about to flunk out because you didn't avoid the first four failure behaviors, just blow it away. There will be plenty of chances to make your fortune. The educators aren't any fun and you don't think they like you anyway. Doing your homework and studying was a drag—you'll show them, you'll just *quit!* Don't take this school thing too seriously.

Master educators will be able to point out to their learners that following these five failure behaviors will surely result in just that, *failure*.

Study Groups

The idea of a **study group** is a simple one. Your students simply seek out a small group of like-minded students, perhaps those who are more studious than they are, to share notes, questioning, discussions, and so forth to prepare for each class or scheduled tests. Your students can organize study groups in numerous ways. Some groups choose to assign the primary responsibility for a single class to one member and alternate leadership roles. One member might be assigned the task of completing supplemental reading and summarizing it for the rest of the group. Alternatively, each member can be responsible for personal reading, research, and reporting for discussion on different areas of the content (Figure 3–7). The following tips are adapted from *How to Study* by Ron Fry:

1. Keep groups to a minimum of four and maximum of six.
2. Seek diversity of experience, but demand common dedication. Best friends are not required, but cordiality and respect among members is important.
3. Avoid members who are inherently unequal (employers and employees, upperclassmen with underclassmen, couples, and others.)
4. Don't just invite friends. If this is really a study group, it is not a social function.
5. Assign leadership for each session. The leader must master the assigned topic or material and share with the remainder of the group.
6. Maintain rigorous formality. Require member commitment to times and assignments. Eliminate those members who are not serious.
7. Appoint a chairperson. This person would be in charge of scheduling sessions and settling disputes.
8. Establish guidelines. Decide early the exact requirements and assignments of each member. Every member should be committed to success and contribute equally to the success of the whole group.

IT'S WORTH REMEMBERING ✳

Courage is not the absence of fear, but taking action in the face of it.

---

study group
a group of like-minded students who get together to share notes, questioning, discussions, and so forth to prepare for each class or scheduled tests.

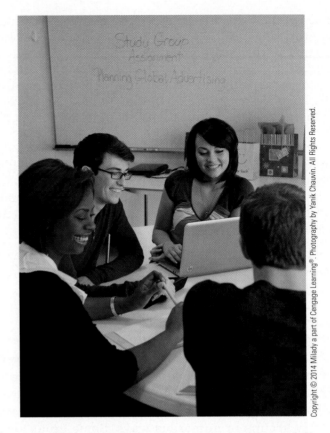

Figure 3–7   Study groups share notes, questioning, and discussions.

☑ Fitness Is a Must

For learning to occur, learners must have a healthy body, mind, and attitude. It is important that learners exercise their brains to become and remain mentally fit. It is also important that they become and remain physically fit. Master educators convey the importance of following a balanced diet, drinking sufficient water daily, getting appropriate weekly exercise, and staying free of drugs and excessive use of alcohol. When they adhere to these healthy behaviors, learners will feel better and their ability to learn will be enhanced (Figure 3–8). Many of the barriers to learning will have been eliminated. Learners may have to study when they are tired or ill. Tell them to begin those study sessions with slow, rhythmic breathing. This will help with their relaxation and improve their circulation.

Teaching Testing Skills

Educators must also think about preparing their students for a state licensing examination, if one is required, and helping graduates secure the position they desire in their chosen field. In addition, you will also

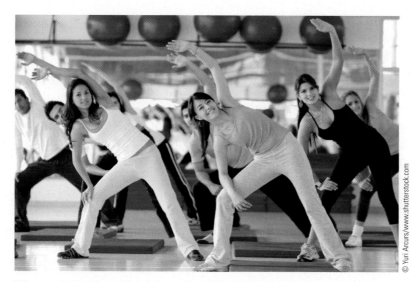

Figure 3–8   By adhering to healthy behaviors, learning will be enhanced.

need to know how to prepare your learners for taking tests effectively. Therefore, we will approach this topic from the perspective of your role as an educator. You can then apply the same principles that you teach to your students to your own licensure preparation, if applicable. Many factors contribute to how well learners perform on tests. These factors include physical and psychological well-being, time management, reading skills, note-taking skills, study skills, learning skills, memory, writing skills, and test-taking skills.

Test-taking skills are important for all learners for three important reasons:

1. If only some of the learners have test-taking skills and others do not, the test results may be invalid. Good students may lose out in competitive situations to weaker students who know less but who achieve higher results because they are test-wise.
2. Test-wise learners may have less test anxiety. These learners may be less intimidated by tests because they have some strategies for dealing with them.
3. Test-wise learners demand better results. Because some of the strategies for taking multiple-choice tests work only on poorly written test questions, test-wise learners force educators to construct better tests.

Master educators present a variety of attitudes and experiences in teaching effective test-taking skills. They should ensure that all learners have an opportunity to:

- Clearly understand the purpose of testing.
- Be experienced in using test-taking materials: pencil, test booklet, and answer sheet.
- Have experience in following directions similar to those that will be used in the test.
- Practice completing requested information, working in columns and rows, filling in responses, and asking for information.

CONSIDER AND CONNECT

The first and foremost way for any learner to do well on any test is to be thoroughly familiar with the course content.

- Gain an awareness of ways to make efficient use of time.
- Recognize the need to read carefully.
- Prepare for the testing process, both mentally and physically.

☑ Preparing for the Test

Much of the preparation for a test begins with the daily habits and time management that are part of effective study habits. In other words, part of successful test taking results from having a planned, realistic study schedule, reading and actively studying, creating a well-organized notebook, developing a detailed terminology list, taking effective notes during class, organizing and reviewing handouts, reviewing past quizzes or tests, and so forth (Figure 3–9). Learners must listen carefully in class for the cues or clues that the educator will give them regarding what can be expected on the test. In addition, before learners actually take the test, they should:

- Begin to get mentally and physically ready. They should develop a positive attitude toward taking the test.
- Know what to expect; learn ahead of time what type of test they will be taking, the date and time of the test, and what materials are needed.
- Follow a healthy diet to ensure that the body and mind are clear and ready.
- Plan to exercise regularly in the weeks preceding the test.
- Get plenty of rest the evening before the test.
- Dress comfortably (if unsure of the weather or temperature, they should dress in layers to adapt to a changing environment if necessary).
- Expect some anxiety; being concerned about the test results may improve results.
- Avoid cramming the night before an examination.

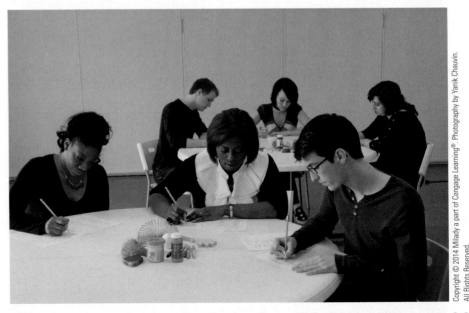

Figure 3–9   Properly preparing for test day will facilitate more successful results.

On Test Day

After learners have taken all the necessary preliminary steps in test preparation, they can adopt a number of helpful strategies for the day of the actual examination. They should:

* Relax and try to slow down physically; take slow, deep breaths to calm themselves.
* Review the material lightly on the day of the examination, if possible.
* Arrive early with the correct self-confident attitude; be alert, calm, and ready for the challenge.
* Read all written directions and listen carefully to all verbal directions before beginning. Ask the test examiner questions about anything that seems unclear.
* Skim the entire test before beginning to answer the questions.
* Budget their time to ensure that they have ample time to complete the test; for example, they should not spend too much time on one question.
* Wear a watch to monitor the time allotted.
* Begin work as soon as possible and mark the answers in the test booklet carefully but quickly.
* Answer the easiest questions first to reserve time for the more difficult ones; reviewing all the questions first may give them clues to the more difficult questions, which can then be returned to.
* Mark any questions that are skipped so that they can be easily identified later.
* Read each question carefully; make sure that they know what the question is asking so that they can answer all parts.
* Answer as many questions as possible; for questions of which they are unsure of the answer, they should guess or estimate.
* Look over the test when it is completed to be sure that they have read all questions correctly and answered as many as possible.
* Make changes to answers only if there is a good reason to do so.
* Check the test booklet carefully before turning it in.

Deductive Reasoning

Another technique that a master educator will share with learners for better test results is deductive reasoning. **Deductive reasoning** allows learners to reach a probable conclusion by employing logical reasoning. Some deductive-reasoning strategies are discussed next.

    Eliminating Incorrect Options. The more answers that are eliminated as incorrect, the better chance the learner has of identifying the correct one. In addition, the following deductive strategies are helpful in test taking:

* Rapidly define the problem or question. This strategy enables the test taker to analyze and evaluate the different possible solutions or answers.
* Watch for key words or terms. The test taker should look very closely for any qualifying conditions or statements. Look for such words and phrases as *usually, commonly, in most instances, never, always,* and so forth.

Deductive reasoning
this process allows learners to reach a probable conclusion by employing logical reasoning.

- Study the question stem, which will often provide a clue to the correct answer. Look for matches between the stem and one of the distracters or options.
- Watch for grammatical clues. If the last word in a stem is "an," the learner will know that the answer must begin with a vowel rather than a consonant.
- Look at similar or related questions. Questions covering the same material may provide clues.
- In answering essay questions, watch for such words as *compare*, *contrast*, *discuss*, *evaluate*, *analyze*, *define*, or *describe* and develop the answer accordingly.
- For reading tests that contain long paragraphs followed by several questions, read the entire questions first; this technique will help in identifying the important elements in the paragraph.
- When charts or graphs are provided to answer a group of questions, first read the stem questions, identify the elements in the chart or graph relating to the stem, and then answer the question.
- Watch for questions that contain several qualifiers—they are usually the correct choice.
- Try to determine the test writer's intent while taking care not to make incorrect assumptions.

Test-Taking Strategies

There are a few test-wise tips that educators can provide their learners. The tips apply to specific types of test questions. Because master educators will never design a test or examination for the purpose of "tricking" the learner or ensuring failure, they will want to share these tips with all learners.

True/False Questions. When teaching students to take tests that contain true/false questions, you will want them to consider the following advice:

- Watch for qualifying words (e.g., *all*, *most*, *some*, *none*, *always*, *usually*, *sometimes*, *never*, *much*, *little*, *no*, *equal*, *less*, *good*, *bad*, and so forth). Absolutes are generally not true.
- For a statement to be true, the *entire* statement must be true.
- Long statements are more likely to be true than short statements (because it takes more detail to provide the truthful, factual data).
- Be careful not to consider wild exceptions to the statement.

Multiple-Choice Questions. When teaching your learners to take tests that contain multiple-choice questions, you will want them to consider the following advice:

- Read the entire question carefully, including all the foils or distracters.
- Look for the best answer; more than one choice may be true.
- Eliminate incorrect responses by crossing them out (if taking the test on the test form).
- When two answers are close or similar, one is probably the correct choice.
- Do not use an answer that is grammatically incorrect (remember the "a" versus "an" example).
- The *all of the above* type of response is likely to be the correct response.

- The longest, most inclusive answer is generally correct.
- Do not spend too much time on difficult questions; mark those to be returned to later.
- Pay special attention to words such as *not*, *except*, and *but*.
- Guess if you do not know the answer (if there is no penalty).
- Eliminate obviously wrong or silly answers.
- When two options are identical but phrased differently, both must be wrong.
- When two options are opposites, one is probably wrong and the other is probably correct, depending on the number of distracters.
- The answer to one question may be found in the stem of another question.
- When you have no idea what the correct answer is, the middle options are more likely to be correct on *nonstandardized* tests.

Matching Questions. Strategies that your students should consider when completing test questions that require matching two columns of information, such as key terms and their definitions, are as follows.

- Read all items in each list before beginning.
- Check off items from the right-hand list to eliminate choices.

Essay Questions. An essay question is one wherein the scoring of the student's response may vary from educator to educator. When teaching your learners to take tests containing essay questions, present the following strategies:

- Be aware that educators generally think that reasoning ability, factual accuracy, relevance, organization, completeness, and clarity are the most important qualities.
- Brainstorm before beginning to write your response.
- Outline your response before you begin writing.
- Organize your answer according to the cue words used in the question.

Educator Strategies

As a master educator, you will want to adopt certain attitudes in regard to test taking and convey them to your learners. A few are provided here for your consideration:

- Encourage learners to pace themselves; some will spend too much time on the first part of the test or on the more difficult questions.
- Treat each test as a learning experience for students. Spend time teaching them how to mark answer sheets correctly and how to skim questions and answer the easiest ones first.
- Be positive and enthusiastic with students when discussing the test-taking process.
- See that the very best testing environment is provided—for example, proper temperature control, adequate ventilation, appropriate desk arrangement, and controlled noise level.

Remember that, as a master educator, the success of your learners is a direct manifestation of your success. Therefore, you will want to make sure that all your students learn the best possible study and test-taking skills to increase their chances of success. As a student in training to become an educator, you will want to practice the same strategies and techniques, which will result in the best possible achievement in your course of study and in your licensing examination, if applicable. After you have obtained that certification or license to teach, you can pursue your career in education with vigor and continuous learning.

Wrapping It Up

Educators will want to give strong consideration to beginning every course of study with the strategies and techniques shared in this chapter. Doing so will enable students to learn success behaviors at the beginning of the program, thus eliminating or greatly reducing the withdrawal rate at our nation's schools. By developing effective study techniques and test-taking skills and avoiding the five failure behaviors, learners will be able to work cooperatively with their educators to reduce barriers to learning and achieve the career success that they seek.

In Retrospect

1. List and explain reading skills.

2. List note-taking and highlighting skills.

3. List and explain 15 strategies for effective studying.

4. List and explain the five failure habits that should be avoided at all costs.

5. What are some key elements that should be followed when developing a study group?

6. Why is it important to train students in test-wise strategies?

Basic Learning Styles and Principles

Objectives (Desired Performance Goals):

After reading and studying this chapter, you should be able to:

- List the four important steps in learning.

- Explain eight distinct intelligences and how they impact learning.

- List the benefits of identifying learning styles for students.

! CRITICAL CONCEPT

Traditional academia has taught in ways that appeal to basically two intelligences: verbal/linguistic and logical/mathematical. A master educator will, however, deliver content in a manner that reaches all intelligences and allows learners to use their full brain power.

Why Learning Styles Are Important

TODAY'S CLASSROOMS are filled with students who possess a variety of learning styles. Learners are as different as tomatoes growing in a garden. Each needs to be properly prepared, tended, and treated as unique.

As educators, we need to be able to reach a diverse group of students with a variety of backgrounds, experiences, cultures, and learning styles. This chapter is designed to assist you in doing just that.

The Role of the Educator

Chapter 1, "The Career Education Instructor," pointed out that a teacher today is more focused on being a facilitator of learning for students. We might take that concept even further and describe a teacher as a *catalyst* for learning. *Merriam Webster's Collegiate Dictionary*, Tenth Edition, defines a *catalyst* as "an agent that provokes or speeds significant change or action." When we think about it, isn't that exactly what we want to do as educators? Don't we want to create circumstances within which learning is provoked or takes place at a faster rate? Teachers today cannot effectively teach with the old attitude of superiority.

Instead, we must consider how the brains of our adult students learn best and then take whatever steps necessary to facilitate or become a catalyst for that learning. We must become knowledgeable of a variety of learning profiles and models as well as the use of multiple intelligences. We must offer our adult learners choices and master a medley of delivery methods that make learning fun and inspire a love of learning in our students.

Learning Styles Defined

When our students have difficulty learning what we are teaching, it may be because they are processing the information outside their natural learning style. A learning style is an individual's preferred method of thinking, understanding, and processing information. For example, when you are teaching bacteriology, some students would prefer to learn by listening to a lecture, some would prefer to research and study the information on their own, others would prefer to watch a video, and yet others would actually prefer to work in a laboratory setting discovering for themselves what it all means. Research tells us that we must integrate teaching strategies that meet the needs of a more multicultural student body with a variety of learning styles.

Learning-Style Profiles

A wide array of learning-style profiles is available for teachers to consider. Many are very similar and others are quite different, depending upon their perspective on the cognitive process. For example, in the previous edition of this text, an entire chapter was dedicated to Bernice McCarthy's 4MAT learning model, which identifies the four learner types as Imaginative, Analytical, Common Sense, and Dynamic (Figure 4–1). Figure 4–2 charts comparable learning styles.

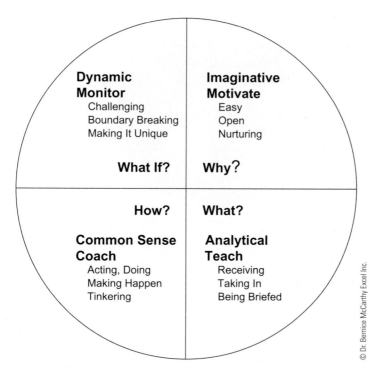

Figure 4–1   The 4MAT learning model.

© Dr. Bernice McCarthy Excel Inc.

Interactive Learners (Comparable to Imaginative Learners)	These learners do best when they ask "Why?" They learn by watching, listening, and sharing ideas. They appreciate instructors who can involve them in the learning experience and who are supportive, sympathetic, and friendly. They like to have discussions with other students and study well with a group of people.
Reader/Listener Learners (Comparable to Analytical Learners)	These individuals ask "What?" They learn best by reading and hearing new ideas, then mulling over information in their minds. They are eager to find the reasons for things, and are excellent at remembering facts and details. They work well with instructors who answer their questions freely and who keep them focused on the subject matter.
Systematic Learners (Comparable to Common-Sense Learners)	When these learners sit down to study, they get more out of the information when they can connect what they are studying to real-life situations. They tend to ask "How?" They study best by themselves because they can concentrate better. Their favorite instructors are those who challenge them to "check things out," and who are down-to-earth and fair.
Intuitive Learners (Comparable to Dynamic Learners)	These learners ask "What if . . . " They like to learn through trial and error. When they are studying, they actually want to try out what they are reading about. They appreciate instructors who understand their need to be stimulated with new ideas and who do not insist on just one way of doing something.

© Dr. Bernice McCarthy Excel Inc.

Figure 4–2   Comparable learning styles.

A great deal of research has been conducted with respect to sensory learning styles, and it indicates that 35 percent of people are mainly visual learners, 25 percent are mainly auditory learners, and 40 percent are mainly **kinesthetic learners** (Figure 4–3). Visual learners, for example, process information through what they see. They tend to think in pictures and have vivid imaginations. Auditory learners, on the other hand, process information through what they hear. They like to listen and talk things through. Kinesthetic learners process information by the physical experience of doing and touching. They like to feel and manipulate things for themselves. They prefer to be involved physically and may not learn well just by listening. Sensory learning styles may best be summed up by the ancient sage Confucius, who said, "I hear and I forget, I see and I remember, I do and I understand." Probably the most important thing to remember

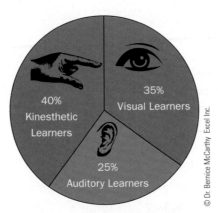

Figure 4–3   Sensory learning styles.

when considering learning styles is that the human brain does not learn in just one way. As human beings we are far more complex and use a variety of styles depending on our needs and the situation.

Four Steps in Learning

Regardless of a student's learning style, he will likely learn new information in four important steps, as follows:

1. **Desire.** Before we learn anything, we have to want to learn. We must want to understand something or know how to do a particular task for it to be meaningful to us.
2. **Input and Environment.** Students must receive information about the subject matter (the how to, for example) in an environment that is conducive to learning. This is the step that creates jobs for teachers!
3. **Assimilation.** Next, students must process and understand the information and/or how the task is performed.
4. **Repetition.** Once a student has the desire to learn, receives the information in an environment conducive to learning, and, finally, understands it, he must repeat or practice either the underlying theory or the practical application until the information or task has been mastered.

When you think about it, these four steps are how we have learned most of what we know, such as how to walk, how to drive, how to play the piano, how to speak, how to cut hair, and so forth.

Multiple Intelligences

Howard Gardner of Harvard University, in his book *Frames of Mind: The Theory of Multiple Intelligences*, outlines a theory regarding learning that encompasses a broad spectrum of learning profiles and steps in learning.

Gardner defines two fundamental concepts of the multiple intelligence theory: First, he states that intelligence is not fixed; humans have the ability to develop intellectual capacity (a process that educators can facilitate). Second, he establishes that education is not unitary; there are many ways in which our students can be smart. Since there are many intelligences, everyone benefits from each intelligence to some degree. He has identified nine to date, eight of which will be discussed in this chapter.

In defining each intelligence, Gardner determined that three prerequisites must be met, as follows:

1. It must require skills that enable an individual to resolve genuine problems.
2. It must require the ability to create an effective product.
3. It must have the potential for finding or creating problems.

For example, an Australian Aborigine may not score high in intelligence if measured by the ability to function in New York City, but he may be considered highly intelligent in his native environment. In the same light, a New York City stockbroker who is highly successful on Wall Street might not be able to survive in the remote outback of Australia. This example speaks to the theory of *how* we are smart as opposed to how smart we are. Gardner, in his research, determined that people can succeed in the eyes of their own culture even if there is no apparent link to formal education.

Gardner believes that all people possess at least eight specific intelligences, and that we have developed some intelligences more than others. If we subscribe to his theory, when students find a task or subject area easy, they are likely using a more fully developed and preferred intelligence. Conversely, if they are struggling with a topic or task, they may be using a less-developed intelligence. Gardner says that although they are not necessarily dependent on each other, these intelligences seldom operate in isolation. Every normal individual possesses varying degrees of each of these intelligences, but the ways in which intelligences combine and blend are as varied as the faces and personalities of individuals. Gardner's theory has become the framework for many current educational strategies that are proving successful in enhancing student success.

STUDENTS ARE SMART IN MANY WAYS!

Verbal/Linguistic	Musical/Rhythmic
Bodily/Kinesthetic	Interpersonal
Logical/Mathematical	Intrapersonal
Visual/Spatial	Naturalist

Verbal/Linguistic Intelligence

The **verbal/linguistic intelligence** is the ability to communicate through language, which includes listening, reading, writing, and speaking. When applying the verbal/linguistic intelligence, students show they are "word wise." They have an extensive vocabulary. They tell great stories. They are good with puns and playing on words. They always seem to know what to say and when to say it. They learn best through verbal presentations, reading, writing, discussions, conducting interviews, and listening to lectures.

verbal/linguistic intelligence the ability to communicate through language, which includes listening, reading, writing, and speaking.

People who are word wise may choose a career as an author, poet, public speaker, translator, talk show host, attorney, judge, politician, or teacher. Famous people considered to be word wise include Charles Dickens, William Shakespeare, Abraham Lincoln, Sir Winston Churchill, John Steinbeck, Jane Austin, Martin Luther King, Jr., Connie Chung, Emily Dickinson, and Geno Stampora.

Teaching Ideas and Activities for the Verbal/Linguistic Intelligence

- Using interesting graphics, slogans, and posters (Figure 4–4).
- Creating opportunities to read and discuss
- Listening to tapes and lectures
- Employing word games, mnemonics, and affirmations
- Using metaphors, similes, and paraphrasing
- Assigning journaling activities
- Implementing games for vocabulary development such as Password, Wheel of Fortune, Jeopardy, and Scrabble

Study Tips for the Verbal/Linguistic Intelligence

- Working in study groups to explain and discuss
- Reading text and highlighting 20 percent or less (Figure 4-5)
- Rewriting notes
- Outlining chapters in chosen format (linear or mind mapping)
- Reciting information
- Writing scripts for role-plays
- Debating

Learners who are more developed in the verbal/linguistic intelligence are often highly interpersonal and will remember much of what they hear and more of what they hear and then say. Asking the students for their opinions or to explain their perspectives will give them the opportunity for open participation.

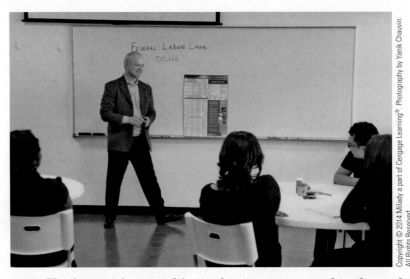

Figure 4–4   Use interesting graphics and posters to appeal to the verbal/linguistic intelligence.

Learners who are more developed in the verbal/linguistic intelligence are very often highly interpersonal and will remember much of what they hear and more of what they hear and then say. Asking the students what there opinion is or why they are saying something will give them the opportunity for open participation.

Visual Spatial Intelligence
The Visual/Spatial Intelligence is the ability to understand spatial relationships and to comprehend and create images. When applying the visual/spatial intelligence, students show they are space wise. These students have a flair for color and style.

Figure 4–5 Teach learners to highlight no more than 20% of the text.

Visual/Spatial Intelligence

The **visual/spatial intelligence** is the ability to understand spatial relationships and comprehend and create images. When applying the visual/spatial intelligence, students show they are "space wise." These students have a flair for color and style. They have good artistic skills and are good at drawing, art, and creative projects. They relate best when they can understand concepts by drawing diagrams, reading through flowcharts, and performing demonstrations. These students will be frequent volunteers. They can parallel park, get more dishes in a dishwasher than anyone else, or design and decorate a room. People who are space wise might choose a career as an architect or artist, photographer or sculptor, designer or landscaper, movie director, pilot, or someone in the beauty and wellness industry. Famous people considered to be space wise are Pablo Picasso, Frank Lloyd Wright, Peggy Fleming, Steven Spielberg, Nancy Kerrigan, Dan Marino, John Elway, and Vidal Sassoon.

visual/spatial intelligence the ability to understand spatial relationships and comprehend and create images.

Teaching Ideas and Activities for the Visual/Spatial Intelligence

- Using visual aids and hands-on experience
- Using mind mapping and window paning (Figure 4–6).
- Rearranging the classroom and changing the teacher location
- Designing graphics, logos, and flyers
- Using ball-toss reviews
- Employing dancing and physical energizers
- Making a mobile
- Creating a collage, montage, or historical timeline
- Implementing visualization techniques
- Playing with geometric shapes
- Creating visual aids such as a human skeleton

Study Tips for the Visual/Spatial Intelligence

- Mind-mapping notes using diagrams, graphics, and arrows
- Color-coding notes so each topic is in the same color
- Organizing notes from main points to supporting facts
- Working with other visual/spatial learners
- Working in a group to find and solve problems

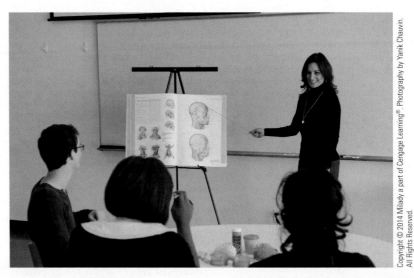

Figure 4–6   Mind mapping notes highly effective for the visual/spatial learner.

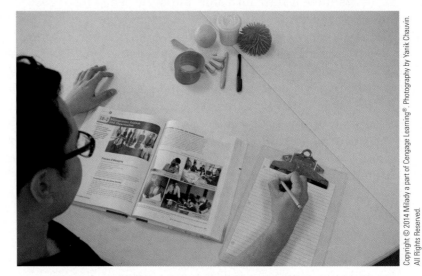

Figure 4–7   Students who favor visual/spatial intelligence thrive in a picture-rich environment.

Students who favor the visual/spatial intelligence love a picture-rich environment full of posters, mobiles, and art (Figure 4–7). You will often find them doodling and fidgeting. You can catch their attention by asking them to imagine or picture something relevant to the topic being covered. They tend to forget spoken words and ideas.

Logical/Mathematical Intelligence

logical/mathematical intelligence the ability to understand logical reasoning and problem solving in areas such as math, science, sequences, and patterns.

The **logical/mathematical intelligence** demonstrates the ability to understand logical reasoning and problem solving in areas such as math, science, sequences, and patterns. Logical/mathematical thinkers can think things through in a logical, systematic manner. When applying the logical/mathematical intelligence, students are showing that they are "logic wise." These students are good with numbers and computations, usually love games, and generally follow the rules. They are able to quantify, analyze, sequence, evaluate, synthesize, and apply (Figure 4–8). They often ask the "why" and "how" questions. They like to understand the reasons for doing something. They want to classify, sort, understand, predict, and fix things. People who are logic wise might choose a career as a lawyer, banker, teacher, astronomer, inventor, engineer, scientist, computer programmer, or detective. Famous people who are logic wise include Albert Einstein, Plato, Isaac Newton, Marie Curie, Bill Gates, and Ted Koppel.

EXPENSES	Percent of Total Gross Income
Salaries and commissions (including payroll taxes)	53.5
Rent	13.0
Supplies	5.0
Advertising	3.0
Depreciation	3.0
Laundry	1.0
Cleaning	1.0
Light and power	1.0
Repairs	1.5
Insurance	0.75
Telephone	0.75
Miscellaneous	1.5
Total expenses	85.0
Net profit	15.0
Total	100.0

Figure 4–8   The logical/mathematical intelligence likes quantifying, sorting, and categorizing information.

Teaching Ideas and Activities for the Logical/Mathematical Intelligence

- Evaluating ideas
- Playing on strong critical-thinking skills
- Sequencing events (such as steps in a procedure)
- Conducting experiments (such as chemistry or hair color formulas)
- Brainstorming ideas
- Classifying and categorizing information
- Synthesizing ideas
- Playing number games
- Making charts and graphs
- Discovering patterns and trends
- Using graphic organizers
- Playing Jeopardy-type games
- Explaining algorithms (e.g., the pH scale)

Study Tips for the Logical/Mathematical Intelligence

- Studying in a quiet setting
- Pausing to ponder over what has been read
- Taking one-minute reflection period for introspection
- Thinking about why material is important and what it relates to
- Considering the causes and effects of the information
- Journaling key points and what the information means to the student

The learner who is strong in the logical/mathematical intelligence likes things in place and order and experiences stress over confusion and chaos. Repetitive seatwork will bore these students. You can grab their attention by asking how they would solve something or what the experts would think of the matter. They are motivated by challenges, problems, and projects.

Intrapersonal Intelligence

intrapersonal intelligence the ability to understand one's own behavior and feelings.

The **intrapersonal intelligence** reflects the ability to understand one's own behavior and feelings. These learners have the ability to quietly contemplate and self-assess their accomplishments, reviewing their behavior and innermost feelings. When applying the intrapersonal intelligence, students show they are "self wise." These learners were once considered to be antisocial. They tend to be loners and think best on their own instead of bouncing ideas off others. They retain information better after they have had time to think about it. They like self-assessment, reflection, and planning. They enjoy tasks in solitude and use their intuition. You may find them daydreaming or meditating. They are very much into self-discovery learning. People who are self wise might choose a career as an author, philosopher, theologian, psychiatrist, psychologist, researcher, backpacker, sailor, or artist. Famous people who are self wise include Sigmund Freud, Mahatma Gandhi, Eleanor Roosevelt, Socrates, Confucius, and Thoreau.

Teaching Ideas and Activities for the Intrapersonal Intelligence

- Assigning workbook activities
- Having students recall personal feelings or memories
- Arranging Internet research projects (Figure 4–9).
- Setting goals and priorities and drafting an action plan
- Giving alternatives and letting the student choose

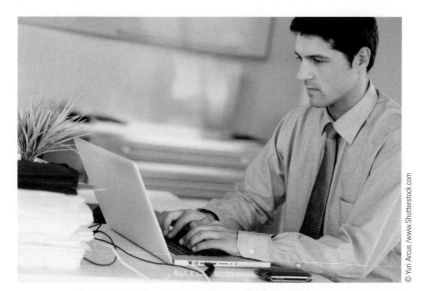

Figure 4–9   Assign Internet research projects to the intrapersonal intelligence.

- Scheduling reflection and introspection
- Avoiding teacher-directed activities
- Assigning self-paced, independent projects

Study Tips for the Intrapersonal Intelligence

- Studying in a quiet setting
- Pausing to ponder over what has been read
- Taking one-minute reflection period for introspection
- Thinking about why material is important and what it relates to
- Considering the causes and effects of the information
- Relating content to personal experiences
- Journaling key points and what the information means to the student

You can best instruct these students by giving them more silent reflection time to think about what has been learned. Involve these learners with individual needs, frustrations, questions, and goals. Involve these students by asking what they would do in a certain situation or how the situation makes them feel. These students are motivated by being allowed to manage their own work.

Bodily/Kinesthetic Intelligence

The **bodily/kinesthetic intelligence** indicates the ability to use the physical body skillfully to solve problems, create products, or present ideas and emotions as well as take in knowledge through bodily sensation such as coordination or working with the hands. Students who are strong in this intelligence are known as "body wise." Learners who prefer this intelligence are able to unite their body and mind to master physical performance and manipulative skills. They use their bodies to communicate, dance, act, and perform athletic tasks. They often learn best when there is movement or the information is presented through a physical demonstration or hands-on involvement (Figure 4-10). You might recognize learners of this preferred intelligence as the "wiggle worms" who can't sit still in class. They are always in motion. People who are body wise might choose a career as a dancer, athlete, surgeon, carpenter, clown, astronaut, sheep

bodily/kinesthetic intelligence the ability to use the physical body skillfully to solve problems, create products, or present ideas and emotions as well as take in knowledge through bodily sensation such as coordination or working with the hands.

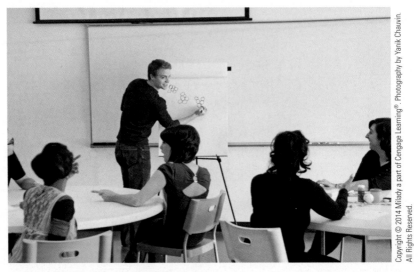

Figure 4–10   Bodily/kinesthetic learners enjoy role-playing and using physical gestures.

shearer, barber, or cosmetologist. Famous people who are body wise include Charlie Chaplin, Babe Ruth, Michael Jordan, Martina Navratilova, Madonna, Steven Segal, and Mikhail Baryshnikov.

Teaching Ideas and Activities for the Bodily/Kinesthetic Intelligence

- Having students role-play
- Building models and labeling them
- Creating simulations
- Playing charades or Pictionary
- Choreographing a movement or procedural sequence
- Using physical gestures
- Practicing skills applications
- Conducting experiments
- Assigning projects that appeal to touch and feel
- Using CD-ROM technology for hand–eye coordination
- Inserting energizers and stretching activities

Study Tips for the Bodily/Kinesthetic Intelligence

- Employing group study with alternating discussion leaders
- Pacing and reciting while you study
- Peer coaching the material to another student
- Using flashcards with a fellow student
- Applying the course material in a practical manner
- Acting out the information
- Designing games that apply to the material

Students who are strong in the bodily/kinesthetic intelligence dislike having to sit for long periods of time. They prefer to be able to get up on their own schedule and stand, walk around, or stretch as needed. They like to apply the information to real-world experience in their own actions. One way to grab the attention of these learners is to ask how they feel about something or how they would respond to a specific issue.

Interpersonal Intelligence

The **interpersonal intelligence** reflects the ability to relate to others, noticing their moods, motivations, and feelings. Students who are strong in this intelligence are known as "people wise." People-wise students are sensitive to the moods, motives, and feelings of other people. They are good leaders and organizers. They are good mediators. They practice empathy by putting themselves in the shoes of the other person and seeing things from their perspective. They make and maintain friends easily. Learners who prefer this intelligence have the ability to persuade, get along with, and influence others. You might recognize them as the social butterflies on the team. They enjoy bouncing their ideas off others and making friends. They relate best through interaction with other students (Figure 4–11). Students who are people wise might choose a career as a coach, teacher, customer service representative, politician, actor, sociologist, philanthropist, religious leader, salesperson, or therapist. Famous people who have exhibited strength in interpersonal intelligence include Ronald Reagan, Mother Theresa, Mahatma Gandhi, Oprah Winfrey, Sir Winston Churchill, John F. Kennedy, and Martin Luther King, Jr.

interpersonal intelligence the ability to relate to others, noticing their moods, motivations, and feelings.

Teaching Ideas and Activities for the Interpersonal Intelligence

* Forming teams for group interaction
* Requiring teams to determine a name, slogan, and logo
* Using team-building activities
* Assigning team presentations
* Role-playing
* Having students practice active listening
* Assigning peer-coaching activities
* Resolving case studies
* Involving students in mediation and motivation
* Assigning students to plan competitions or events

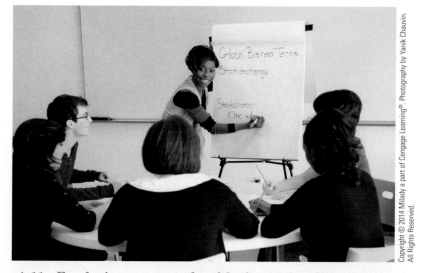

Figure 4–11 Employing group study with alternating discussion leaders works well for the interpersonal intelligence.

Study Tips for the Interpersonal Intelligence

- Employing group study with alternating discussion leaders
- Peer coaching the material to another student
- Using flashcards with a fellow student
- Designing games that apply to the material
- Studying with a partner
- Developing cooperative games for the content
- Conducting partner or team research

Students who are strong in the interpersonal intelligence also like to apply the information to the real world, much like bodily/kinesthetic learners. They prefer to work with others and find working alone distasteful. They enjoy small groups and workstation projects. These learners can be reached by asking what can be done next or what was learned today. You will recognize these learners because their workstations are where socializing will take place.

Musical/Rhythmic Intelligence

musical/rhythmic intelligence the ability to comprehend and/or create meaningful musical sounds. This intelligence indicates an understanding and appreciation of music and ability to keep rhythm.

The **musical/rhythmic intelligence** is the ability to comprehend and/or create meaningful musical sounds. This intelligence indicates an understanding and appreciation of music and ability to keep rhythm, although it does not necessarily mean that an individual has a great singing voice. It's a talent obviously apparent in musicians, composers, and recording engineers, but most of us have a musical intelligence that can be developed. Students who are strong in this intelligence are known as "music wise." Music-wise students are always humming, whistling, singing, or listening to music. They respond to music and learn through rhythm and sound, writing lyrics or jingles, playing music, and so forth (Figure 4–12). Students who are music wise might choose a career as a cheerleader, kindergarten teacher, musician, jingle-writer, choir director, theater director, composer, recording engineer, or singer. Famous people who are music wise include Ludwig van Beethoven, Barbara Streisand, Mozart, Leonard Bernstein, Paul Simon, and Ray Charles.

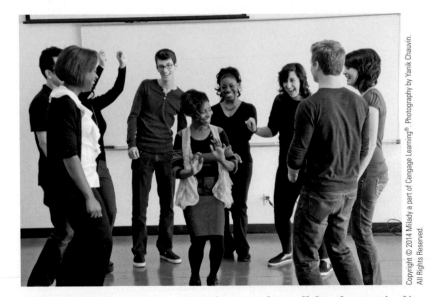

Figure 4–12   Using dance as an energizer works well for the musical/ rhythmic intelligence.

Teaching Ideas and Activities for the Musical/Rhythmic Intelligence

- Creating music in the classroom
- Using music to call students back from breaks
- Having students write and perform musical jingles
- Putting vocabulary into music or jingle format
- Implementing musical and dancing energizers during class
- Playing music in the background during group activities
- Developing team cheers
- Creating sounds for the subject being taught
- Doing "clap and slap" memory games
- Assigning essays that are turned into a musical
- Composing a musical or rap review drill
- Having students perform a song when late for class
- Writing a song that includes facts about the subject matter

Study Tips for the Musical/Rhythmic Intelligence

- Playing background music while studying
- Creating rhymes out of vocabulary words
- Beating out rhythms while studying
- Playing upbeat music on study breaks
- Writing a rap about the study topic

Those individuals who have a fully developed musical/rhythmic intelligence have strong memories for rhymes and can be energized through music. These learners are sensitive to pitch, timing, tone, timbre, and rhythm of sounds. They enjoy making melodies and learn through rhythm and sound, whether the sounds are from the human voice, musical instruments, or those of nature. Most students, however, can learn through music or rhythm—recall how you learned the alphabet, the names of all the states, or the months that have only 30 days.

Naturalist Intelligence

The **naturalist intelligence** suggests the ability to make consequential distinctions in the natural world and to use this ability productively such as in farming or biological science. Those students who prefer the naturalist intelligence are known as "nature wise." They have a keen awareness of the flora and fauna of nature and its phenomena. These individuals can discriminate both natural and nonnatural items. For example, they know one plant or bird from another, but they also can identify brands of cars, planes, sneakers, or handbags. They learn best when the content can be sorted and classified or is related to the natural world. They have keen observational skills (Figure 4–13). Students who are nature wise might choose a career as an ecologist, oceanographer, zoologist, marine biologist, forest ranger, or holistic skin care therapist. Famous personalities who are nature wise include Charles Darwin, Henry Davis Thoreau, Jacques Cousteau, Martha Stewart, and Horst Rechelbacher.

naturalist intelligence the ability to make consequential distinctions in the natural world and to use this ability productively such as in farming or biological science.

Teaching Ideas and Activities for the Naturalist Intelligence

- Observing and recording observations (such as aging skin)
- Classifying and categorizing (such as hair color levels)
- Listing natural ingredients in products

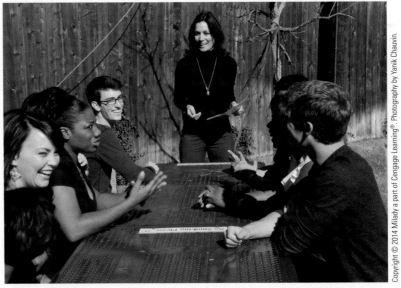

Figure 4–13   Spark interest in your naturalist intelligence learners by taking the class outdoors.

- Teaching aromatherapy
- Teaching natural hair techniques
- Observing characteristics and changes
- Recording changes in hair, skin, or nails
- Logging information on client record cards
- Journaling observations
- Classifying by color, size, function, or form
- Collecting specimens (bacteriology and infection control)
- Growing things (bacteria)
- Conducting a seven-minute nature walk as an energizer
- Teaching outdoors occasionally
- Taking outdoor field trips where appropriate
- Using analogies that show a relationship between nature and the topic

Study Tips for the Naturalist Intelligence

- Sorting and classifying subject matter
- Studying outdoors when practical and not distracting
- Exploring aspects of the content that reflect a love of nature
- Relating abstract information to something concrete in nature
- Taking a nature walk during study breaks
- Rewarding study accomplishments with things enjoyed in nature
- Playing nature sounds while studying (e.g., birds, jungle sounds, ocean sounds)

Those students who have highly developed naturalist intelligence learn best when the subject matter or content can be sorted and classified and related to the natural world. They have a strong interest in environmental balance and the ecosystem and probably recycle. They seek relief of stress through natural environments. You might get this student's attention by asking what would be the most natural solution to a problem or how something could be separated into more limited categories.

The Benefits and Importance of Identifying Learning Styles

There are numerous benefits for identifying learning styles, both for the students and the educator. By knowing how they learn and relate to the world, students can make smarter choices. They will be able to look for a work environment that best suits them, which will facilitate more success on the job. In addition, they will be able to target areas that need improvement and pinpoint areas that are more difficult in the learning environment. Further, knowing their learning style will allow them to develop study techniques that complement their style and result in better grades and achievement.

As for educators, by knowing your students' intelligence preferences and learning styles, you will be better equipped to create lesson plans and classroom environments that appeal to all their needs, thus facilitating a greater degree of success for all students. You will be able to formulate classroom presentations that offer extra focus in areas where students are weakest. As educators we must extend our supply of teaching methodologies to encompass all intelligences. We must make the content accessible to all our students, thereby giving all students an equal opportunity to succeed.

How to Identify Preferred Intelligences

There are a number of ways to ascertain which intelligences students favor. For example, you might pose a problem and have the group go about resolving it. Some students may approach it from a highly logical perspective, whereas others might try to physically "act out" the situation to achieve the answer, while yet others will want to have a group discussion and brainstorm about the topic. Another option would be to ask the students to build a model of something. Some will sit and think about it for awhile; others will draw a diagram; others will jump right in and begin building it.

To help you and your students identify their most effective intelligences, a questionnaire is provided in (Figure 4–14). This will help you as a teacher focus your presentations on those that most appeal to your learners. In addition, it will allow your learners to focus on making sure they are making the most of their existing abilities and recognizing opportunities for developing others. Please remind your students that they will manifest a mixture of intelligences, with some being more developed than others. No purpose is served in trying to label a student as one type only. Have students check each statement in the questionnaire that applies to them and then add the totals. Upon completion, have students compare the totals to see which intelligences are the most and least developed. The higher the score, the more the student prefers that particular intelligence.

Place a check mark at each statement that applies to you in each box and add the total. Compare the totals from all eight intelligences to see where you are strongest and to identify that which could be developed. The higher you score, the more you favor that intelligence.

___ You talk through problems, ask questions, and explain solutions.

___ You refer to things you've heard or read in your conversations.

___ You read books, magazines, newspapers, product labels.

___ You enjoy making puns; tongue-twisters; limericks.

___ You learn through listening: lecture, cassettes, CDs, radio.

___ You are good at debating and winning arguments.

___ You're a good story-teller, you express yourself well in writing and verbally.

___ You like crosswords, scrabble, other word puzzles.

___ You sometimes have to explain a word you have used.

___ In school, you preferred English, history, social studies.

___ L – TOTAL

___ You don't mind dancing and may even enjoy it.

___ You are known as a good "do-it-yourselfer."

___ You enjoy thrilling rides at the theme park.

___ You enjoy sports or regular physical exercise.

___ You prefer "hands-on" learning rather than reading a book or manual.

___ You enjoy "rough housing" when playing with your children.

___ Your comprehension is increased when you can physically handle something.

___ When communicating, you use gestures and body language to get your point across.

___ You walk or pace when thinking problems or situations through.

___ In school, you preferred PE and handicraft, hands-on classes.

___ B – TOTAL

___ You prefer the step-by-step and systematic approach to problem solving.

___ When considering things people say and do, you look for logical flaws.

___ You consider yourself a "numbers person" and enjoy doing mental calculations.

___ It's helpful to quantify or categorize things to understand their relevance.

___ You have a natural interest in new scientific discoveries and advances.

___ You are good at finding specific examples to support a perspective or point of view.

___ You love brain teasers and puzzles that tap into your logical thinking skills.

___ Your vacations follow a pre-planned itinerary.

___ In school, math and science were your favorite subjects.

___ M – TOTAL

___ You doodle when taking notes or thinking something through.

___ When reading, you prefer subject matter filled with illustrations.

___ You enjoy the arts: theater, film, art, music, etc.

___ You are able to visualize how things look from various perspectives.

___ At family gatherings or special events, you're recording it for history with a camera or camcorder.

___ You support your position or point with drawings and diagrams.

___ You find games like Pictionary or jigsaw puzzles and mazes appealing and enjoyable.

___ You are skilled at taking things apart and putting them back together.

___ You are an adept navigator and read maps well.

___ In school, you preferred arts and crafts classes and geometry to algebra.

___ V – TOTAL

R: Musical/Rhythmic	I: Interpersonal	S: Intrapersonal	N: Naturalist
___ You may manage to sing and carry a tune.	___ You enjoy and are effective at mentoring others.	___ You work independently or have contemplated doing so.	___ You could see yourself as a farmer or even a fisherman.
___ You remember tunes after hearing them just a couple of times.	___ Working with a group, team, or committee is preferable to working alone.	___ You like to spend "quiet time" reflecting on important issues in your life or just life itself.	___ You can identify many different types of trees, flowers, and plants.
___ You actually play at least one musical instrument.	___ When solving a problem, you tend to seek advice and input from others rather than trying to solve it yourself.	___ You keep a daily journal or log to record your innermost thoughts.	___ You like pets.
___ You prefer music in the background when working or studying.	___ Others tend to come to you when they need advice or a good listener.	___ You have established your personal goals and a plan of action for achieving them.	___ You have an interest and good knowledge of how the body works or you keep abreast on health issues.
___ You are often caught humming or whistling.	___ When it comes to sports, you prefer team sports rather than individual sports.	___ You have a personal interest or hobby that you keep to yourself and don't share.	___ You consider conservation of resources and achieving sustainable growth are important issues of our age.
___ When you hear music, you tap in time.	___ You don't hesitate to take the lead or show others how to accomplish something.	___ The ideal vacation to you is an isolated mountain cabin or bungalow on the beach rather than a busy resort.	___ When out walking, you notice animal tracks, nests, and wildlife and can "read" weather signs.
___ You can't visualize life without music.	___ When it comes to close friends, you have many.	___ You like hiking or fishing alone. You are comfy with self.	___ You are intrigued by psychology and human motivations and social issues.
___ You can identify different musical instruments.	___ You are a good communicator and helpful in resolving disputes.	___ You are an independent thinker and can make up your own mind.	___ You are interested in astronomical developments and the evolution of life in general.
___ You often listen to music at home and in your car.	___ You enjoy games that require participation with others such as board games.	___ You have attended self-help seminars or read books to learn more about yourself.	___ You like to garden and know one plant from another.
___ Commercial music or even theme music often pops into your head.	___ You prefer to be at a party than at home watching television.	___ You know your own strengths and weaknesses.	___ You are interested in global environmental issues.
___ R – TOTAL	___ I – TOTAL	___ S – TOTAL	___ N – TOTAL

L: Verbal/Linguistic

M: Logical/Mathematical

V: Visual/Spatial

B: Bodily/Kinesthetic

R: Musical/Rhythmic

I: Interpersonal

S: Intrapersonal

N: Naturalist

Figure 4–14   What is your strongest intelligence?

Developing Intelligences

Gardner tells us that we do not have a "fixed" intelligence. As previously stated, we may have abilities in all intelligences, but have developed or prefer some more than others. If we look at our lives and how development progresses, we might recognize that a three-year-old is going to be low in all the intelligences, but from age three to six, children will develop substantially in the verbal/linguistic, musical/rhythmic, and visual/spatial intelligences. It is also understood that we can progress in the bodily/kinesthetic intelligence all the way up to age 70, but there is likely no age limit for an individual to develop in the interpersonal, intrapersonal, and logical/mathematical intelligences as long as the brain is still functioning. The main thing to remember is that the most successful people have likely developed an intelligence area that they were weak in at one point in their lives.

Combining Intelligences

We noted earlier that we must integrate teaching strategies that meet the needs of a more multicultural student body with a variety of learning styles. Consider that if we present material that strictly addresses only one intelligence—for example, the verbal/linguistic intelligence—we might reach as little as 5 percent or as much as 75 percent of the student body. However, if we were to design our classes to include methods that appeal to all intelligences, we have a much better chance of 100 percent success. We are told in adult education that we should focus on at least three to four intelligences in every class we teach and should address all the intelligences during the course of a week of study.

Wrapping It Up

Traditional academia has taught in ways that appeal to basically two intelligences: verbal/linguistic and logical/mathematical. If you consider what a standard IQ (intelligence quotient) test measures, it is generally an individual's ability with words and numbers. So students who are naturally strong in verbal and logical skills will likely do well on a standard IQ test. In these cases, the IQ score will be a fairly good predictor of success in school because the way traditional education teaches (through lectures) and the material students receive (logical and sequentially developed textbooks) depend heavily on those two intelligences. If we think about it, teachers are generally born from students who do well in school, thus creating a self-perpetuating system designed to reach only those two intelligences. As a master educator, you have the opportunity to deliver content that reaches all intelligences and allows your learners to really begin to use their full brain power.

Remember that there is no "best" way to learn. There are many different learning styles and intelligences, and different styles are suited to different people and/or situations. Every normal individual possesses varying degrees of the eight different intelligences, but the ways we combine and blend the intelligences vary as much as the personalities of those applying them. We need to remind our students that they are a mixture of styles and preferences and that their preferences may change depending on the circumstances or subject matter. By teaching our students about their individuality and valuing multiple intelligences, we validate all students. As a result, students enjoy their own self-worth and develop a love of life-long learning.

In Retrospect

1. List and explain the four important steps in learning.

2. List the eight distinct intelligences and explain the characteristics of each.

3. List the benefits of identifying learning styles for students.

Objectives (Desired Performance Goals):

After reading and studying this chapter, you should be able to:

- Define *teaching*.
- Explain what is meant by *teaching methods*.
- Explain what is meant by *learning methods*.
- Explain the purpose and use of interactive lectures, demonstrations, group discussions, peer coaching, and role-playing in learning.
- Discuss why window paning is an effective method of learning.
- Explain the purpose and benefits of field trips and using guest speakers in learning.
- Demonstrate mind mapping and explain why it is an important learning method.
- Explain the use and purpose of projects, workbooks, partially complete handouts, case studies, and concept connectors.
- Explain the purpose and benefits of visualization and the use of stories and anecdotes in the educational process.
- Explain the use of mnemonics, energizers, characterizations, experiments, humor, games, and group synergy.

! CRITICAL CONCEPT

A master educator believes in his students...he leads and teases and pushes and nudges students to the next level of understanding...never stopping until the lightbulb turns on.

About Teaching and Learning

A MASTER EDUCATOR has the responsibility of making sure that all students understand that learning is a life-long endeavor—that it doesn't end with completion of any given course of study. Therefore, it is vital that master educators have a thorough understanding of the teaching and learning processes. That means being aware of the many different teaching methods that lead to learning. Educators must also convince students that when they enter the work force, they must be prepared to invest time and money in continuing education throughout their careers if they are to attain and maintain success. Until graduation, however, the educator will accompany the learner through the teaching and learning process.

Teaching is the act of imparting knowledge or instructing by precept, example, or experience. It is any manner of communicating information or skills so that others may learn. Learning occurs when skills or knowledge are acquired by instruction (teaching), study, or experience or when a behavior is modified as a result of gaining knowledge or understanding through instruction, study, or experience. Teaching and learning occur through many means, and not all students learn in the same manner or at the same time. Therefore, the master educator must develop skills in a wide variety of teaching methods and techniques to maximize the potential for all learner types.

There is a plethora of activities and teaching tools or aids that may be used by the master educator to ensure that every learner type is reached. Learner-centered education will dominate education in the twenty-first century. This will be accomplished when educators incorporate a variety of learner-centered activities into the process, generating maximum learner involvement. Many of the tools and techniques discussed in this chapter include learner-centered activities.

As we learned in Chapter 4, there are four principal steps in learning:

- Desire: First, we have to want to know something.
- Information: Second, we have to obtain the necessary information (the how to) about the subject matter.
- Assimilation: Third, we have to understand the information or how the task is performed.
- Repetition: Fourth, we have to practice the task—either using the underlying theory or the practical applications—until we have it mastered.

It shouldn't be so difficult for us to apply learning to our most important life goals. Everything we do is habit forming if it is repeated often enough, and that definitely applies to learning.

Teaching and Learning Methods

A teaching method represents the manner in which the educator uses the material and resources available to produce or achieve desired educational objectives and facilitate learning for all students. Even the most sophisticated curriculum and comprehensive lesson plans for any course of study will be fruitless if not delivered with effective teaching methods that render the desired results. Teaching methods must be appropriate for the type of lesson and the types of learners in the classroom. The more varied the methods within any given class, demonstration, or presentation, the more likely that every learner will ultimately "get it." Learning methods refer to the various ways that learners hear, comprehend, and retain information. In many cases, teaching and learning methods are the same. In this chapter, we will consider a wide array of teaching and learning methods for use and consideration by those in pursuit of becoming a master educator.

☑ Interactive Lecture

Traditional education is generally composed of an extensive amount of lecturing. Though lecture does have its place in our classrooms, it will only be highly effective with certain types of learners. Lecture is a discourse or formal presentation given before a group of learners especially for the purpose of instruction. It is a system of conveying information, explaining facts or details, or describing practices and procedures. Lectures should be kept brief and to the point. They will be more effective if used in conjunction with other methods and techniques so that frequent variation of the stimuli occurs—otherwise known as interactive lectures.

In Chapter 7, "Effective Presentations," we will discuss with great specificity how to prepare for and deliver a powerful classroom presentation. All those techniques relate directly to preparing for the interactive lecture method of teaching. The master educator will develop powerful openings for each lecture and build thorough content for the substance of the lecture. He will vary the stimuli for the learners by using techniques explained in Chapter 7 and others that will be discussed later in this chapter. He will develop expert skills in questioning during the interactive lecture that will achieve the best possible results for the learners. And, finally, he will incorporate a closing for the presentation that has a high impact on the learners. Basically, there is merit in the interactive lecture method of teaching if it is not overused, if it is combined with other methods, and if it *supplements,* rather than replaces, the textbook (Figure 5–1).

> ⌒ **CONSIDER AND CONNECT**
>
> Master educators must take care when using the important technique of interactive lecture because it is not the most effective delivery method for today's adult learners.

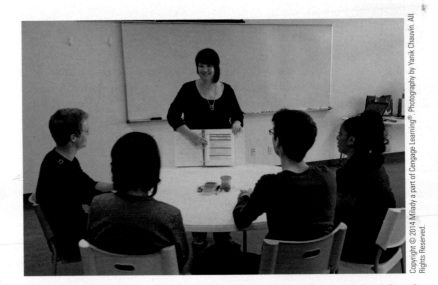

Figure 5–1   Interactive lecturing is more effective when used with other teaching methods and techniques.

Demonstration and Practice

Master educators use the demonstration method of teaching to bring the lesson or presentation to life. It provides educators with the opportunity to perform an actual skill or procedure that will be later performed by the students. The demonstration is used to help clarify and instill the underlying theory of a procedure into the minds of the learners. This method can be used to illustrate how to use implements and equipment and to solidify correct procedures.

When the demonstration method is called for, the educator must follow certain steps to ensure that it is effective and that learning objectives are met. These steps are discussed next.

Preparation. This occurs prior to delivering the demonstration. It includes identifying the objectives of the lesson to be certain that the demonstration will achieve them. It includes preparing the students for the lesson and motivating them to observe, listen, and learn. It involves gathering and organizing all materials and tools necessary for the demonstration ahead of time. It also requires the educator to take the necessary steps to ensure that all students can see and hear the demonstration clearly.

Demonstration. Master educators avoid distractions while showing and explaining a single fundamental procedure completely by going through a step-by-step process. They will perform the demonstration at an appropriate speed, ensuring students do not miss key points or steps (Figure 5–2). Emphasis is placed on special techniques. Safe practice will be demonstrated and emphasized. Students will be questioned during the demonstration to verify their understanding. Master educators observe nonverbal Cues from the students that indicate how they are responding to the demonstration and take appropriate action. For example, if students appear quizzical or uninterested, the educator may vary the stimuli by changing the activity. A master educator will not pass an object around for student consideration during a demonstration. To do so will distract the learners from the important steps in the demonstration. Master educators will involve the learners in the demonstration whenever possible. For example, the educator may "show and tell" a specific procedure and then ask one of the students to perform the procedure while he narrates the steps. Further, another student might perform the step while yet another student narrates the procedure.

> **CONSIDER AND CONNECT**
>
> Demonstrations are highly effective in illustrating a manipulative procedure or clarifying a principle.

> **CONSIDER AND CONNECT**
>
> New terms introduced during a demonstration should be explained and written on the board for later discussion.

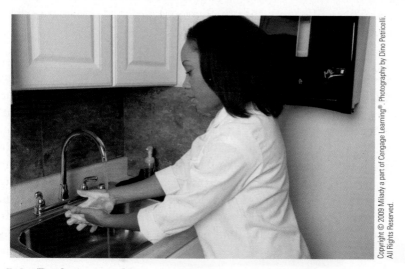

Figure 5–2   Perform step-by-step procedures to ensure learner understanding.

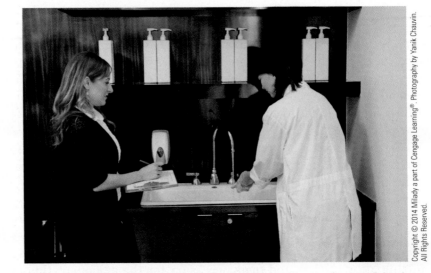

Figure 5–3   Assessing student practice is key to the student achieving acceptable skills.

Practice or Application. This has also been called the "return demonstration." After the educator has completed his demonstration, students must have the opportunity to practice the skill or procedure under educator supervision. This practice should occur as soon after the demonstration as possible Figure 5–3. Students should use the same implements and equipment as those used by the educator to ensure consistency in the application. Practical application of procedures allows students to acquire skill and to progress at a rate most suited to their learning style. It provides the opportunity for learners to correct individual mistakes and take pride in their achievement. It is a known fact that repetition causes learning to occur. Therefore, multiple practice sessions should be held for each practical skill demonstrated.

Evaluation or Assessment. Master educators closely supervise student practice of a skill and evaluate their performance according to the school's published grading policy and predetermined performance criteria. They will give immediate feedback and assistance to those students participating in the practice session to ensure their work achieves the standards required. This will ensure that the learners' practice makes a perfect procedure permanent.

☑ Group Discussion and Discovery

Through discussion and discovery, learners are provided the opportunity to work in a group environment and share their own opinions, judgments, and perceptions. It allows learners to become actively involved in the learning process. Very often the group activity is led or guided by the educator, who provides information and facts and then questions the groups in a manner that facilitates their arrival at the correct answer or conclusion. Another approach, which is more open-ended, uses the educator more as a facilitator. The groups of students decide which questions to ask and how to find the answers, rather than the educator. This type of learning is extremely advantageous because it requires a high degree of learner participation (Figure 5–4),

---

IT'S WORTH REMEMBERING ✳

Master educators perform demonstrations that reflect the highest quality of workmanship and skills ability that exemplifies the performance standards expected of their students.

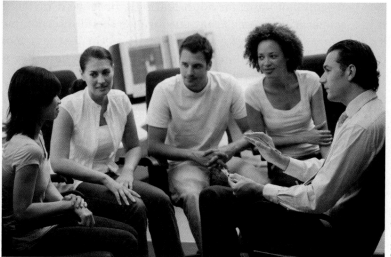

Figure 5–4 **Group discussion requires a high degree of student participation.**

THE TOP 10 WAYS TO ENSURE THE BEST RESULTS IN GROUP DISCUSSION AND DISCOVERY ARE TO:

1. Involve all learners.

2. Avoid interrupting learners and groups when at work.

3. Provide ample time and opportunities for learners to experiment and discover.

4. Allow for choices among all learners.

5. Ensure that each activity is based on problems or questions that are solvable.

6. Ensure that all learners know and understand their individual role in the process.

7. Allow for differences of opinions among learners.

8. Use visual aids as frequently as possible.

9. Require that opinions and statements brought forth by the learners be supported by evidence and facts.

10. Teach with enthusiasm and ensure that the process enriches knowledge rather than shares ignorance.

which is a powerful motivator for adult learners. Because it involves group work, it is a cooperative process that encourages social interaction among students. This method does make more demands on the learners, mostly because there is a lack of immediate feedback to show them how they are progressing toward a given objective.

With good leadership by the educator, the group discussion and discovery method will be kept on track and can stimulate thought and analysis, encourage interpretations of the facts, and change old behaviors and attitudes into new and improved ones.

☑ Role-Playing

position role-playing
the learner plays the part of a particular position (such as any practitioner, manager, or educator), rather than the part of a specific individual.

character role-playing
the learner plays the part of a specific person and acts as that person would in the given situation.

role-reversal role-playing
learners assume the roles of other persons with whom they interact on a regular basis. For example, the student might play the educator or a client.

Role-playing is an important learning tool that deserves special attention. The purpose of role-playing is to help learners understand the views and feelings of other people as well as to explore one's own behavior and motivations with respect to a wide range of personal and social issues (Figure 5–5). By acting out situations in which people are in conflict, students can begin to better understand other points of view and perspectives on an issue. The educator's purpose in role-playing is to structure the scenario and lead the follow-up discussion. All class members are involved, either as role-players or as observers who analyze the enactment and take notes for later discussion. In adult career education, role-playing can be highly beneficial in determining how various conflict situations should be handled, including both client conflicts and peer conflicts.

When role-playing, the student takes on the attitude and behavior of another person in a particular situation. The results of role-playing seem to be more effective in smaller groups when the entire group participates in the analysis and follow-up discussion. Learning can be just as effective for the observers as for the participants if the activity is properly conducted and directed. There are three basic types of role-playing: *position role-playing*, *character role-playing*, and *role-reversal*. Position role-playing requires

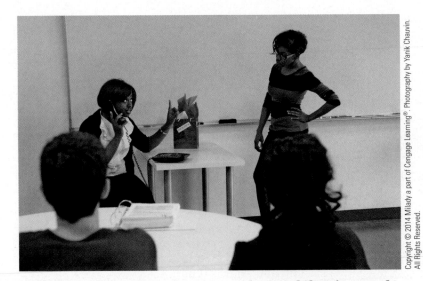

Figure 5–5   Role-playing helps learners understand the views and feelings of other people.

the learner to play the part of a particular position (such as any practitioner, manager, or educator), rather than the part of a specific individual. In character role-playing, the learner plays the part of a specific person and acts as that person would in the given situation. In role-reversal, however, learners assume the roles of other persons with whom they interact on a regular basis. For example, the student might play the educator or a client.

Role-playing can be more effective if a coach is used who also becomes a "tag team" member of the activity. In other words, the coach may be asked to step in and take over a particular part at any given time. Some helpful hints in making sure that role-playing is highly effective include:

- using volunteers only, whenever possible.
- never role-playing situations that involve the learner's own personal problems.
- selecting situations that will not embarrass any of the learners.
- integrating the role-play activity into the context of a larger lesson.

Role-playing also helps learners adjust to and bond with the other students with whom they interact. It is a fun way to acquaint learners with possible problems they will encounter in their careers and with possible solutions for dealing with those problems. It provides examples of behavior that can be most effective in a given scenario. Role-playing can also be beneficial in helping learners develop their own style of self-expression. It is a great way to show students how they might react in real-life circumstances before they even occur.

Role-playing can be useful when teaching client consultation skills, how to deal with a dissatisfied client, and how to interview for employment. Many situations can be clarified and resolved through the activity of role-playing. Learners should be able to suggest several scenarios based on their own training experiences. The role of the master educator in role-playing is to ensure that all learners leave the experience with a feeling that there is likely more than one solution to any conflict or problem and with some thoughts on how those solutions can be achieved.

Window Paning

Window paning is the process of transferring key elements, points, or steps in a lesson to visual images that are then hand-sketched into the squares or "panes" of a matrix. The mind thinks in pictures or images when the right brain cortex is more active than the left. With that in mind, master educators incorporate the use of pictures or images whenever possible to help learners grasp ideas more quickly and retain them for longer periods of time. Research indicates that people can retain in their short-term memory an average of seven "bits," or pieces, of information, plus or minus two bits. Therefore, it is recommended that master educators use window panes containing no more than nine panes for a given topic.

Effective use of the nine panes within the window allows the learner to absorb nine critical bits of information in a manner that is much easier to recall than the written word is (Figure 5–6). For example, if the educator were teaching learners how to perform cardiopulmonary resuscitation (CPR), he could list all the steps in writing or he could have the learners interpret each step by drawing their perception of it.

CONSIDER AND CONNECT

Role-playing is effective in stimulating learner interest and participation by giving learners insight into the various roles they will be playing throughout their lives and encouraging consideration of how those roles should be played.

window paning
the process of transferring key elements, points, or steps in a lesson to visual images that are then hand-sketched into the squares or "panes" of a matrix.

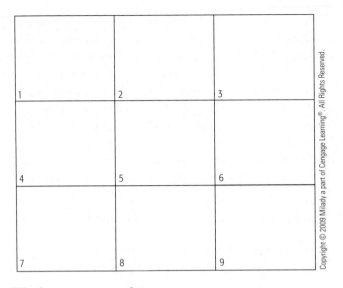

Figure 5–6   Window pane template.

The first window pane suggests that you must first become aware that there may be a need to administer CPR. The second pane suggests that you tilt the head back, lift the chin, and open the victim's airway. The third pane indicates that you must determine whether the person is breathing by looking, listening, and feeling for a breath. The fourth pane shows that you must give the victim two full breaths into his mouth. The fifth pane indicates that if breathing is still blocked, you should administer the Heimlich maneuver. The sixth pane indicates that you should administer rescue breathing. The seventh pane indicates that if there is still no pulse, you should administer chest compressions. The final pane indicates that you should continue until help arrives.

In contrast, the educator could simply provide the learner with a written procedure that states the following:

Steps in Cardiopulmonary Resuscitation

By learning to administer CPR—a simple, life-saving technique—you may literally save the life of a victim whose airway has been blocked (Figure 5–7).

1. Victim should be lying flat on his back on a firm surface so that you can shake his shoulders and ask loudly, "Are you OK?" If the victim doesn't respond, call 911 and proceed.
2. Open the victim's airway by tilting his head back and lifting his chin upward.
3. For 5 to 10 seconds, look, listen, and feel for breathing.
4. If the victim is not breathing, pinch his nose and give two full breaths into his mouth using a microshield, if available. If air does not go in, reposition his head and try again.
5. If breathing remains blocked, adjust the victim's position and perform abdominal thrusts (also known as the Heimlich maneuver).
6. Check the victim's carotid pulse at the side of his neck for 5 to 10 seconds.

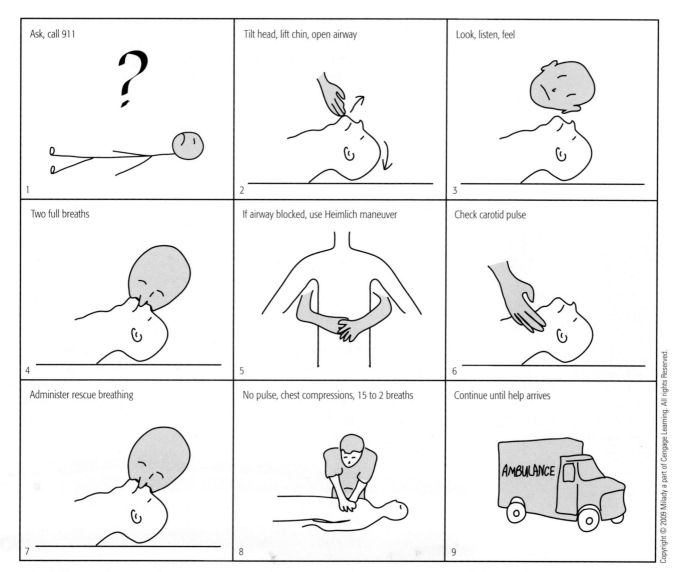

Figure 5–7 Window paning allows the student to transfer key elements, points, or steps into visual images in a matrix.

7. If the victim has a pulse but is still not breathing, administer rescue breathing by giving one breath every five seconds, averaging 12 breaths per minute.
8. Depress the lower part of the victim's sternum about 1.5 to 2 inches. Place the heel of one hand on the lower part of the sternum and place the other hand on top of the first hand for added pressure. Perform 15 compressions to every two breaths. Recheck pulse after one minute.
9. Proceed until help arrives or you feel too exhausted to continue.

Can you see how much easier it would be for learners to grasp and retain the steps by actually drawing them and then studying the images that represent the various steps? Learners can recall the images that trigger specific concepts in a procedure much more simply than they can memorize the written steps. Master educators will remember to limit window panes to no more than nine images. They will encourage learners to use their own simple, hand-sketched line drawings, which may be dissimilar to yours. Finally, encourage learners to develop and create their own window panes for any given topic with which they are struggling. By creating their own panes that address the steps or information they need to recall, they will have a much greater opportunity for retention and remembering. This visual "chunking" of information has proved highly successful in achieving learner results. When using window paning as a learning method, educators should ensure that all learners have mastered all the panes in the first matrix before moving on to the next one.

☑ Field Trips

We have placed a great deal of emphasis throughout this text on the importance of learner involvement and self-discovery in the educational process. Incorporating field trips into the routine class schedule accomplishes both. Excursions into the workplace at various venues provide students with an opportunity for *active* learning. In addition, excursions encourage the students to explore the marketplace and discover for themselves various aspects of the career path they have chosen. Master educators involve the students in determining which types of field trips are appropriate and most beneficial. In a cooperative effort with the students, a determination will be made prior to the field trip as to what objectives are to be achieved during the trip. Students will be directed to share responsibility in gathering and recording information about the observations they make during the trip. Upon return to class from a scheduled field trip there should be an organized review of the event and an in-depth discussion regarding the students' observations. Master educators will be able to tie those observations to the initial objectives identified as important for the field trip. Such discussion and evaluations should occur immediately after the conclusion of the field trip if they are to have the greatest value.

The advantages of incorporating field trips into career education include the following. They may:

- broaden the understanding of the professional career being pursued by each learner.
- build interest in the chosen field of study.
- add variety to learner activities and reduce the occurrence of monotony or boredom.
- strengthen important images and impressions by learners.
- provide broader "real-world" experience than is available in the classroom or lab.
- may provide opportunities for skills practice.

As previously stated, the master educator involves the learners in determining which types of trips are desired and significant, because many are options available. Trips that might be considered relevant include visits to:

- Professional service facilities. Learners get to observe the skills and abilities of those already working in their chosen field. They are able to get a feel for the professional environment and atmosphere. This can be especially beneficial for soon-to-graduate students who will be seeking employment in the near future (Figure 5–8).

IT'S WORTH REMEMBERING ✳

For maximum results, master educators incorporate window paning with demonstration, application, evaluation, *and* written procedures handouts.

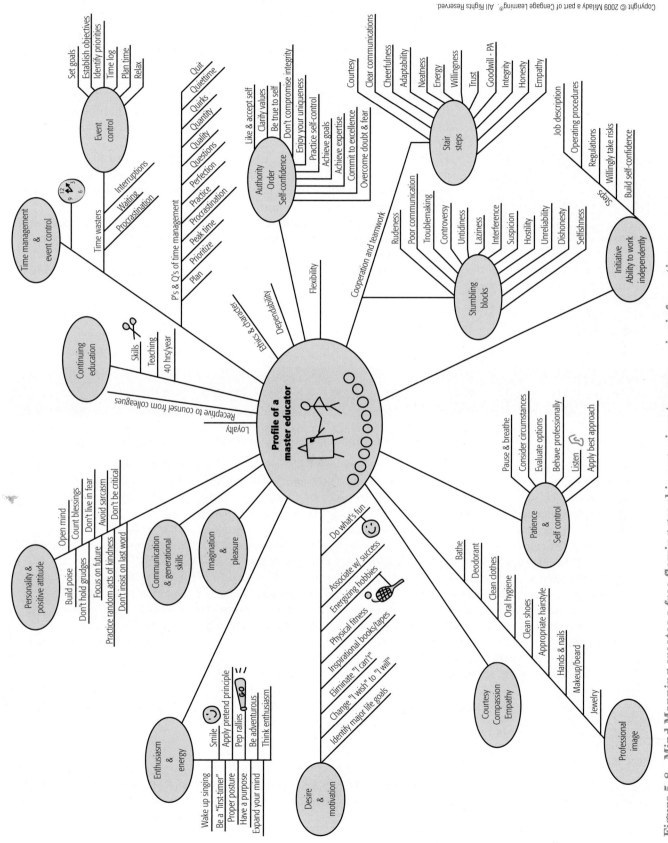

Figure 5–8   Mind Mapping creates a free-flowing graphic organizer to summarize information.

- Professional product-distribution centers. Learners have the opportunity to see first hand the retail side of their chosen field as well as to consider the wide array of products, tools, and implements that will be available to them in the workplace.
- Trade shows. Learners can observe professional technicians presenting and introducing the latest products that will enhance their professional work.
- Manufacturers of industry products. Learners can observe how products are actually formulated and manufactured. This can be highly beneficial in helping them to understand the chemistry behind the products they may use daily.
- High school career days. Learners have the opportunity to actively share with potential students what their experience as a career-education student has been. It gives them the opportunity to fine-tune their own communications and interpersonal skills.
- County fairs and community events. Learners may have the opportunity to demonstrate to the visiting public the skills they have learned so far in the course of study .
- Civic club meetings. Various professional clubs or organizations may be interested in a presentation on your professional field.

A number of other opportunities are available for curriculum-related field trips for students.

IT'S WORTH REMEMBERING ✳

Never burn your bridges; rather, build a network of contacts who have a favorable opinion of you.

PROFESSIONAL SERVICE VISIT CHECKLIST

When you visit a professional service facility, observe the following areas and rate them from 1 to 5, with 5 being the best.

_____ **Business image**: Is the establishment image consistent with and appropriate for your interests? Is the image pleasing and inviting? What is the decor and arrangement? If you are not comfortable or if you find it unattractive, is it likely that clients will also?

_____ **Professionalism**: Do the employees present the appropriate professional appearance and behavior? Do they give their clients the appropriate levels of attention and personal service or do they act as if work is their time to socialize?

_____ **Management**: Does the establishment show signs of being well managed? Is the phone answered promptly with professional telephone skills? Is the mood positive? Does everyone appear to work as a team?

_____ **Client service**: Are clients greeted promptly and warmly when they enter? Are they kept informed of the status of their appointment? Are they offered a magazine or beverage while they wait? Is there a comfortable reception area?

_____ **Prices**: Compare price for value. Are clients getting their money's worth? Do they pay the same price in one establishment but get better service and attention in another? If possible, take home brochures and price lists.

_____ **Retail** (if applicable): Is there a well-stocked retail display offering clients a variety of product lines and a range of prices? Do the employees promote retail sales?

_____ **Internal marketing**: Are there posters or promotions found throughout the establishment? If so, are they tasteful and of good quality?

_____ **Services**: Make a list of all services offered by each establishment. This will help you decide what earnings potential you might have at the establishment.

Establishment Name: _____

Establishment Manager: _____

Keep this checklist on file for future reference and comparison to other establishments. Even if you did not like the establishment or wouldn't consider working there, write a brief note thanking the manager for his or her time.

Guest Speakers

Using guest speakers in the classroom environment can be extremely motivating for learners. Guest speakers can also provide a perfect solution for disseminating information to your students on topics about which you may have limited knowledge. None of us can achieve expert levels in every topic related to the various disciplines we teach. Therefore, inviting a guest speaker who is an expert can provide a great learning opportunity for students.

Master educators recognize, however, that having a guest speaker does not reduce or eliminate their responsibility to be present and participate in the classroom presentation. Without the proper groundwork being laid in advance of the presentation, the event can do more harm than good. Guest speakers have been known to be disorganized, talk too long, have a negative attitude toward the training the learners are receiving, dislike the products used by the institution, or just be poor speakers in general. Therefore, master educators will work with the guest speaker ahead of time to plan the program. A preliminary meeting with any guest speaker is recommended. This will allow you to lay the ground rules for the speaker's presentation. You can establish the time frame that he will be required to adhere to. You can set forth any parameters appropriate for the topic, including the objectives of the presentation. After all, how can you expect the guest speaker to deliver the material needed if he does not understand his purpose? Ask for an outline of the presentation prior to the scheduled event. Review of the outline may indicate that a personal discussion with the speaker is needed. While the speaker may be an expert on the topic of the day, he may not be skilled as an educator or presenter. Therefore, you may want to give him some tips about how to get the learners involved with the presentation. It is also important for you to be prepared to take control of the class if that becomes necessary. If not, it will still be appropriate for you to ask the class controversial or stimulating questions about the topic to spark discussion. Finally, the master educator will be an attentive listener during the presentation and be prepared to close the class with a summary of the information and review questions that will reinforce the learners' retention of the material.

Mind Mapping

Mind mapping is another method of learning that has not been part of the traditional educational process or experience. It is used for developing an innovative and more creative approach to thinking. It is highly effective for visual learners. Mind mapping creates a free-flowing, graphic organizing system to outline material or information (Figure 5–9). It is easy to learn, and when students master the technique of mind mapping, they will be able to organize entire projects in a matter of minutes. Student creativity will be immediately increased. Mind mapping engages both hemispheres of the learner's brain and improves recall abilities in all learners. Mastering the art of mind mapping has allowed students who were barely passing to become "straight A" students when they used it to outline chapters or

mind mapping
another method of learning that has not been part of the traditional educational process or experience. It is used for developing an innovative and more creative approach to thinking.

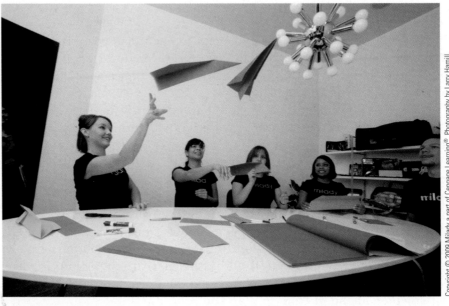

Figure 5–9   Excursions into the work place provide students with first-hand observations of their potential future.

Several steps are beneficial when developing mind maps:

1. *The primary image in the center should be in color.* Remember, a picture is worth a thousand words. The image chosen should encourage creative thought while also increasing the learner's memory.
2. *Depict images or pictures throughout the mind map.* Images will aid in recall and will also help to stimulate both sides of the brain.
3. *Words used in mind mapping should be printed, not cursive.* Printing is more photographic in your mind and provides for more comprehensive feedback when it is needed.
4. *Print words on lines that are connected to other lines.* This ensures that the basic structure of mind mapping will remain intact.
5. Whenever possible, there should only be one word per line. This gives the learner more flexibility in developing and mapping the topic.
6. *Colors should be used throughout the mind map to increase recall.* Color stimulates the correct cortical process while also delighting the eye. This aids in retention.
7. *Keep the mind as open and uncluttered as possible.* If the learner stops to think about where a line or word should go, the entire process will be hindered. The learner should not worry about the organization or order of the map; it will usually take care of itself.

The example of a mind map in Figure 5–9 depicts the qualities and characteristics of a master educator as outlined in Chapter 1, "The Career Education Instructor."

key information for testing. Mind mapping has proved more effective than the linear form of note taking taught in traditional education. When mind mapping, the central or main idea is more clearly defined. The map lays out the relative importance of each idea or element of the subject matter. For example, the more important ideas or material will be nearer the center and the less important material will be located in the outer parameters. Proximity and connections are used to establish the links between key concepts or ideas. All of this results in review and recall occurring more quickly and being more effective. Because the mind map begins in the center and grows outward, new points can be easily added at any time. As learners develop the art of mind mapping, they will see that each one takes on a unique appearance, which adds to the learners' recall ability of different topics or subjects.

Mind mapping is nothing more than putting ideas on paper using headings, color, drawings, symbols, and connecting elements to identify relationships between concepts, topics, or ideas. The result is a colorful design that becomes a comprehensive map of the subject matter.

Peer Coaching

In today's climate of adult learners, **peer coaching** or peer tutoring can be extremely effective. In a career-training environment, where learners have such diverse backgrounds and learning styles, a method that provides for one-on-one, personalized instruction such as peer coaching can increase learning results in the classroom. By teaming up two students to work together and "coach" or tutor each other, learners can set their own pace and receive individualized feedback on a regular basis (Figure 5–10). This can be highly motivational for both learners. The one-on-one interaction provides the opportunity for immediate recognition and encouragement

peer coaching a method that provides for one-on-one, personalized instruction that can increase learning results by allowing learners to set their own pace and receive individualized feedback on a regular basis.

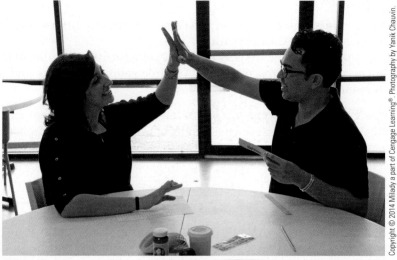

Figure 5–10   Peer coaching allows learners to set their own pace and receive individualized feedback.

when progress is made. When you have helped another individual learn something, you also become motivated and have fun. Some steps that increase the effectiveness of peer coaching include:

- Assign learners to work and study in pairs. Students can either be of comparable ability or a more advanced student can be paired with one who is progressing at a lesser rate and needs assistance. The more advanced student can tutor the slower student or can also receive the benefit of being quizzed by the other learner, if tutoring is not appropriate.
- Prepare instructional materials appropriate for the area that needs improvement. The problems and exercises that need to be worked on must be identified by the educator.
- Provide appropriate training to the student coaches. Like educators, they are not born; they must have some guidance and instruction.
- Monitor learner progress by observing, answering questions, and intervening whenever necessary.
- Monitor and assess the compatibility of the team. If team members are not achieving the desired results or appear unable to work together effectively, reassign the teams.

☑ Projects

Projects are used to allow learners to apply what they have learned either in the classroom or laboratory. This is where they can take the underlying theories of a subject and integrate them with practice and action. Projects can be very effective in helping students develop problem-solving skills. They give learners the opportunity for another type of hands-on experience. Projects can be assigned to individuals, to pairs, to small teams, or to the entire class. Projects may be practical, hands-on-type activities or they may be written essays. Examples of projects that might be assigned by educators include the following:

- Have students write essays on the various topics within the curriculum or associated with the curriculum.
- Have students build a display or create an educational bulletin board using samples, pictures, or labels of course-related products and a statement of how each is used.

The previous suggestions are just a few ideas of projects that can be assigned to students to increase their understanding of a given topic and add to learner retention.

☑ Workbooks and Partially Complete Handouts

Workbooks have long been considered an effective teaching and learning aid. Master educators will take care not to rely so heavily on workbook activities that sufficient instruction does not take place. Workbook assignments should closely follow the lesson or text material being covered. Educators may choose not to assign every single page of the workbook for completion. The material is available to be used at the discretion of the educator. Certainly, workbooks are not as effective for some learner types as others. Educators should also consider developing handouts for learners that include blanks for key terms or information that must be filled in by the learners. As the educator is making the presentation, overhead slides can be projected that include the key terms or words that learners are to fill in. This procedure aids the learners because they do not have to write down everything being covered. It also allows them to stay on track with the presentation and be able to focus on the importance of the lesson.

Case Studies

Another type of teaching and learning method involves two types of case studies useful in adult career education. These case studies provide detailed descriptions of realistic problem situations that require resolution. One type of case study presents only the problem and the learner is challenged with arriving at the appropriate solution. The other type presents both the problem and one possible solution to the problem. The learner is then challenged with analyzing how well the problem was solved and making recommendations, if applicable, for other possible solutions. When an educator develops a case-study project, he must make certain that the case is sufficiently challenging to the learners while also ensuring that it is a worthy problem that can be solved. Case studies should be directly related to the objectives of the lesson and depict interesting situations that are familiar to all learners so that they have appropriate opportunity to resolve the identified problem. Some suggestions for developing effective case studies are as follows:

- Prepare more than one case study for each class. This gives your learners a choice and allows you more flexibility as an educator.
- Avoid gender specificity whenever possible. This allows the learners to be more objective in their consideration of suitable solutions.
- Debrief with questions ranging from the general to more specific. Debriefing questions are different from those developed for the case-study discussion. This allows learners to consider the general problems or challenges first and then move into specific details of a possible solution.
- Give options for answering the discussion questions. If you have developed five questions for learners to consider in the case study, make the first and last one the easiest. Make the second and fourth ones the next easiest, and make the middle question the most difficult. Then allow the learners to consider the questions in any order they choose. When debriefing, vary the order in which you review the discussion questions and possible solutions with the learners. Probably not all learners will have discussed or responded to all five questions. By reviewing them in random order, your learners will either be checking their own answers or taking notes about the ones they had not reached, which creates interest and energy in the debriefing discussion.

Concept Connectors

Concept connectors merely bridge the gap or provide a link between the student and the information being learned. A concept connector will link the learner's experience with the skill or information that is being conveyed. In addition, it will provide a link between the learner's life experiences with the objectives of the lesson or the school experience as a whole. For example, the educator might use the following concept connector to open a class regarding home construction:

> *A chef will tell you that it takes more than knowing what ingredients to use in a recipe to create a perfect soufflé. An architect will tell you that the raw materials don't "build" the structure unless they are used and assembled properly. A floriculturist will say that it takes more than flowers, greenery, and ornamentation to make a beautiful bouquet. In every case, it takes an understanding of how all the components work together to create the artistic outcomes designed by these professionals. By understanding all the parts or pieces of the puzzle of building a house, you will be able to ensure the quality of the finished design and style.*

In this example, the learner can connect what he knows about cooking or flower arranging to the fact that there are many component steps needed and used in building a home as well.

✓ Visualization

visualization the process by which the mind translates the content of a lesson into visual imagery.

Visualization is the process by which the mind translates the content of a lesson into visual imagery. Master educators encourage learners to visualize themselves performing perfect practical skills. When students visualize themselves performing a perfect procedure, and they practice it sufficiently, they will eventually perform it perfectly. Visualization has become increasingly common among athletes. Through visualization, they think about and create their futures. Your students can do the same thing. For example, you might have them perform the following exercise, which will take about 15 minutes. They will need a pen and paper.

1. Find a quiet, comfortable place to relax.
2. Identify the practical skills in your work that you have performed the best recently.
3. Take a deep breath, close your eyes, and allow yourself to imagine all the steps and aspects of that service for about five minutes.
4. Recall specific moments during the procedure, especially when something went well; re-create all the senses you experienced in detail.
5. Pay attention to your personal thoughts, feelings, physical sensations, and actions during the service.
6. Open your eyes and write down all the details you can remember. Study your results.

By identifying the underlying feelings and attitudes during a successful procedure, the learner can practice reproducing those same experiences in future applications. A continual process of visualization and analysis of positive performance will allow the learner to constantly improve the quality of skills.

✓ Stories and Anecdotes

Master educators periodically incorporate stories, brief anecdotes, or testimonials into their classroom presentations. They can be used to describe or explain a specific point or process, but will not always prove it. They do, however, get learners on the same page with the educator and help get their focus directed toward the objectives of the lesson. You will recall that an important characteristic for adult learners is relevance. Students enjoy hearing the human or personal side of a story. So, it is important for every educator to incorporate discussion of the subject matter with talk about your passions, your dreams, your setbacks, and your personal experiences. This a great tool for developing rapport and becoming *real* to your students. Bring the human element into every classroom if at all possible. Just remember to keep a balance between the body, the brain, and the emotions. Students learn best when their bodies are charged emotionally and their brains are engaged.

Mnemonics

Mnemonics are aids that can be used to assist the learner's memory. These aids can be word or phrase associations, songs, or any other method that will trigger in the memory key terms or information contained in a lesson. For example, songs may be used to help students remember the skeletal system, and phrases may be developed to teach various elements of chemistry. The educator can always call upon the learners to create the phrases or mnemonics that will be helpful in remembering and retaining important information. Certainly, if the learner has "authored" the mnemonic, it will have even greater impact.

mnemonics aids that can be used to assist the learner's memory.

Energizers

We will discuss in Chapter 7, "Effective Presentations," the fact that most classes or presentations experience a "spurt–sag–spurt" cycle. It is the job of the master educator to keep the "sag" portion of any class to an absolute minimum. It is a fact that all educators have to deal with heavy content or dry material from time to time. That cannot be avoided. However, when the heavy material creates a "sag" in the lesson, the educator can incorporate a brief energizer to bring new life into the classroom. A change of pace may be just the thing to get the minds of your learners back on track. An energizer is a brief activity that may take only one to three minutes. Energizers provide for both mental and physical breaks, but keep the learners focused for the remainder of the class. A few examples of energizers that could be used to change the pace are as follows:

- Where I'd rather be. You may ask the learners to put down their pencils, close their eyes, and take two minutes to visualize where they would rather be at that exact moment. After the two minutes, you ask the learners to take out colored markers and give them five minutes to draw the scene they depicted. It's a fun exercise and allows the learners to let their minds wander for a few minutes to something they enjoy. Have the students use masking tape to hang their drawings on the wall if they wish. This results in more humor later on when other students have the chance to view the drawings.
- Beach ball babble. Have one student blow up a beach ball and throw it to another learner in the classroom. That learner must then state one point that they have learned so far in the presentation. They then throw the ball to another learner who must do the same thing. The energizer continues until the educator wishes to get back to the topic

IT'S WORTH REMEMBERING ✳

Educational research indicates that educators who talk only about content, and not about people, are failing to deliver.

at hand or until all learners have participated. Learners are allowed to state the same point but are asked to phrase it differently if it has been stated previously. This activity is also a fun way to review at the end of the class.

- Brainstorming. Explain to students that you are going to have a brief brainstorming session regarding the challenges with today's topic. For example, it might be how to handle a difficult or dissatisfied client. The educator then brings a bucket or bowl of ice cubes into the classroom. As each student is called upon or volunteers to discuss the topic, he or she is asked to place his or her hand in the container of ice. When the learner can no longer hold the hand in the ice, he or she can no longer talk. This is a fun way to bring new energy into the classroom and also control those long-winded learners who never want to give up the floor.

☑ Characterizations and Cartoons

characterizations
Translating content into personage, such as cartoons or historical characters, to aid in learning.

By using **characterizations** in the classroom, the educator allows the learners to translate the content of the lesson into personage. Such translation might occur through historical characters or even cartoon characters. When teaching electricity, for example, the educator may reference the many unsuccessful attempts that Ben Franklin made in order to discover electricity in the first place. Cartoons can also be helpful in making important points. The cartoon in Figure 5–11 might be converted to an overhead transparency when teaching students the importance of repaying their student loans and building good credit for their future.

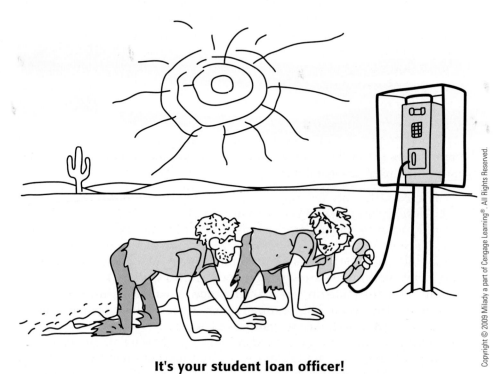

It's your student loan officer!

Figure 5–11   Cartoons can be helpful in making important points in a lesson.

Experiments

An experiment is an operation or procedure carried out under controlled conditions in order to discover an unknown effect or result or to illustrate a known effect or law. Experimentation is a great way to reach intuitive learners in the discovery stage of learning. Experimentation can be highly effective when teaching chemistry, for example. Following are two experiments that can be used when teaching chemistry.

- Have students perform the Alka-Seltzer test at home and report back the combustion results they experienced. Items needed are a small film canister, construction paper, scissors and tape, Alka-Seltzer tablets, and water. Instruct students to make a cone-shaped object that is just a little larger than the film canister at the open end. Have students experiment by placing one Alka-Seltzer tablet in the film canister and adding various levels and temperatures of water. Instruct the students to quickly place the lid on the film canister and then place the paper cone (or rocket) over the canister and wait. Have them record how long it takes for combustion to occur, the lid to pop off, and the "rocket" to go into orbit. Water levels and temperature of the water will affect the degree of combustion that occurs. Instruct the students to perform the experiment outdoors and report back to the class on the outcomes.
- Have students pour a small amount of oil into a transparent container or test tube followed by a small amount of water. Instruct them to place their thumb or other cover over the top and shake the container and write down their observations. Then have them add a small amount of liquid soap and again cover, shake, and write down their observations. Then lead a discussion about the fact that when the soap was added, a milky white emulsion was created. The chemical nature of soap allows it to keep the small drops or globs of oil suspended in the water. This is why soap has a cleaning action. Dirt clings to your skin and clothing because a film of grease holds it there. By experimentation, students learn that the purpose of soap is to break up the film so the dirt can be washed away.

Humor

Use of humor in the classroom can be highly effective. When learners are laughing, they feel good and their minds are open to new experiences and ideas. Using humor certainly does not mean constantly telling jokes. It does mean, however, that you can interject humor into your presentations to make a point. Humor should be timely and natural, not planned in advance (Figure 5–12). When humor is derived from real-life experience, it accomplishes three objectives: It shares a perspective on the topic that the learners have never heard before because it comes from a personal experience; it emphasizes a point; and it causes bonding with the learners because all humans can relate to both the successes and failures of others since they have experienced them as well. Master educators will ensure that the humor in the classroom is relevant and fits naturally and logically into the presentation. They remember that the purpose of humor is to emphasize an idea, not to replace it. They will base the humor on caring rather than criticism, and if there is to be a subject of the humor, it will be the educator, not one of the learners or

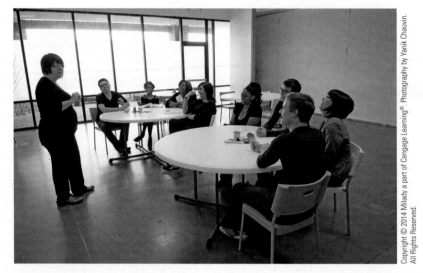

Figure 5–12   Humor in the classroom should be relevant and fit naturally into the presentation.

someone else. Master educators never use offensive language or "off-color" humor in the classroom, and they will never use humorous stories at the expense of any race, religion, sex, or political preference. Master educators know that if they are unsure whether the humor they are considering is appropriate, it is better left unused.

Games, Group Synergy, and Competitions

We've established that the primary role of a master educator is to facilitate, or make easier, student learning. Since statistics show that learners retain only 10 percent of what they read, 20 percent of what they hear, 30 percent of what they see, 50 percent of what they hear and see, 70 percent of what they say, and 90 percent of what they *hear*, *say*, and *do*, it becomes quite evident that involvement on the part of the learner is essential for maximum retention of the material. That brings us to the topic of group synergy. We discussed in Chapter 2, "The Teaching Plan and Learning Environment," the relevance of the classroom arrangement for effective group activities. Master educators will keep the appropriate classroom layouts in mind when planning group activities.

When establishing groups, master educators will limit them to no more than seven members—a higher number will minimize the possibility of all members participating. Group leaders will be established to direct the group through the activity or exercise. The leader will introduce the activity, direct participants through the required behavior, and then summarize the conclusions or discussions of the group. Master educators observe and monitor group activity but will not take over group discussions even when the group appears to be at a roadblock. The primary purpose of the group activity is to allow the learners to work through the material in such a manner that they learn it, retain it, and will be able to apply it in the laboratory or workplace (Figure 5–13). Your learners will gain tremendous self-confidence through the group exploration, struggling, and discovery process. When the insights achieved

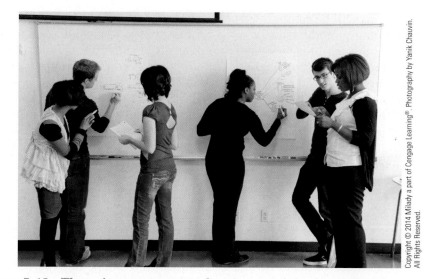

Figure 5–13   The primary purpose of a group activity is to allow learners to manage the material for learning, retention, and application.

come from the learner's own struggle, the new knowledge becomes his and he will retain it much longer than if those insights were simply provided by the educator.

In addition to increasing fun and energy, games and competitions allow learners to measure themselves not only against themselves but also against others in the classroom if they choose to do so. Master educators will incorporate a wide array of games and competitions into the training process. Following are some examples of games and competitions that educators might use:

- ***Pictionary*** activity. Have the class divide into two teams. Create 7–10 cards containing terminology (with corresponding page numbers and definitions) from bacteriology, such as cocci, bacilli, spirilla, diplococci, streptococci, staphylococci, flagella, cilia, contagious, immune, virus, parasite, spherical spores, and so on. Have the artist from the first team select a card and, by drawing on the chalkboard or a flip chart, depict the term on the card. The artist cannot use signs, words, or gestures while drawing. Allow two minutes for the artist's team to guess the correct term. Allow the opposing team an option to answer and score if the artist's team is unable to offer the correct answer within the two-minute time frame. After the term has been identified, offer extra points to the winning team if they can provide the correct definition. If they cannot, allow the opposing team the opportunity to provide the correct definition. (Set up a point scale prior to the activity.) Remind the students that a picture paints a thousand words. If they can remember or associate the picture with what the term means, it will be much easier to remember the name and definition.
- The "Bump" activity. Divide the class into groups of five students. Provide a sheet of flip-chart paper or a large piece of butcher paper to each group. Instruct each group that they have three minutes to write as many household antiseptics and disinfectants (or any topic as may be applicable) as possible. They can work individually within their group,

but items will be compared as a group. The objective is for the group to list as many products as possible that are not listed by another group. After three minutes, ask each group (one at a time) to read aloud all the products they have listed on their sheet. If another group has the same product listed, they will yell out, "Bump!" The group listing the product and all groups having that particular product must draw a line through it. When all groups have read their list, ask each group to count all products that do not have a line through them or have not been "bumped." The group with the most points wins. Small prizes such as tools or candy can be awarded to the winning team.

☑ Wrapping It Up

In this chapter, we have attempted to share not only an extensive list of teaching methods but also various techniques that can be incorporated into the classroom environment for the purpose of inspiring and reaching every learner. We have also provided a number of examples to set the ball in motion for aspiring master educators. A true master educator will never limit his imagination and will work to develop his own creativity so that he can bring more variety, enthusiasm, and energy into his classrooms. He will know that learning is lifelong and that, even as an educator, he must try new things, experience new attitudes, and employ ever-changing techniques if he is to be successful in his role as a master educator.

In Retrospect

1. Define teaching.

2. Explain what is meant by *teaching methods*.

3. Explain what is meant by *learning methods*.

4. Explain the purpose and use of lectures, demonstrations, group discussions, peer coaching, role-playing, and the discovery method of learning.

5. Discuss why window paning is an effective method of learning.

6. Explain the purpose and benefits of field trips and using guest speakers in the classroom.

7. Explain why mind mapping is an important learning method.

8. Explain the use and purpose of projects, workbooks, partially complete handouts, case studies, and concept connectors.

9. Explain the purpose and benefits of visualization in the educational process and how stories and anecdotes can increase learning retention.

10. Explain the use of mnemonics, energizers, characterizations, experiments, humor, games, and group synergy.

6 Communicating Confidently

Objectives (Desired Performance Goals):

After reading and studying this chapter, you should be able to:

- Define communication.
- Identify barriers to communication.
- Listen more effectively.
- Recognize your communication style.
- List key tips for communicating confidently.
- Explain strategies for in-school communication.

! CRITICAL CONCEPT

You may believe you understand what someone said, but what you heard may not be what was meant at all.

Effective Communication Skills

YOU MAY HAVE HEARD it said that knowledge is power. Frankly, *knowledge alone is not power*. You have spent perhaps years accumulating your knowledge, skills, and expertise in one discipline or another. Now you are pursuing the path of becoming an educator in that field with the intention of sharing your knowledge and skills with your learners. The fact is you will remain powerless as an educator if you never develop the skills required to communicate your knowledge effectively to your learners. What greater barrier to learning can there be than those created because learners cannot understand or communicate with the educator? The most successful educators are usually the best communicators.

What Is Communication?

Merriam Webster's Collegiate Dictionary notes that to communicate is to transmit information, thought, or feeling so that it is satisfactorily received or understood (Figure 6–1). The key here is that communication does not occur until the message is received and understood. The transfer of information can occur in a variety of ways, such as through the spoken or written word or nonverbally through body language, gestures, or facial expressions. Because the message must be understood for communication to occur, each information exchange must have a sender and a receiver.

☑ Sending and Receiving Information

When we speak or write something for someone else to read, we send information or ideas to another person or persons. If we listen to someone else speak or read something aloud, we receive information or ideas from them. When the information is written, the sender is the writer and the receiver is the reader. When the information is oral, the sender is the speaker and the receiver is the listener. We also know that we can communicate or send and receive information without the use of words through nonverbal communication. We do this by using gestures, eye contact, facial expressions, voice variation, mannerisms, posture, and body movements. Nonverbal communication can be added

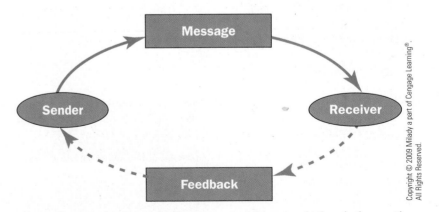

Figure 6–1   Communication is the process of transmitting information so that it is satisfactorily understood.

to spoken communication to change or enhance the meaning. For example, you might smile as you say, "It is a pleasure to finally meet you." By smiling as you make the statement, you are more convincing to the receiver that you are sincere. The same statement said with a frown and sarcasm might indicate you felt the person had been avoiding a personal meeting.

In order for the communication process to be complete, it must be determined if the information has been received and understood, and that requires feedback. Feedback is the receiver's way of acknowledging the message or information. To ensure that your message or information has been received, you must create an information package. The package includes the words spoken or written, the content of the message, and the gestures used (if any). The packaging and controlling of the message is called encoding. For example, you might give one of your students the following message: "Marilyn, please take the first aid kit to Ms. Hollis." How is that message packaged? Is it totally clear? It might be for an advanced student who knows exactly which first aid kit is being referred to and exactly where it is kept. However, for a new student, you might need to alter the message this way, "Marilyn, please take the small first aid kit, which is located on the left side of the top shelf of the classroom storage closet, to Ms. Hollis in her office when she has completed her next class." A master educator must learn to package or encode the information in a manner that is suitable for the learner's background. Failure to do so could cause a barrier to learning.

encoding packing information so that it is understood to achieve the desired results.

To complete the process, the receiver of the information must interpret or decode the message or information and respond or give feedback to the sender. In the previous example, Marilyn might respond with, "Yes, I know exactly which kit you are talking about. I will take it to Ms. Hollis at 9:30 when her class is over." This is an example of successful decoding because

decode to interpret the message or information.

THE COMMUNICATION CYCLE

EDUCATOR:	Packages theory, facts, skills, or information by encoding or translating the information into words, symbols, signs, or behavior that the learner can understand. This may be accomplished by an interactive lecture or practical demonstration.
LEARNER:	Opens the package by decoding the theory, facts, skills, or information by interpreting the words, symbols, signs, or behavior of the educator. This could be achieved through listening and interactive participation in the class.
LEARNER:	Packages a response by encoding or translating his understanding of the message into another message that is sent back to the educator. This could be accomplished by an "aha" statement of understanding or by passing a test or accurately completing an assignment.
EDUCATOR:	Decodes the response to determine whether the theory, facts, skills, or information were, in fact, understood appropriately by the learner. This might be done through observation or testing.

Marilyn responds in the exact manner that you expected. However, the first message, "Take the first aid kit to Ms. Hollis," might have resulted in the following response: "I'll be happy to, but are you referring to the small first aid kit or the large, metal box with first aid supplies? Is that kept in the classroom storage closet or primary stockroom? Do you want me to take it now or after class?" Clearly, the message was not packaged and controlled sufficiently to attain the desired reaction. For communication to be effective, the communication cycle must be completed.

Educators must learn to encode or package their information and lessons so that they are understood and so that the feedback from their learners is what is expected. Mastering the art of communication will greatly reduce any barriers to learning that might otherwise exist in your classrooms.

Barriers to Communication

There is a great line in the classic Paul Newman film, *Cool Hand Luke*, where the warden says, "What we have here is a failure to communicate." The truth of the matter is that people have communication problems all the time. Theologian Reuel Howe suggested that meaning barriers exist between all people, making communication much more difficult than most people realize . . . that it is totally false to assume that if one can talk, one can communicate. Author Robert Throop, in his book *9 Routes to Success for Students, published by Cengage*, says that miscommunication may occur due to a variety of barriers that can be classified as physical, mental, emotional, and cultural.

Physical Barriers. Any disturbing factor in the physical environment that prevents full communication is a physical barrier, such as room temperature, distracting activities and movement, personal discomfort, physical impediments, distracting side conversations (Figure 6–2), or noise.

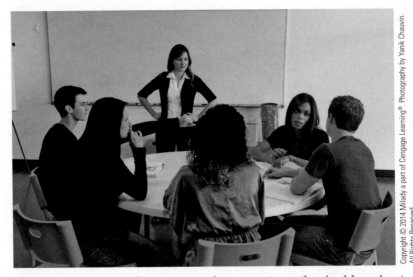

Figure 6–2   Distracting side conversations create a physical barrier to communication.

Mental Barriers. A barrier to communication could be caused by assumptions made based on previous knowledge or experience by one party in the communication process. The assumption may be that the information is going to be interesting or boring, for example. Additionally, communication may not occur due to selective listening (the listener only listens to that which is of personal interest and tunes out everything else). Finally, learning disabilities can create a barrier to learning, as some learning differences cause an inability to concentrate or focus on the content being discussed.

Emotional Barriers. Similar to mental barriers, emotional barriers such as stress and worry, fear, anger, love, and prejudices can restrict effective communication.

Cultural Barriers. Cultural traditions, manners, and habits may create distance in a speaker–listener relationship. Paying close attention to those we communicate with and keeping an open mind may help us to move beyond our own cultural comfort zone and help us communicate with others.

Getting the Message Across

Fortunately, we have more than mere words to deliver our message. Having a profound and eloquent vocabulary will be meaningless if we slur our words or have an offensive, hard-to-listen-to voice. According to research done by Albert Mehrabian, only 7 percent of the message we want to communicate is accomplished through the *words* we speak. Further, he determined that up to 38 percent of our message is communicated through *how* we say the words. It's our tone of voice—the pitch, rate, and tone—that increases the potential for successful communication to 45 percent. The other 55 percent is delivered visually by our appearance and posture, facial expressions, gestures, and eye contact (Figure 6–3).

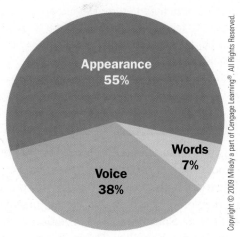

Figure 6–3   Why is our physical presentation so important in communication?

IT'S WORTH REMEMBERING ✳

Based on how communication is accomplished, it is no surprise how ineffective e-mail and text messaging can be, considering that we are trying to communicate without the benefit of as much as 93 percent of our communication tools!

The Spoken Word

A pleasant tone of voice can be one of your greatest assets. A number of factors affect voice quality, such as regional influence. Certain expressions are clearly tied to various regions of the country or world. For example, in the South and Southwest when a person is preparing to do something, he might say, "I'm fixin' to . . ." whereas elsewhere in the country people say, "I'm going to . . ." or "I'm getting ready to. . . ." Emotion also influences voice tone and quality. Our voices can convey whether we are tired, excited, bored, hurt, angry, frustrated, interested, or happy. Our intonation can give the receiver knowledge about the way the message needs to be interpreted. For example, our intonation, pitch, pace, and emphasis can add expression of anger, disappointment, or happiness with the exact same sentence. Finally, articulation, which is the clarity of our speech, will greatly impact the effectiveness of our communication. We must take care to enunciate clearly and pronounce all our words correctly. Tongue twisters can be very helpful in improving articulation skills.

V-O-I-C-E

V – Volume, variety (be heard)
O – Open mouth (be understood)
I – Intonation (be interesting)
C – Concise (use economy of language)
E – Enunciate (be clear)

TONGUE TWISTERS

- A tutor who tooted the flute tried to tutor two tooters to toot. Said the two to the tutor, "is it easier to toot or to tutor two tooters to toot?"
- Whenever the weather is cold, whenever the weather is hot, we'll weather the weather whether we like it or not.

Nonverbal Communication

We have established that as much as 80 percent to 90 percent of the communication process is nonverbal, and nonverbal messages can be more revealing than verbal communication. A great communicator will pay close attention to the nonverbal cues being delivered by others in a variety of ways, as discussed next.

Facial Expressions. Some facial expressions are universal. For example, a smile is a smile whether it's in Paris, Texas, or Paris, France. By the same token, a frown is a frown whether conveyed in London or Los Angeles. The intensity and frequency of facial expressions vary, however, from culture to culture. In Sweden, facial expressions can be more subtle and veiled, while in Italy, they might be highly demonstrative. As previously stated, we can usually determine another person's mood or feelings, such as sadness, anger, hostility, excitement, and happiness, from facial expressions.

Eye Contact. In the United States, we have generally been taught that if someone could not look you in the eye, they were likely lying to you. However, in some cultures, looking downward while speaking to someone is considered respectful. Because that is not the case in this country, we need to practice making effective eye contact with students, supervisors, peers, and clients. Eye contact can also be used to indicate a person's choice. For example, when you are presenting in the classroom and are about to start a review, the student who does not want to be called upon will make sure to avoid eye contract. On the other hand, however, when you enter a place of business and want service, you immediately attempt to make eye contact. When teaching students how to perform a successful client consultation, note the importance of conducting the consultation face to face rather than making eye contact through the styling mirror.

Body Language. Body language can be extremely instrumental when trying to make a positive impression on others. If we are too tense, that may come across in our message. Conversely, we can overdo our gesturing and turn off listeners. As educators, we must make sure our gestures are open and compatible with our message (Figure 6–4). We must use our body movements in a manner that is also consistent with the purpose of the material we are presenting to our students. Gestures can be used to direct the learners' attention to the topic at hand, to add emphasis to the message, and to vary the stimuli for the learners in our classrooms. In addition, gestures can be used to clarify information. For example, a gesture can indicate the size or shape of something and so forth. As with words, gestures can mean different things in different locations or countries.

THE OK GESTURE

This gesture in the United States and the United Kingdom means "OK."
This gesture in Brazil means a vulgar insult.
This gesture in Japan refers to money.
This gesture in France means "worthless."

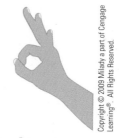

A simple gesture can mean widely different things depending on the country and culture.

When considering our body language, we also need to consider our body positioning and what are known as *comfort zones*. The *social distance zone* between two individuals when measured nose to nose is between 24 and 30 inches. This is the distance at which the average person feels comfortable communicating in a social situation. The *intimate distance zone* is from 10 to 14 inches. In this zone, the communicator invites the other party into close proximity, where space is shared and both parties feel a part of the communicating process. We enter the intimate zone

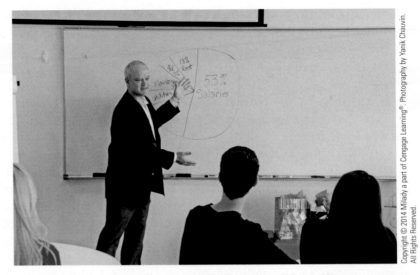

Figure 6–4   Gestures should be open and compatible with our message.

when we touch another person, which creates a new level of communication between the parties.

open closed body posture body language open and listener is accepting of the message being conveyed by the speaker.

There are two groups of body language postures: open/closed and forward/back. When a person is expressing open body language, his hands and arms are open and his legs are uncrossed. He is fully facing the speaker and has both feet planted on the ground with no barriers placed between him and the speaker. The person with open body posture is generally accepting of the messages being conveyed. However, if a person's body language is closed, his arms are likely folded or crossed and he may even turn away from the speaker, signaling that he is rejecting the message being delivered.

forward/back body posture indicates that the listener is actively accepting the message.

The forward/back mode of body language refers to whether people are actively or passively reacting or responding to the message. When a listener leans forward and faces the speaker, he is actively accepting the message. When he is leaning forward and pointing at the speaker, he may be actively rejecting the message. When a listener is leaning back, looking up at the ceiling perhaps, or doodling on a pad, cleaning his glasses, or twiddling his thumbs, he is either passively absorbing or passively ignoring the message. These various posture groups combine to create four basic modes of body language, which are known as responsive, reflective, combative, or fugitive, and are described as follows (Figure 6–5):

responsive the open/forward mode indicates the listener is actively accepting the message.

- **Responsive.** The open/forward mode indicates that the listener is actively accepting the message. This would be the appropriate time to ask for agreement or request a concession. If you were in sales, this would be the time to go for the close (Figure 6–6).

reflective the open/back mode indicates the listener is interested and receptive, but not actively accepting the information.

- **Reflective.** When a person is in the open/back mode, they are interested and receptive, but not actively accepting the information. You would not want to try to close a sale if the client were in this mode—it might drive the client away and into the "fugitive mode" (described next). Instead, this is the time to present further facts and incentives. Or you may want to keep quiet and let the listener think about the presented information.

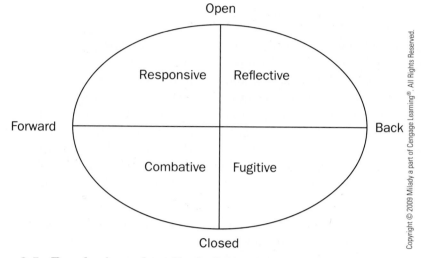

Figure 6–5   **Four basic modes of body language.**

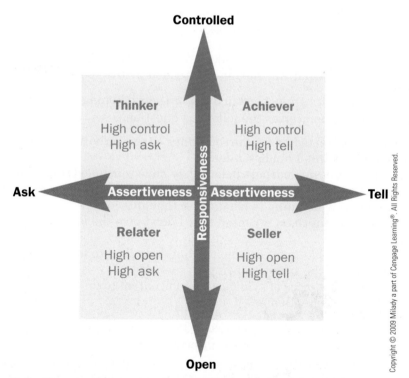
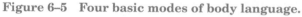

Figure 6–6   **Responsiveness and assertiveness affect communication style.**

IT'S WORTH REMEMBERING ✳

Our most valuable discoveries are accomplished through effective listening.

- **Fugitive.** The closed/back mode suggests that the listener is trying to escape, either physically through the door or mentally from boredom. If this body language is identified, make every effort to spark interest in any way you can. You may have to use tactics or comments that are not even relevant to the initial message.
- **Combative.** In this closed/forward mode, the listener is likely to present active resistance. The speaker will need to defuse the listener's anger and make every attempt to avoid contradiction and outright argument. The goal in this mode is to steer the listener into the reflective mode.

fugitive the closed/back mode suggests the listener is trying to escape, either physically or mentally.

combative in this closed/forward mode, the listener presents resistance.

Effective Listening

Educators often tend to be better speakers than they are listeners. This creates a problem for two reasons. First, we have established that communication requires both speaking and listening. Second, we spend much more time listening than we do speaking. Therefore, we must learn to listen and listen well. You will have the opportunity to create more successful graduates if you learn about them—their situations, their preferences, and their needs. This information will allow you to serve them better. **Active listening** is an effective way to communicate and can be useful when dealing with conflict situations as well as with student counseling situations. As an active listener, you will:

active listening active listening means being with the speaker, concentrating on what is being said; not interrupting; repeating what the speaker has said and paraphrasing it to make certain you have understood; establishing that what you repeated was what was meant.

- Be with the speaker. You will concentrate on what is being said and not let your attention be diverted.
- Wait until the speaker finishes before speaking. You will not interrupt or interject. You will wait until the speaker has concluded his remarks before responding.
- Repeat what the speaker has said. You will reflect upon what has been said and restate it or paraphrase it to make certain you have correctly understood the meaning.
- Gain agreement from the speaker. You will establish that what you repeated was what was meant or intended by the speaker.

Master educators may need to monitor their listening skills on a regular basis by asking themselves the following questions:

- Do I get distracted by my surroundings or the activities going on around me while I am listening?
- Do I interrupt my learners before they have concluded their remarks?
- Do I leap ahead of the learner, anticipating his next thoughts rather than actually listening to what those thoughts are?
- Do I have so much on my mind that I don't give the learner my full attention?
- Do I reject or block out comments that don't fit into my conception or perception of the situation being discussed?
- Do I allow one piece of evidence or information to unduly influence my opinions or perceptions?

The art of listening is not easy. It requires an open mind and an appreciation of the contributions your peers and your learners have to make. Master educators will be receptive to learners' ideas and attentive to their needs and feelings. By listening attentively and appreciating the opinions of others, you will gain the trust and respect that is essential for effective communications.

✓ Communication Styles

We each possess a particular communication style, and we can become better communicators if we learn to recognize the styles of other people. Researchers David Merrill and Roger Reid discovered that people essentially show two major forms of behavior when they communicate: responsiveness and assertiveness. **Responsiveness** is the degree to which a person is open

responsiveness the degree to which a person is open in interactions with others.

in interactions with others. Someone with a low degree of responsiveness may be guarded or even quite closed to interactions with others. On the other hand, someone with a high degree of responsiveness will readily show emotion and will almost always be perceived by others as being friendly. **Assertiveness** is the degree of boldness or confidence one has in dealing with others. Assertive behavior can range from merely asking questions (low assertiveness) to more forcefully telling others what is expected of them (high assertiveness). These two modes of communication styles can be represented in a diagram, as shown in Figure 6–6. By placing the two behaviors of responsiveness and assertiveness at right angles to each other, we create a model with four boxes. A person's degree of responsiveness and assertiveness will place him in one of the boxes, each of which correlates to a communication style: Thinker, Achiever, Seller, and Relater.

- **The Thinker.** People who tend to be guarded in their interactions with others are thinkers. They are not outgoing. Self-control is very important to them and they generally are very reserved when it comes to revealing personal information. Instead, they choose to deflect attention from themselves by asking questions of those with whom they are communicating.
- **The Achiever.** Like Thinkers, Achievers score high in the self-control department and resist the impulse to reveal much about their inner selves. Unlike Thinkers, however, Achievers are very assertive people. They do not hesitate to express their expectations clearly.
- **The Seller.** The Seller is a "people" person. Touchy, feely, warm, and outgoing with others, the Seller is also assertive and given to forthright expression, often telling you about his accomplishments and ambitions.
- **The Relater.** Relaters are usually warm and friendly in their interactions with others. They are less concerned about themselves than they are about their receivers. Relaters ask questions that are sometimes quite personal in nature.

Identifying Your Communication Style

None of us communicates in only one communication mode. For example, when we communicate with a close friend or spouse, we may be very open and personal, in the same manner as a Relater. However, when we communicate with our boss, we might tend to be self-controlled and unassertive, like the Thinker. However, Merrill and Reid note that we tend to favor one style over another in most of our interactions and communications with others. Find out your dominant style by checking off each of the communication characteristics that apply to you in the accompanying questionnaire. The box with the most checkmarks represents your preferred style.

You can use your knowledge of communication styles to improve the quality of your communication. By identifying your own style and the style of the person with whom you are communicating, you can identify potential communication problems. Once you understand the problems, you can take action to improve your rapport, and, consequently, your communication, with the other person. If you determined you were a Type One communicator, you are a Thinker. If the most checks were in Type Two, you are an Achiever. If you had the most checks in Type Three, you are a Relater and, finally, if you chose more qualities of the Type Four, you are a Seller.

assertiveness the degree of boldness or confidence one has in dealing with others.

thinker thinker communicators are guarded in interactions with other thinkers; they are not outgoing; self-control is important to them.

achiever achiever communicators score high in self-control and resist impulses to reveal much about their inner selves; they are very sensitive and express their expectations clearly.

seller seller communicators are a "people" persons; they are touchy, feely, warm, and outgoing with others and assertive.

relater relater communicators are warm and friendly and less concerned about themselves than others; they can ask questions of a personal nature.

COMMUNICATIONS STYLES QUESTIONNAIRE

Type One

_____ Quiet, level tone of voice
_____ Leans back or away
_____ Limited eye contact
_____ Stiff posture
_____ Uses big words

Type Two

_____ Factual speech
_____ Leans forward and faces others
_____ Limited facial expressions
_____ Limited body movements
_____ Fast-paced speech

Type Three

_____ Little emphasis on detail
_____ Touches others
_____ Smiles, nods
_____ Casual posture
_____ Talks about relationships

Type Four

_____ Dramatic or loud tone of voice
_____ Animated facial expressions
_____ Direct eye contact
_____ Lots of body and hand motions
_____ Uses voice to emphasize points

✓ Establishing Trust and Rapport

Merriam Webster's Collegiate Dictionary defines *trust* as: (1) assured reliance on the character, ability, strength, or truth of someone or something; (2) one in which confidence is placed. Certainly, this is the type of relationship educators will want to have with their students. Additionally, we will want to help our students establish trusting relationships with their colleagues and clients. Once trust has been established, the next step is building rapport. People build rapport by being more alike in their communication styles through a technique called *mirroring* (Figure 6–7). We all mirror others to a certain degree without even being aware of it. If you pay attention to two people who are deep in conversation, you are likely to notice that their postures are similar or that they are both speaking in a similar manner, either softly or vibrantly, depending on the nature of the conversation. We can take this unconscious process further by paying attention to another person's behavior and mirroring it. We want to take care not to imitate another person's behavior to the extent that it is noticeable. Mirroring should be accomplished through subtle, small adjustments to closely match the communication style of your companion. This behavior will create harmony and make the other person more comfortable.

Mirroring can be achieved with both body movements and words. If you are talking with someone who is relaxed and laid back, you may want to relax your posture to more closely match that position. If they smile and nod, you can respond in kind. If they lean forward, you might do the same in a casual way. Another way to mirror a person's communication style is to match their use of words. People tend to use words that reflect how they perceive the world. You can often tell which one of the senses is preferred by another individual by his use of words. You can determine if someone is more visual than auditory by their choice of words. For example, if they say, "I can see that," rather than, "I hear what you are saying," they are likely more visual than auditory. You might then want to use visual words when communicating with this person. We also should remember the importance of

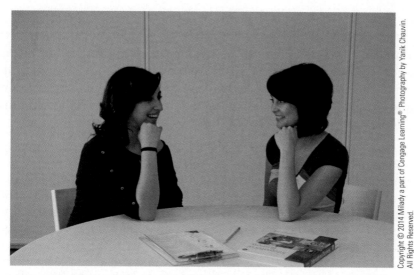

Figure 6–7 Mirroring body language establishes rapport.

restating and confirming in the communication process. This is exactly what we teach our students to do in the consultation process. When communicating with others, make sure you have a complete understanding of what they are saying by paraphrasing what they have said and repeating it back to them. This simple process will help eliminate many major failures to communicate.

Steps for Increasing Personal Awareness

Some steps the master educator should consider for increasing personal awareness of learners, their cultures, and their backgrounds follow.

Maintain Clear and Open Communication. Communication is the key to opening doors and resolving cultural and social barriers.

Speak Clearly and Concisely. When teaching students whose first language is not your own, it is important to avoid slang—it may not be understood.

Observe the Nonverbal Language of Other Cultures. Behaviors and mannerisms vary from culture to culture. Be especially cautious in your interpretation of a learner's nonverbal messages. Politely inquire about other cultures so you can ensure more accurate interpretation of behavior.

Consider Causes of Conflict. When misunderstandings arise, consider the possibility that they may be based on cultural perspectives or differences.

Accept Different Cultures. Understand that different cultures have different perspectives, values, and traditions. For example, discussing your personal accomplishments or knowledge might be considered a sign of confidence in one country while being considered pompous, egotistical, and condescending in another.

Explain Your Own Philosophy or Culture. Learners from other cultures may think that respecting those in authority, such as their educator, means not asking questions or disagreeing. You will want to ensure that your learners are encouraged to ask questions to obtain the maximum benefit from their training.

By following these simple guidelines, you will attain awareness of the diversified cultures represented at your institutions. Once that awareness has been achieved, you will be better equipped to prepare for your daily presentations.

Tips to Communicating Confidently

An important step in communicating more confidently is building our own self-confidence. Once we have achieved a higher level of self-confidence, we can apply that confidence to all of our endeavors, including communication skills. The following strategies are beneficial in building confidence:

- **Make Yourself Feel Good.** Feeling good has been tied to hormonal elements and the body's rate of endorphin production. If you can remember a time when you had a great self-confidence, think about that. An alternative is to think about a time when you were extremely happy and satisfied. This process of taking deliberate control of your thought content has an impact on your self-confidence, as well as other areas of your life.
- **Overcome Self-Consciousness.** When you feel self-conscious, you begin to feel anxious. The best thing to do is to take the focus off yourself. Concentrate on your purpose, whatever it might be at the time. If occupied with a task, you can't feel too self-conscious.
- **Minimize Self-Criticism.** Studies have shown that negative behaviors are habit-forming. If that seems unreasonable, think about what you say to yourself when you trip and fall or break something. You probably call yourself a name that describes you as stupid, such as "klutz" or "moron." How does that make you feel? Creating a positive self-talk statement is a much better strategy.
- **Perfect Your Speech.** Learn to speak properly and it will give you great confidence. Take control when feeling angry or frustrated and keep your speech calm. This will cause people to respect you even more and your self-confidence will soar.
- **Curb Anger and Cool Down Emotionally.** When things cause you to feel anger, wait a few days to cool down. Let the rage pass with time. As the time passes, you will be able to be more objective about the issues and the truth of the matter (Figure 6–8).
- **Develop and Deliver Powerful Anecdotes.** Build a repertoire of powerful anecdotes that have an impact on others. Practice their

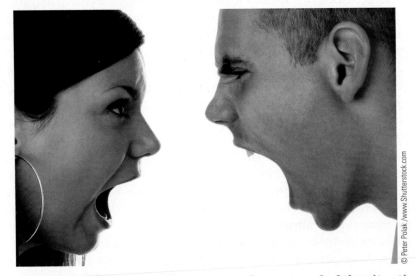

Figure 6–8   When you react with anger, you lose control of the situation.

delivery so they can be used for emphasis. Reuse them whenever necessary. People will feel entertained and supported by your effort to become a good storyteller.

- **Don't Ask, "How Are You?"** Everyone does that. Why not come up with your own "how are you" that will spur an honest answer and create a genuine connection with the other person? Instead, for example, you might ask, "How is your day going?" or "Are you having a great day?"
- **Develop a Unique Response.** When everyone else asks you how you are, instead of saying, "Fine," create your own special response. Perhaps you will say what Steve Martin of Austin, Texas, says: "It's a great day to be alive."
- **Ask Provocative and Pleasing Questions.** This strategy will draw people out. Your sincerity will convince people to open up and share. It may take several questions to get them to open up.
- **Talk Less, Listen More.** You can become the most popular person at the party by asking open-ended questions and then closing your mouth. People really appreciate those who listen to them.
- **Use Brief Responses.** When a speaker is sharing something that is important to him, don't make him feel derailed by a long response. Let him be the center of attention.
- **Is It Feeling or Fact?** Make an attempt to determine whether the speaker is expressing facts or feelings. Take care to respond with sensitivity when the speaker is coming from the more sensitive domain of emotion.
- **Give Positive Reinforcement.** When communicating with others, interject phrases such as, "I agree" or "You're right." This tactic can be especially useful during a disagreement.
- **Do Not Gossip.** Gossiping breaks down trust, and trust is the most important ingredient in successful relationships—whether it is a relationship between an educator and student or a coworker—and in successful business.
- **Share Hugs.** As an educator, you will need to exercise caution with regard to hugging students, but be aware that doctors are even prescribing hugs to help people get over illness. A hug is a powerful tool, and when you make someone else feel better, you feel more confident, and that will be reflected in your communication.

In-School Communication

Behaving in a professional manner is the first step in making meaningful communication possible. The school community is usually a close-knit one in which people spend long hours working side by side. For this reason, it is important to maintain boundaries regarding what you will and will not do or say at the school. Remember, the school is your place of business and, as such, must be treated respectfully and carefully.

Communicating with Coworkers

As with all communication, basic principles should guide your interactions with coworkers. In a work environment, you will not have the opportunity to handpick your colleagues. There will always be people you like or relate to better than others and people whose behaviors or opinions you find yourself in conflict with. These people can try your patience and your nerves, but they are your colleagues and are deserving of your respect. Here are some guidelines to keep in mind as you interact and communicate with fellow staffers:

- **Treat Everyone with Respect.** Regardless of whether or not you like someone, your colleagues are professionals who contribute to the bottom line of the school. As professionals, they have information they can offer you. Look at these people as having something to teach you, and hone in on their talents, knowledge, and techniques.

- **Remain Objective.** Different types of personalities working side by side over long and intense hours are likely to breed some degree of dissension and disagreement. In order to learn and grow, you must make every effort to remain objective and resist being pulled into spats and cliques. When one or two people in the school behave disrespectfully toward one another, the entire team suffers because the atmosphere changes. Not only will this be unpleasant for you but also the tension will be felt by the students and clients, who may decide to take their business elsewhere if they find the atmosphere in your school too tense.

- **Be Honest and Sensitive.** Many people use the excuse of being honest as license to say anything to anyone. While honesty is always the best policy, using unkind words or actions with regard to your colleagues is never a good idea. Be sensitive. Put yourself in the other person's place and think through what you want to say before you say it. That way, you will not use any negative or hurtful words.

- **Remain Neutral.** Undoubtedly, there will come a time when you are called on to make a statement or to "pick a side." Do whatever you can to avoid being drawn into the conflict. If you have a problem with your colleagues, the best way to resolve it is to speak with them directly and privately.

- **Avoid Gossip.** Gossiping never resolves a problem; it only makes it worse. Participating in gossip can be just as damaging to you as it is to the object of your gossip.

- **Seek Help from Someone You Respect.** If you find yourself in a position where you are at odds with a coworker, you may want to seek out a third party—someone who is not involved and who can remain objective—such as the manager or a more experienced educator. Ask for advice about how to proceed and really listen to what they have to tell you. Since they are not involved, they are more likely to see the situation as it truly is and can offer you valuable insights.

- **Do Not Take Things Personally.** This is often easier said than done. How many times have you had a bad day, or been thinking about something totally unrelated, when a person asks you what's wrong or wonders if you are mad at them? Just because someone is behaving in a certain manner and you happen to be there, do not interpret the words or behaviors as being meant for you. If you are confused or concerned by someone's actions, find a quiet and private place to ask the person about it. The person may not even realize he was giving off any signals.

- **Keep Your Private Life Private.** There is a time and a place for everything, but the school is never the place to discuss your personal life and relationships. It may be tempting to engage in that kind of conversation, especially if others in the school are doing so, but that is what friends are for.

Communicating with Managers

Another important relationship for you within the school is the one you will build with your manager. The school manager is generally the person who has the most responsibility for how well the school is run, in terms of daily maintenance and operations and student and customer service. The manager's job is a very demanding one.

Your manager is probably the one who hired you and is responsible for your training and for how well you move into the school culture. Therefore, your manager has a vested interest in your success. As a school employee, you may see the manager as a powerful and influential person, but it is also important to remember that the manager is a human being. He is not perfect, and he will not be able to do everything you think should be done in every instance. Whether he personally likes you or not, his job is to look beyond his personal feelings and make decisions that are best for the school as a whole. The approach you should take is to try to understand the decisions and rules that the manager makes, whether you agree with them or not.

Many school professionals have inappropriate expectations of their school managers, such as requesting that they solve personal issues between staff members. Inexperienced managers, hoping to keep everything flowing smoothly, may make the mistake of getting involved in petty issues. You and your manager must both understand that the manager's job is to make sure the business is running smoothly, not to babysit temperamental employees. Following are some guidelines for interacting and communicating with your school manager:

- **Be a Problem-Solver.** When you need to speak with your manager about some issue or problem, plan some possible solutions beforehand. This will indicate that you are working in the school's best interest and are trying to help, not make things worse.
- **Get Your Facts Straight.** Make sure that all your facts and information are accurate before you speak to your school manager. This way, you will avoid wasting time solving a "problem" that really does not exist.
- **Be Open and Honest.** When you find yourself in a situation you do not understand or do not have the experience to deal with, tell your school manager immediately and be willing to learn.
- **Do Not Gossip or Complain About Colleagues.** Going to your manager with gossip or to "tattle" on a coworker tells your manager that you are a troublemaker. If you are having a legitimate problem with someone and have tried everything in your power to handle the problem yourself, then it is appropriate to go to your manager. But you must approach your manager with a true desire to solve the problem, not just to vent.
- **Check Your Attitude.** The school environment, although fun and friendly, can also be stressful, so it is important to take a moment periodically to "take your temperature." Ask yourself how you are feeling. Do you need an attitude adjustment? Be honest with yourself.
- **Be Open to Constructive Criticism.** It is never easy to hear that you need improvement in any area, but keep in mind that part of your manager's job is to help you achieve your professional goals. The manager is supposed to evaluate your skills and offer suggestions on how to increase them. Keep an open mind and do not take criticism personally.

☑ Wrapping It Up

The goal of effective communication is mutual understanding. We can communicate more confidently when we keep that goal in mind. When we take care to speak less and listen more, we let others know we care about what they have to say. Achieving mutual understanding is easier said than done, and most of us were not taught in school how to communicate. With a little effort, however, we can become great communicators, and we can make others feel special in the process. We need to remember that the greatest communication skill of all is giving value to others. We should practice communicating our enthusiasm, self-esteem, self-confidence, energy, and appreciation of others. If people are made to feel important, they will reciprocate in kind with openness, cooperation, and mutual respect. Communication will happen!

In Retrospect

1. Define communication.

2. Identify barriers to communication.

3. Describe how to listen more effectively.

4. Explain communication styles.

5. List key tips for communicating confidently.

6. Explain strategies for in-school communication.

Effective Presentations

Objectives (Desired Performance Goals):

After reading and studying this chapter, you should be able to:

- Explain what is meant by the acronym C-R-E-A-T-E with respect to education in the classroom.

- Identify the various components of powerful presentations.

- Explain the 10 methods used for inspiring learner motivation.

- List 10 elements important to powerful openings.

- Explain the purpose of closing all presentations with impact.

- List five methods used to strengthen the body or major content of a lesson.

- List six effective methods used to facilitate transitions.

- State five methods for varying the stimuli within a lesson.

- Explain the difference between lower-order and high-order questions.

- Explain why reinforcement during a lesson is important.

! CRITICAL CONCEPT

Preparing an effective presentation allows you to navigate around the mental roadblocks that may exist in your students.

Communication Skills

STUDENTS JUDGE EDUCATORS by what they hear from them. You may be the most efficient, intelligent, and accomplished educator within your institution, but neither your efficiency nor intellect will serve you well if you cannot communicate your knowledge and accomplishments to your learners. Your success as a master educator depends on your ability to influence the students in your classrooms. You will need to speak or present material in a manner that ensures your learners understand the message. As we established in Chapter 6, "Communicating Confidently," , master educators will take many steps to become more aware of their learners—their cultures, and their backgrounds—in order to improve and enhance the learning process (Figure 7–1). In this chapter, we will focus primarily on listening and speaking skills as well as the use of nonverbal communication skills.

C-R-E-A-T-E

With respect to education in the classroom or speaking in public, the six Ps refer to *Proper Preparation and Practice Prevent Poor Performance*. A more positive approach for the six Ps is *Proper Preparation and Practice Promote Positive Performance*. Either way, proper planning will make all the difference in your classroom presentations. The master educator will take every step necessary to present an effective, stimulating, and memorable class that includes a powerful opening, an impressive body, and a dynamic closing. Many educators have learned to follow a reliable formula called C-R-E-A-T-E. Each letter represents one building block in the foundation of a good lesson, as described next.

C—Consider the Topic

Limit your class to a specific area within the subject matter being taught. Certainly, it will be critical for you to have knowledge of how much your students already know about your chosen topic. You will also need to

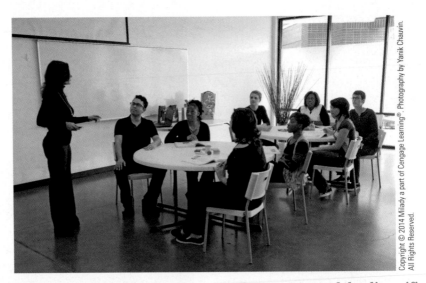

Figure 7–1   Educators should strive to attain awareness of the diversified cultures represented in the classroom.

determine how much time has been set aside for your presentation. The master educator will ask questions that might have a bearing on the content of the lesson or the physical environment in which the lesson will be presented. Once those questions have been answered, the first block in the construction of a good lesson will have been laid.

R—Research the Topic

The master educator will become a subject-matter expert in every category within a program or course of study for which she is responsible. It will certainly never be the intention to mislead or misinform students. Therefore, trusting to memory the technical information to be conveyed could be disastrous. Thus, a well-prepared lesson plan is crucial. Other considerations in planning the material include questions about what the students want and need to know as well as what type of humor can be added to make learning more fun. What types of activities will interest students, and what will antagonize or bore them? When you have answered these questions, your research can begin. As an educator, you will already have general knowledge about any topic you are scheduled to teach. A master educator, however, will conduct further research and study additional reference materials available to bring more than just the basics into the classroom.

E—Examples for Clarification

Throughout any presentation, a master educator provides examples that bring clarity and meaning to the points delivered. Remember to keep examples appropriate. They must make the needed point and be related to the topic at hand. Examples should be understood by every learner. Being aware of cultural differences will help ensure that examples, anecdotes, and analogies are understood by all.

A—Analyze Your Learners

While setting up and preparing for the class presentation, spend some time analyzing the students. Watch them, listen to them, and pay attention to their reactions and their body language. Are they noisy and restless, are they distracted and preoccupied, or are they quiet and respectful? This analysis can be valuable in helping you determine what approach to take with this particular class presentation. The more you have prepared your presentation, the more flexibility you may employ to adapt to different learner moods or classroom environments. After you begin the presentation, you will begin to *feel* the students and begin to bond with them. Take your cues from them and adjust your presentation accordingly.

T—Teach with Poise

Once you have researched the content of your class and prepared the detailed lesson plan, it is time to prepare for the actual presentation. An educator must effectively address classes each day, so fine-tuning of speaking and presenting skills will come much faster than for those who do so only occasionally. However, whether it will be your first class or your thousandth class, you should prepare physically for the presentation. Consider practicing in front of a mirror where you can observe your gestures, your eye contact, how you use your notes, and your posture. Do you project confidence and exhibit authority? Also consider recording your presentation so you can hear what your students will hear. Consider your rate, pitch, and tone of speech. Do you pronounce words clearly and correctly? As you become a more seasoned educator and have taught certain classes numerous times, preparation to this extent will not be necessary. Just remember that you must convey poise and confidence in the classroom if you are to have credibility with your learners.

E—Enjoy and Be Enthusiastic

If you have thoroughly prepared prior to your presentation, which is necessary to promote positive performance, you will have nothing to worry about. You can approach the classroom with confidence and ease. If you relax and begin to enjoy yourself in the classroom, so will your learners. If you are tense and nervous, they will likely mirror your feelings. Learn to enjoy presenting and you will become a great presenter. Be at ease, enjoy your students, and you will be in demand as a master educator and receive rave reviews from your students. A master educator will believe in what is being taught and be enthusiastic about it! Enthusiasm is contagious and can build a lasting, positive impression in the minds of your learners.

C-R-E-A-T-E: THE BUILDING BLOCKS OF A GOOD LESSON

C: Consider the Topic

R: Research the Topic

E: Examples for Clarification

A: Analyze your Learners

T: Teach with Poise

E: Enjoy the Experience

✓ What Makes a Powerful Presentation?

Any class you present that enables your learners to expand their skills, reinforce their ideals, change their attitudes, and gain new knowledge will be a powerful presentation. None of that will occur, however, if the learners aren't listening. If you are broadcasting or sending your message to any station other than WII-FM (What's In It For Me?) or MMFI-AM (Make Me Feel Important About Myself), it is unlikely that it will be heard or received. You might compare it to tossing a golf ball at a dart board. You may have the best aim and hit the bull's eye on every try, but the ball doesn't stick, does it? (Figure 7–2). Likewise, you may have the ability to speak well, but is what you are saying "sticking"? Is it being heard? You must first decide what you want to hit before you decide what you're going to throw at your learners.

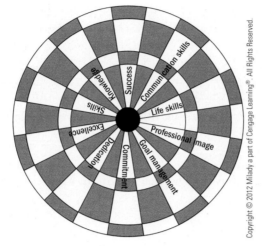

Figure 7–2 **Make sure the message you are conveying addresses station WII-FM and is hitting the target for the student.**

Powerful Motivation

When planning to develop an effective opening, it might be helpful to consider the 10 basic desires or needs that your adult learners have as human beings. Every individual has both psychological and physical needs and will do whatever is necessary to achieve them.

THE TOP 10 BASIC DESIRES OF ADULTS

1. **Personal Power.** Everyone needs to feel a certain degree of control or mastery over themselves and even others.

2. **Pride and Importance.** People need to enjoy ego gratification and a feeling of importance.

3. **Financial Security.** Humans want to know that their personal needs and wants will be met.

4. **Approval and Recognition.** Everyone needs to experience social or group approval and acceptance by one's peers; we want recognition when we put forth effort; we need to be reassured of our value and worth.

5. **Sense of Belonging.** We all need to feel we belong to a place or a group or a family; we need a sense of roots.

6. **Desire to Win.** Humans all have a competitive nature and want to be first or to be the best.

7. **Feeling of Accomplishment and Need for Creative Expression.** We all need to have the opportunity to express our creativity and feel we have contributed something worthwhile.

(Continued)

THE TOP 10 WAYS TO FACILITATE MOTIVATION (*Continued*)

8. **New Experiences.** Everyone has a sense of adventure, however small; we need to experience new things and feelings.

9. **Freedom.** Humans seek liberty and desire a certain degree of privacy without intrusion.

10. **Self-Esteem, Love, and Emotional Security.** We all need to respect ourselves, experience love in all forms, and be emotionally secure.

It is helpful for the educator to consider these basic human needs when developing classroom presentations. In career education, it is easy to appeal to your learners' need for financial success, need for new experiences, need for creative expression, and need for feelings of accomplishment. Throughout the educational process, you also will have the opportunity to appeal to their needs for ego gratification, recognition of efforts, acceptance, and self-esteem as well.

Creating Motivational Circumstances

We have noted that motivation is internal, but educators can create circumstances or situations within which students can become motivated. There are a number of ways an educator can accomplish this, as discussed next.

THE TOP 10 WAYS TO FACILITATE MOTIVATION

1. **Establish Strong Personal Contact.** Arrive for class early and make yourself available to learners during breaks and after class for personal discussion. Learn to relate to your students.

2. **Get Learners in an Active Mood.** For example: encourage questions; be aware of room environment and comfort; vary the stimuli during the presentation; use partial handouts that learners complete during the class for presented information to be useful.

3. **Humanize the Content.** Support your content with personal examples and illustrations to strengthen the objectives of the lesson. Show learners how the information will work for them. Sharing stories about your passions and experiences builds rapport with learners and balances the cognitive and emotional elements of the learning process.

4. **Give Praise, Recognition, and Approval.** Take care to avoid criticism of any type in a public situation or in front of peers. Praise, however, tastes even sweeter when others hear it.

5. **Encourage Questions and Feedback.** Never make a learner feel embarrassed for asking a question. Encourage questions and learn how to address incorrect responses from students in a manner that does not humiliate or embarrass them.

6. **Encourage Personal Competition.** Learners improve greatly when they learn to compare where they are at a given point in time with where they would like to be. *They* determine how they can improve their personal performance.

7. **Display Enthusiasm and Excitement.** Your learners can hardly be expected to get excited about a topic or lesson if the educator is not. By being available before and after class, you convey your interest to students. Concentrate on eye contact with students during the presentation; this tells the learners you are "with" them.

8. **Identify Long-Term Benefits and Stress the Value of Internal Motives.** Help your learners understand how they will benefit in the future as they master the information or skills you are presenting. Encourage them to seek out their own personal desires or objectives, which may be even more motivational to them. Remember, adults concentrate on the individual steps of a project or task only after they have seen the big picture and how it will benefit them.

9. **Encourage Interpersonal Relationships.** As an educator, you may not be able to connect with each and every learner in every class on an individual basis. However, by encouraging interaction among the learners, you have expanded their network, their relationships, and the support they have available to ensure that they get maximum benefit from the education provided.

10. **Offer Choices.** This correlates to the human need to be in control. By offering learners choices that they can make, they feel they have control. When developing exercises, projects, and activities for a given class, provide two or more and allow learners to choose which ones they would like to complete rather than making specific assignments. By giving them the opportunity to choose, they not only feel in control, but also find themselves in a more personal motivational environment.

IT'S WORTH REMEMBERING ✳

Educational research shows that learners enjoy hearing the human side of any story.

Powerful Openings

As stated earlier, we communicate by speaking, listening, reading, and writing. Studies have shown that only 7 percent of our communication is verbal (the words we use) and 38 percent of our communication is vocal (how we speak those words). So if what we say and how we say it represents only 45 percent of our speaking communication, what represents the remaining 55 percent? The answer is visual communication. Our overall appearance, facial expressions, body language, posture, and gestures represent 55 percent of the message we are delivering to our learners. Each

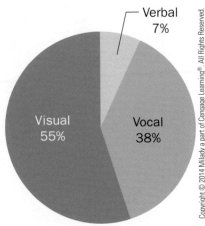

Figure 7–3   Critical Elements of Communication

element is important and all elements are critical if effective communication is to occur (Figure 7–3).

A powerful opening for your class informs your learners that their time will be used well, that you understand who they are, that you respect them because you are prepared, and that you know the material through education and practical experience.

Be Enthusiastic, Energetic, and Animated. You will not hold the attention of any learner for long if you present a dull, disinterested attitude. Use vitality and excitement to challenge your learners.

Never Say You Are Sorry. A master educator prepares so thoroughly that there will never be a need to apologize to a class. However, if an apology is appropriate, it should be timely and sincere.

Be Sincere and Focus on Your Learners. Take focus off yourself and place it on your learners. By concentrating on delivering your message and influencing your learners, you will not need to be worrying about whether or not you are giving an effective presentation. Your students will appreciate your sincere and honest effort to benefit them.

Maintain Eye Contact. Avoid looking over the heads of your learners or gazing at the walls, ceiling, or floor. Nothing can convey your sincerity and interest better than making one-to-one, personal eye contact with all learners throughout the presentation. Move about the room and direct your interest to many different learners.

Tell Them What You're Going to Tell Them. Give students a general overview of the day's lesson at the beginning. Let them know what they can expect from the class. Chart the course of the lesson.

Direct Learners' Attention. Ask learners specific questions that will focus their attention on the important matters of the day's lesson.

Convey Visual Integrity. Since 55 percent of your impact on learners will be through your appearance, facial expressions, posture, and body language, your visual appearance is critical to the presentation process. The first impression that learners form of you can impact whether they are receptive to your message or will generally reject it.

- Clothing—Does your clothing reflect the image desired by the institution and promote the importance of professionalism?
- Facial expressions—Do your expressions convey an attitude of interest and animation?
- Gestures—Are your gestures open and compatible with your message?
- Posture—Are you at ease? Do you stand straight and proud?
- Body movements—Are your movements consistent with the purpose of the material you are presenting? Do they direct learner attention to the topic at hand?

Consider Your Voice Quality. Remember, 38 percent of how your message will impact your learners is based on your voice—*how* you say what you are telling them. The best voice is clear, pleasant, and natural without affectations.

articulation
the act or process of pronouncing distinctly and carefully; enunciation.

- **Articulation**—Are your words slurred or are they distinct? Can your students understand what you are saying? Practicing tongue twisters, such as *the whispering watchman waited while the woman whined*, helps you limber up your lips, teeth, and tongue for clearer speech.
- **Pitch**—Do you vary your pitch frequently in each sentence to ensure a pleasant and friendly sound?

- Emphasis—Do you emphasize key words to put power behind them? By changing the emphasis within a given statement, you can change its entire meaning.
- Pace—Do you vary the speed at which you speak and use timed pauses? By varying your speed and utilizing appropriate pauses, you can show emphasis and action.
- Tone—Do you smile as often and as sincerely as possible? Your facial expressions, such as a smile or frown, will give a different tone to your voice, even when saying the same thing. Try asking, "Why haven't I seen you lately?" first with a smile, then with a look of happy surprise, then with a look of shock, and then with a frown. You'll quickly notice that each expression gave a different tone to your voice and a different meaning to the question.
- Vocabulary—Do you use terminology suitable for the learning level of your students? Do you pronounce technical terms properly? Take care not to talk over their heads or to appear condescending by defining words they already know.

Use the first 15 minutes of class time to inform and excite your learners. Getting their attention will increase their retention. Your opening will be powerful if you make the effort to establish and maintain a sincere rapport with your learners. A couple of examples of activities that can be used to create a dynamic opening for your classes are provided for your consideration.

COMPOSITION CHALLENGE ACTIVITY

1. Divide the class into two or more teams with at least five students or more on each team.
2. Inform the teams that they will perform the exercise one group at a time and will be timed.
3. Inform the students that they cannot talk to each other prior to or during the competition.
4. Instruct the students that they are to compose a complete sentence on the board relevant to the day's lesson, one word at a time. (For example, you might guide them to complete a sentence about the most important thing they want to get out of today's lesson.)
5. Each student in the team will approach the board one at a time and write one word. Students cannot preplan or discuss their sentence ahead of time. They cannot insert words between words already written on the board. Every student must write at least one word. Rotation of team members will continue until the sentence is completed.
6. The sentence must contain a subject, verb, and proper punctuation.
7. As each team completes its sentence, the time will be called and the sentence recorded for later discussion. The board is then erased for the next team.

By allowing the teams to compete one at a time, the other team or teams get to observe the interaction of the other students. At the conclusion of the competition, the educator can lead a discussion on the importance of being alert, observing what is going on, thinking an idea through to completion, and teamwork. She can also repeat the sentences created to lead into the day's lesson.

ASSOCIATES FOR HIRE ACTIVITY

This exercise is appropriate for opening a class on securing employment or job hunting.

1. Divide the class into groups with at least six students each.
2. Give each group a large sheet of flip-chart paper and assorted colored markers.
3. Direct the group to compose a collective resume for a specific position assigned by the educator appropriate to the career field the students are pursuing. (Vary the positions somewhat for each group.)
4. Remind the group that the average time a manager takes to scan a resume and determine if the applicant should be granted an interview is only 20 seconds. Therefore, they get *20 Seconds to Sizzle* in their group resume.
5. The resume should present the group's collective abilities, accomplishments, education, and experience.
6. Allow the students to use their imaginations and compose *dream data* that will sell the group even if it hasn't occurred yet.

Give the groups 10 to 15 minutes for the assignment and then have each group read their resume to the remainder of the class. Allowing them to create accomplishments and experiences that have not yet occurred adds humor to the activity. The educator can easily lead into a discussion on how to write an effective resume, which is necessary in the early stages of job hunting.

Building Powerful Content

The objectives of the lesson will drive the overall content and points that are to be presented. After you have created a dynamic, powerful opening, you will need to present the core of the lesson. The structure of the lesson must be logical, simple to follow, and relevant to the needs of the learners. A number of structure formats can be considered when planning a classroom presentation.

The *Problem/Solution Structure*. This structure is common in business when a challenge or problem is followed by a proposed solution. The educator might use this format to outline a situation that has caused problems or concerns, such as frequent violations of a standard of conduct set forth for students. The educator would then lead discussion and suggest proposed solutions.

The *Chronological Structure*. This method allows the educator to present key points in a natural time sequence or historical order. This might be an appropriate structure for the educator to follow when discussing the history or evolution of a specific topic, for example. Following a sequential pattern in presenting material doesn't allow you to present the material in order of importance. However, during your summary and review, you can place emphasis on the points that are most significant.

The *Topical Structure*. This qualitative structure allows you to list your points in order of significance, with the most important being discussed at the beginning. This structure might be useful when presenting directly after lunch, when learners may not be able to concentrate through the entire presentation. Generally, a learner is most alert at the beginning of the class.

The *Spatial Structure.* An educator would use this type of format to begin with general subject matter and progress to the specific, or vice versa. This might be effective for a class on infection control, in which a general overview of the importance of infection control is discussed followed by specific instruction on the individual products and steps used in infection control procedures.

The *Theory/Practice Structure.* This format is probably the most frequently used by educators in career education. The educator uses this structure to outline the theory of any given subject and then demonstrate how it works in practice. It is beneficial for the educator to link the theory to what the learners already know and then progress to the less familiar subject matter.

By choosing which structure is preferred for the material, the educator can place the information and ideas to be presented in the most suitable order.

An important facet of the body of your presentation or lesson is that you must build support for the key points. This will help learners to understand the material and overcome doubt or skepticism, especially when you are presenting a topic that is difficult to understand.

Strengthening the Content

A variety of methods can be employed by the master educator to strengthen the body or major content of a lesson.

Facts, Figures, Statistics, and Authorities. Using numerical representations of facts, noting verifiable statements or quotes by third parties, citing direct observation, and providing explanation of factual relationships based on statistical information can add importance and credibility to the information being presented.

Defining Key Terms. Explaining key terms leads to understanding the nature of something, often by moving from the general to the specific. For example, a faradic current (term) is an electrical current (general class) that is an alternating, interrupted current capable of producing a mechanical reaction without a chemical effect (particular qualities).

Anecdotes. Relating stories or experiences will help to clarify a point or show real-life application of the material. Anecdotes may not necessarily prove your statement, however.

anecdote
a short account of some interesting or humorous incident.

Examples and Illustrations. These may be used to not only clarify but also to prove a general statement or detailed points within the presentation. Remember, they also bring the human element to the presentation.

Analogies. Describing a set of similar or related conditions through analogy can make a concept more understandable. For example, you might compare the wrapping of a spiral perm to that of wrapping a ribbon around a pencil in a candy-cane approach from end to end.

analogy
similarity in some respects between things that are otherwise dissimilar.

Closings with Impact

The most powerful opening and the most well-prepared body of a lesson can be lost if at the end of the class, you simply trail off or rush to complete the class on time at the expense of valuable summary and review.

It is important to end each class with a *powerful punch*. The master educator will *summarize* the general lesson and *restate the key points*. She will then *present a challenge* for action or performance on the part of the learners. For example, when closing a class on presentation techniques that has been presented to student instructors, you might present the following challenge to action: "Involvement and learner activity are important in building retention of the subject matter and ensuring that learners will be able to successfully apply required skills on the job. You've experienced the importance of learner involvement in this week's lessons. You've actively discovered ways to involve your learners in your presentations. You are now able to create that same energy and excitement in the classes you teach if you continue to apply those same techniques."

Another approach in closing with a powerful punch is to use *humor, quotes, poems,* or *anecdotes*. Humor can be especially beneficial if the subject matter has been complicated. Humor can lighten the mood and allow you to end on a high note. Quotes from notable sources can bring meaning to your entire presentation as well. For example, when teaching a class on teamwork, you might close with, "Giordano Bruno, an Italian philosopher and astronomer, once said that the hammers must be swung in cadence, when more than one is hammering the iron. When you become a member of a team, you will learn the importance of working, or hammering in cadence, with the other team members." Poems and anecdotes can accomplish the same results. When closing a class on goal setting or building self-esteem, the following poem, whose author is unknown, might be read:

"I Promise Myself
To be so strong that nothing can disturb my peace of mind.
To talk health, happiness, and prosperity to every person I meet.
To make all my friends feel that there is something special in them.
To look at the sunny side of everything and make my optimism come true.
To think only of the best, to work only for the best, and expect only the best.
To be just as enthusiastic about the success of others as I am about my own.
To forget the mistakes of the past and press on to the greater achievements of the future.
To wear a cheerful countenance at all times and give every living creature I meet a smile.
To give so much time to the improvement of myself that I have no time to criticize others.
To be too large for worry, too noble for anger, too strong for fear, and too happy to permit the presence of trouble.
My attitude is my life."

From the: "The Optimist Creed" (Christian D. Larson, 1912)

Another important element of bringing a presentation to closure is the educator's responsibility to assess and evaluate student learning and progress. During the summary and review process, the educator will be able to identify the level of the students' understanding of the content. Later in this chapter, we discuss more fully the effective use of questioning during the class as well as at the time of closure. It is appropriate, however, for written and practical testing to occur for each unit of study.

Connecting All the Parts

We've spent a significant amount of time on how to prepare lessons that contain a powerful opening, a strong body, and a closing with impact. You may be wondering how you move from one part of the lesson into another. The techniques you use to connect all the parts are called transitions. These are moments during a lesson when the educator controls the instructional behavior of learners by shifting from one activity to another. Transitions must be managed in such a way that learner involvement in the class is not decreased. There are a number of ways transitions can be used effectively.

Pause. Silence can be powerful. It can be used to stress a point or to indicate that you've completed one part of the presentation and are about to move to the next.

Incorporate Q & A. Instruct learners to think about the material that has been presented and formulate questions, either alone or in pairs or small groups. A brief question-and-answer period can serve as a helpful review as well as a transition into the next part of the lesson.

Physical Activity or Movement. This could indicate movement by the educator from one part of the classroom to another. It could also suggest physical activity or movement by the learners. You might have learners stand, stretch, and rub the shoulders of the nearest student, and then switch roles, for a few minutes. This serves as a controlled energizer and also serves as a smooth transition into new material.

Introduce Visual Aids. When you incorporate some type of educational aid into your presentation, you have signaled a transition.

Change the Educational Aid. If you began with the overhead projector and transparencies, you may want to move to a flip chart to stress a different part of the information. This indicates a transition.

Redirect Attention. It is not uncommon for learners to get sidetracked from the original topic or point of the lesson. The master educator will easily redirect the attention back to the appropriate point in the lesson without embarrassing the learner. You might simply ask, "Now where were we before Suzette offered those comments?" It's a simple task to then resume your presentation or discussion as outlined.

Varying the Stimuli

Certainly, a major goal we have as educators is to arouse or incite our students to activity. We hope to excite them into growth and learning. It has been estimated that our adult learners can listen with *understanding* for 90 minutes, but can only listen with *retention* of the information for 20 minutes. Therefore, the master educator needs to plan a complete change of pace within the lesson at no less than 20-minute intervals to create a new cycle of learning and retention. How can we accomplish this? In our discussion of how to build a powerful presentation, we have already discussed many skills and techniques that are used to bring variety into the classroom. We will recap some of those techniques here and add more to strengthen your presentations.

Gestures. The use of gestures is a form of varying the **stimuli**. Demosthenes, when asked to identify the first requisite of good speaking,

stimuli
anything causing or regarded as causing a response; something that incites or rouses to action.

responded, "Action!" When he was then asked what the second and third requisites of good speaking are, he responded, "Action!" Clearly, Demosthenes felt that effective speaking is speaking with the whole body. When you use gestures with your hands, your body, or your head, you portray an attitude. One of the best ways to relax the body muscles and help overcome stage fright is by using gestures. Educators must be able to recognize the difference between effective gestures and mere movements. Some might release energy by playing with pocket change, toying with a pencil, or fidgeting with eye glasses, rings, necklaces, or some other object. Such movements do not emphasize relevancy of the message, but instead distract learners from the meaning. An educator will learn proper use of body actions in order to retain the value of the action while making the action serve as an aid, rather than a hindrance, to the learners. A master educator utilizes sufficient purposeful action so that it will not be necessary to indulge in any other action or movements solely for the purpose of draining off excess nervous energy. Gestures have at least three additional purposes:

Clarify the educator's meaning. Gestures can be used to indicate the size, shape, or position of an object. When enumerating a series of points, the educator might hold up the applicable number of fingers as the points are presented. You have often heard that *actions speak louder than words.* Gestures may speak louder than words to reveal the meaning of the educator's message.

Help reveal the educator's attitudes. If an educator wishes to convey an attitude of intimate relationship with learners, she will step forward and lean into the group. If she is denouncing something, she might push away from the group by pushing her hand away from herself with the palm down. Doubt might be conveyed by holding her hands palm up, waist high, while shrugging the shoulders. These are just a few examples of how gestures can convey an attitude. In order to use gestures effectively, practice in front of a full-length mirror. Many of the nation's most effective speakers have practiced for long and useful hours before a mirror; the rewards are great and recognizable.

Lend emphasis. Most presentations or classes experience a "spurt, sag, spurt" cycle. The attention of your learners is certain to lag at times during a presentation. When you reach a point of primary importance, you want to be certain that the learners are paying close attention. Use of effective gestures can help accomplish this. Such gestures might include clapping the hands together, pounding a fist on the desk, pointing a finger at the learners, or any number of other effective movements. Emphatic gestures can suggest forcefulness. Take care not to make the same ones habitual or they will lose value. Use skill when applying emphatic gestures to ensure that they do not take away from the meaning of the message (Figure 7–4).

By moving about the room while teaching, you create interest in your presentation. Students pay close attention to see what you are going to do next.

Voice. A master educator will also learn to use her voice to create excitement and enthusiasm. She will avoid monotone at all costs. She will vary the use of soft and loud expressive tones and both high and low pitch for emphasis and variety. If you are projecting with a strong, forceful voice during a key part of your presentation and suddenly drop your voice to a whisper, it will definitely get the attention of every learner in the classroom, even those whose minds may be wandering. At the same time, if you are

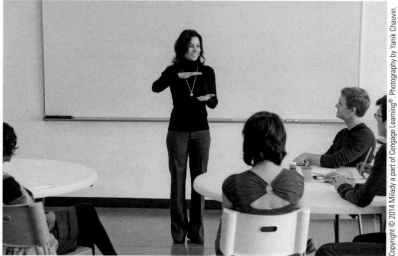

Figure 7–4   Gestures are used to clarify meaning, reveal attitudes, and lend emphasis.

speaking at a steady rate and suddenly increase your rate of speech significantly and use a higher pitch, you create excitement and your learners pay close attention to what is coming next. These changes in your presentation are all variations of the stimuli.

Attention Grabbers. Another technique a master educator will use to vary the stimuli is to use *attention grabbers*. These can range from using a "shocking" opening statement to simply paraphrasing information. An opening statement such as, "You're wasting your time in this class today unless you are willing to put into practice the procedures we are going to discuss," will definitely get the attention of your learners. During the class itself, you might find it appropriate to restate something a learner has contributed by paraphrasing it. You might begin by saying, "So, in other words . . ." or "Let me see if I understand you correctly, what you're saying is. . . ." Another attention grabber is focusing or directing the attention of the learners simply by saying, "Look!" You might even suggest that they listen closely or watch what you are about to demonstrate. Pausing is another simple procedure that will get the attention of your learners in a hurry.

Energizers and Stress Relievers. As previously stated, it is not uncommon for a presentation or class to experience a "spurt, sag, spurt" cycle. Another technique that master educators employ is the use of energizers and stress relievers at a point when the class needs a lift and change of pace. There are times when the material you are presenting is heavy and not always that interesting. Your learners' minds will begin to wander. At that point, you need a change of pace, but there may not be sufficient time for a break. An energizer is a one- to three-minute activity that gives learners a mental break but keeps them focused (Figure 7–5). Energizers are appropriate when the class goes into mid-afternoon "sag." Energizers are more effective if they match or correlate to the topic.

Oral/Visual Switching. Another way to vary the stimuli for learners is to switch from oral teaching methods to visual teaching methods. To assist you in identifying the various techniques that can be used in oral/visual switching, review Table 7–1.

CONSIDER AND CONNECT

Cease teaching for 8 to 10 seconds and watch what happens. Your learners will be sitting on the edge of their seats waiting to see what you are going to do or say next.

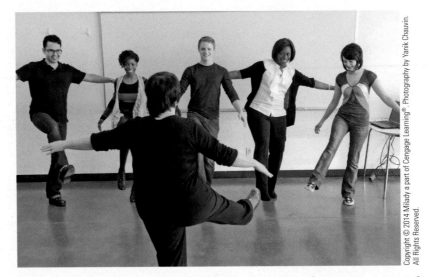

Figure 7–5   An energizer is a brief activity that gives learners a mental break, but keeps them focused.

Table 7–1

ORAL/VISUAL SWITCHING

ORAL	VISUAL
Lecture	Demonstration
Audiotapes	Videotapes
Discussion	Role-Plays
Anecdotes	Pictures
Testimonials	Chalkboard, Other Boards
Analogies	Games
Guest Speaker	Models, Mannequins
Metaphors	Laser Disc
Riddles	CD-ROM
Music	Projects
Poems	Posters
Humor	Energizers
Questions	Slides
Trivia	Tricks
Oral Quizzes	Contests
Summary	Slides
Quotes	Completion

☑ Using Technology

Another method for varying the stimuli for the learners is to integrate the use of technology in the classroom. Technology can range from incorporating PowerPoint slides; to utilizing student CD-ROMs that contain activities, tests, and games; to watching YouTube videos or introducing online tools such as topic specific CourseMate products, and so much more. For more detailed information on how to do this, please refer to Chapter 11.

Questioning

Enthusiasm can be a tremendous ally when you are conducting your oral review at the end of the lesson. Of course, when asking students questions, displaying empathy is another key ingredient. Never make light of a question or disregard it. Put yourself in the place of your learner and you will be able to patiently consider all questions and give them the attention they need and deserve. Never become defensive with your students. If you do not know the answer to a question, offer to obtain it and get back to them. On the other hand, if you have completed your research and preparation thoroughly, it is unlikely that there will be more than a few questions that you, as a master educator, cannot answer.

Fine-tune your ability to ask questions effectively. It has been determined that approximately 93 percent of the questions that educators ask in their classroom merely require the recall of knowledge or facts presented in the classroom. Relatively few questions require higher mental process of the learner.

Asking Questions. The objectives of each lesson and the prior knowledge of the learners will guide the educator in the formulation of questions suitable for the class. Your questions should be planned in advance and you should know at what point you want to ask them. It's important that each question have a purpose. Generally, they will elicit either information or opinions on a variety of topics that should go from general to specific. It is helpful to relate questions to the learner's background or point of reference. Keep the questions as simple and to the point as possible, and make logical transitions between the questions. If you are leading a group discussion with the class, direct your questions to the entire class first and then to individual learners.

There are two types of questioning: low order and high order.

Low-Order Questioning. Low-order, recall-type questions encourage students to keep up with their work and provide for assessment of factual knowledge. They also enable educators to establish whether learners have adequate background knowledge before moving to more complex issues. Lower-level questions will contribute to the academic achievement of learners if they are asked at appropriate difficulty levels, if they are equitably distributed among all learners, and if they result in a high percentage of correct answers. Lower-level questions are either open ended or closed. Open-ended questions require a specific, informational response. They can be directed at either a group or an individual learner. Closed questions are generally directed at only one learner and can be answered with either a yes or a no. Closed questions are typically not as effective as open-ended ones. Examples of low-order questions are as follows:

- Can anyone tell me how long learners can listen with interest?
- Lisa, is it essential to get learners in an active mood at the beginning of a class?

High-Order Questioning. Research shows that higher-level questioning may lead to improved achievement for learners. Higher-level questions require the learner to have knowledge and comprehension, the ability to analyze data, the ability to synthesize information, and the ability to

---

> **CONSIDER AND CONNECT**
>
> Research shows that educators ask questions frequently while presenting their lessons, but the questions fail to challenge the minds of the learners.

> **CONSIDER AND CONNECT**
>
> Don't answer your own questions before your learners have had an opportunity to answer them. Once you have asked a question, allow the learner to respond completely without interrupting.

evaluate information and draw conclusions. Essay-type questions are considered high-order questions. Examples of high-order questioning are as follows:

* Can you distinguish between a galvanic current and a Tesla high-frequency current in terms of their function and effectiveness? (Analysis)
* If you were asked to create a collage of pictures and symbols that reflect your personal values, what would it include? (Synthesis)
* Now that you have read the Standards of Conduct required for employment at three different establishments, which one do you feel has the best policies and why? Please be prepared to defend your choice. (Evaluation)

There are three methods for questioning: group questioning, direct questioning, and redirect questioning (Figure 7–6). The group method is used when the educator asks a question to the entire class or group and anyone can answer. The direct method is used when the educator wishes to solicit an answer from an individual learner. The redirect method is used when a question is asked of a specific student and another student is asked to comment on the first student's response. The educator would then clarify any comments made by either learner. The redirect method may also occur when a student asks a question of the educator, who then asks if another member of the class would like to respond first. The educator will always paraphrase or restate the correct response to ensure that all learners in the classroom hear the correct answer.

Answering Questions. Effective listening is an important part of answering questions. You must really *hear* a question before you can respond to it. Listen for what is being asked as well as what is meant by the question. You'll be able to discern certain emotions or feelings behind the question. Restate or paraphrase the question to ensure you understand it correctly. After responding, verify that you have satisfied the questioner. If not, be prepared to offer additional information, support, or clarification. It's important to be responsive to all questions without indicating that you feel one has been inappropriate or ill-timed. Focus on the questions specifically and stay on track rather than getting sidetracked with unrelated stories. Two students may ask very similar questions, but it is important that you treat each one separately and give each individual attention.

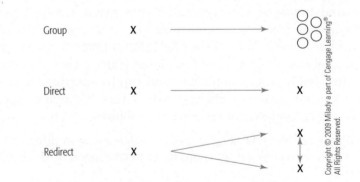

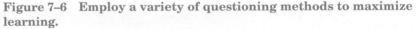

Figure 7–6   Employ a variety of questioning methods to maximize learning.

Reinforcement

Another tool used for creating powerful presentations is the educator's ability to use positive reinforcement during the lesson (Figure 7–7). We have established that all human beings have an innate need to be appreciated and receive recognition for their performance or contribution. Therefore, the educator must be prepared to give positive feedback to students throughout the educational process. Some verbal words of reinforcement include *okay, good, great, wonderful, terrific, fantastic, perfect, phenomenal,* and *outstanding.* Some verbal phrases of reinforcement include the following: I knew you could do it! That's exactly what I was looking for! You have made major progress! It couldn't be any better! Consistent with the importance of nonverbal communication, nonverbal reinforcement can be accomplished through gestures such as smiling, nodding in approval, shaking hands, and giving a high-five or a thumbs-up signal.

It's important for the master educator to know what kinds of reinforcement are acceptable. For example, in today's climate, certain touching—such as hugging—can be considered illegal or harassment if the student is not forewarned of the action. Students must be given the opportunity to allow or refuse the hug.

Wrapping It Up

We have stressed the importance of the educator's ability to communicate effectively with the great diversity of students found in today's classrooms. The master educator will practice steps to increase personal awareness of learners' cultures and backgrounds and follow the reliable C-R-E-A-T-E formula when building daily lesson plans. She will **c**onsider the topic, **r**esearch

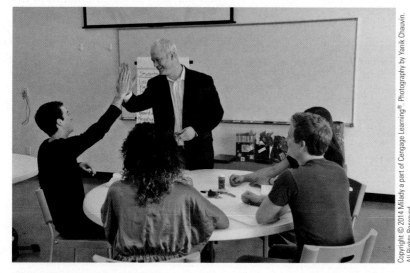

Figure 7–7   **Use positive reinforcement to show appreciation and recognition of student performance.**

the topic, use *e*xamples for clarification, *a*nalyze the learners, *t*each with poise, and enthusiastically *e*njoy the educational experience. She will consider the psychological and physical needs of her adult learners when preparing the motivation for learning the lesson. She will practice a variety of methods for creating circumstances or situations by which her students can become motivated. The master educator will know the importance of structuring each presentation with a powerful opening, a strong body or core content, and a high-impact closing. She will master the art of making smooth transitions within the lesson that will not decrease learner involvement. She will vary the stimuli used to gain the interest and attention of the learners and increase their retention of the material presented. She will plan her questioning of the learners in advance of the class and incorporate both high-order and low-order questions as appropriate. She will also give positive reinforcement, both verbal and nonverbal, to learners throughout the educational process. The master educator will aim to create a comprehensive conceptual and practical framework for generating learner results through participant discovery and involvement in each classroom presentation.

In Retrospect

1. Explain what is meant by the acronym C-R-E-A-T-E model for preparations.

2. Identify the various components of powerful presentations.

3. Explain 10 methods used for inspiring learner motivation.

4. List 10 elements important to powerful components.

5. Explain the importance of closing all presentations with impact.

6. List five methods used to strengthen the body or major content of a lesson.

7. List six effective methods used to facilitate transitions.

8. State five methods for varying the stimuli within a lesson.

9. Explain the difference between low-order and high-order questions.

10. Explain why reinforcement during a lesson is important.

Objectives (Desired Performance Goals):

After reading and studying this chapter, you should be able to:

- Explain low-profile and direct, high-profile control techniques that are used in dealing with learner misconduct.

- Explain specific techniques used in remedying misconduct.

- Explain the difference between a situational barrier to learning and a chronic barrier to learning.

- Describe various difficult learner behaviors and explain methods for managing them.

- List and explain four enemies of conflict management.

! CRITICAL CONCEPT

The trickle-down effect of a teacher's influence impacts the lives of many for years into the future.

Promoting a Positive Environment

AS WE DISCUSSED IN CHAPTER 2, "The Teaching Plan and Learning Environment," a positive learning environment is critical to student success and optimal learning. Various physical and psychological considerations are important in creating an atmosphere of collaboration, cooperation, and inclusiveness. A dedicated educator will consider everything from how colors are used to the motivational content of posters; from the music played in the classroom to ensuring that every learning style is addressed; from creating dynamic presentations to making sure every student is involved in discovery-oriented learning. Ultimately, however, the educator must convey to every learner a sincere attitude of caring. When that is accomplished, the learning environment will be one of motivation, energy, enthusiasm, and excitement. The teacher will enjoy teaching and the learners will enjoy learning.

Professionalism in the Classroom

The educator's image, attitude, and actions are often mirrored by learners. Therefore, it is important that the educator project the best possible image and professionalism at all times (Figure 8–1). She must also develop and maintain a positive enthusiasm for the learning process. The master educator knows that by establishing her own credibility and authority, she will be more effective at maintaining order and control in the classroom. That professionalism will also earn her the respect of the learners, which will generate a high degree of cooperation in the learning environment. It is important for career education instructors to make the transition from professional practitioner to educator. Young, new educators must acknowledge their new role as teacher and fully accept that they cannot interact socially with their adult learners.

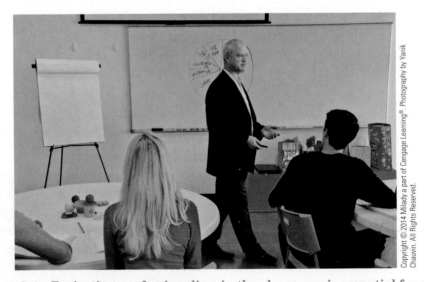

Figure 8–1 Projecting professionalism in the classroom is essential for an educator's credibility.

Principles of Managing Learner Behavior

Master educators will respect adult learners and establish the guidelines that will be followed in the classroom. By setting well-defined goals, guidelines, and expectations for learner behavior early on in the educator–learner relationship, future conflicts and misunderstandings may be avoided. The master educator might even use the transfer technique and involve the learners in the process of establishing the guidelines for professionalism within the classroom environment. Learners are more likely to commit themselves to standards they have helped develop.

The guidelines established should set forth, in a specific document, the rules of conduct as well as the consequences for noncompliance with those rules or standards. The document should be explained and discussed in the new-student orientation process to ensure that all students know what is expected of them, both in behavior as well as performance. Effective guidelines will help prevent learner behaviors that might detract from the educator's ability to facilitate the learning process.

Behavioral psychology shows that learners will react more favorably and desired behaviors can be shaped more quickly and permanently through positive rather than through negative means. Educators will achieve more cooperation from learners by focusing on the positive. All misconduct *cannot* be eliminated by establishing standards to follow; therefore, disciplinary policies must also be established to effectively handle those situations of noncompliance that will occasionally occur. Master educators model and teach students to develop self-control. They restrain anger and frustration and use behavioral conduct techniques that are discreet, relatively unobtrusive, and under control. Hostility, ridicule, sarcasm, and verbal abuse are counterproductive to the objectives of the institution as well as to the purpose of good discipline. Techniques that are consistent with the maintenance of good discipline in the classroom are discussed next.

Preventing behaviors that detract from the educator's abilities to facilitate the learning process is achieved through the following steps:

- Maintenance of high behavioral standards.
- Consistent enforcement of rules and application of consequences.
- Modeling of appropriate behaviors.
- Continual monitoring of learner conduct.

Low-Profile Intervention. This method uses the least amount of force necessary to deter or control misbehavior. Minimal force is associated with minimal time and effort. The more quickly and easily the educator can control misconduct, the more quickly she can concentrate on productive learning activities. The more forceful the response to an act of misconduct, the more disruptive it is to the entire class, which results in loss of educational time.

Uniformity and Consistency. Consistency has been defined as behaving the same way on repeated occasions when the circumstances are the same or similar. Uniformity deals with consistency among different parties or learners. Surveys of students across the country indicate that the unfair application of policies and procedures among learners is one of their significant concerns. Similarly, surveys of institutions across the nation indicate that the educator's ability to fairly and uniformly apply and implement policies and procedures is a characteristic in great demand in the hiring of new educators. In the absence of consistency and uniformity, learners receive conflicting messages and may be unsure of what *is* and *is not* acceptable behavior at any given time.

High-Profile Intervention. This method requires more force and may require more time and effort on the part of the educator. There are occasions when it is necessary to be very direct and assertive when dealing with chronic misconduct.

There is no single approach or method of controlling misconduct that is best for *all* educators and *all* learners at *all* times. Therefore, it is important for the master educator to become familiar with a variety of methods and learn when it is necessary to be direct and assertive and when a low-profile, less direct approach is more effective. Several factors determine how the educator will respond:

- the seriousness of the violation;
- the timing and circumstances surrounding the misbehavior;
- the behavioral history of the learner;
- the nature of the activity under way at the time of the misbehavior;
- the attitude and personality of the learner in violation; and
- the operational style and personality of the educator.

All methods of dealing with misbehavior will be more effective if the educator maintains a high degree of professionalism and decorum during the process. Some low-profile control techniques that can be employed in the classroom to help minimize disruptive behavior are discussed next.

Ignore It. If the behavior is minor, paying no attention to it may be an acceptable strategy. Often the learner's misbehavior is for no other purpose than attracting the attention of the educator or other students. Any response, even a disapproving one, may be reinforcing the attention-seeking behavior. If the conduct is of short duration and relatively insignificant, ignoring it may be the preferred control technique.

Name Dropping. This method might be used when a student is talking to another student during a presentation, for example. Name dropping is an unobtrusive procedure because most learners are unaware of what is being done except for the student(s) whose behavior needs to be controlled. During the presentation or group discussion, the educator might insert the name of the learner in an instructional statement. For example, "We need to remember, Sharon, that it is important as an educator to model the behavior we expect of our students." Sharon, who has otherwise been inattentive, gets the message that the educator is aware of her behavior and that she should refocus her attention.

Close Proximity. A powerful means of controlling misbehavior is to physically move toward the learner who is in violation of the standards. The closer the educator gets to the learner, the more likely it is that the learner will cease the misbehavior due to the educator's awareness and presence.

Eye Contact. Eye contact can be used with little effort on the part of the educator and can be a powerful control strategy for minor misconduct. It is normally used in conjunction with other techniques, but can be applied independently. The learner must recognize from the look in the educator's eyes that the misconduct needs to cease immediately.

Verbal Desists. This technique involves the use of a verbal cue or command to stop the behavior. It can take on many forms, from simply saying the learner's name, such as in the name-dropping technique, to a complex command indicating precisely which behavior is to stop. The master educator will take care not to convey hostility or sarcasm when using verbal desists. If the educator must convey anger, it must always be directed to the situation and not to the character of the learner, if favorable results are to be expected.

Managing Chronic Misconduct

The primary purpose of employing the control procedures previously discussed is to achieve immediate cessation of misbehavior by learners in the classroom. The secondary purpose, however, is to permanently eliminate misconduct. Educators hope their strategies will stop the acts of noncompliance and also deter their recurrence. However, that is not always the case. The master educator recognizes that there are a few students who will chronically violate the rules even in the face of increasingly forceful and punitive control measures. Thus, we will discuss a few general principles that should be considered in the management of remedial strategies.

Specific techniques used in remedying misconduct are selected on the basis of school policies, personal style of the educator, nature of the misconduct, availability of outside help if needed, and the time allowed to address the issues. The educator must decide whether techniques should be applied immediately or whether they should be applied later, for example, at the end of the day or after the scheduled class. The educator must determine whether the action should occur in front of other students, in private, or with another educator or staff member present. For the purposes of discussion here, we will concentrate on direct interactions between the educator and the learner, which are considered high-profile intervention methods.

Reprimands. One of the most common remedial techniques is the use of reprimands. They can be applied with ease both publicly and privately, depending on the circumstances. They should occur as soon after the misbehavior as possible. The educator should explain how she feels about the misconduct and remind the learner how to behave appropriately. The exchange should conclude with the understanding that the same mistakes are not to occur again. Clarification and caring must precede confrontation if a resolution of a problem is expected.

Change the Consequences. If it is determined that the established consequences are not effective and do not work in resolving rule violations, they should be changed. If consequences fail to produce satisfactory results, it is usually because they lack sufficient deterrent force. It may be necessary to exact a higher cost for those who chronically violate the rules.

CONSIDER AND CONNECT

The key to successful use of eye contact is that it must convey to the learner that failure to remedy the misbehavior will result in negative consequences.

CONSIDER AND CONNECT

A master educator plans a variety of learning-appropriate activities to ensure learner involvement and cooperation.

THE TOP 10 GUIDELINES FOR EFFECTIVE REPRIMANDS

1. Be brief and specific.

2. Focus on the behavior, not the learner.

3. Reprimand as soon after the misconduct as possible.

4. Be professional, but firm.

5. Back up the reprimand with consequences, if appropriate.

6. Provide a statement of appropriate behavior in the reprimand.

7. Remain calm and in control.

8. Always avoid embarrassing the learner.

9. Keep to the point; do not remind the learner of past indiscretions.

10. Observe and determine that the learner has accepted the reprimand.

Agreements or Contracts. Verbal agreements are commonly used to follow up on violations of classroom rules. When you believe students will live up to their word, it is appropriate to remind them of your contract. A written contract will add meaning to the agreement made between the educator and learner. A simple written agreement or contract is prepared and signed by the educator and the learner. A signed agreement carries a greater commitment to the agreed-upon behavior (Figure 8–2). This agreement can be as simple as stating the conditions and length of the agreement in the comments section of a regular counseling form used by the institution.

Conferences. A private conference between the educator and the learner gives both parties the opportunity to discuss the problem and potential solutions. The educator must carefully prepare for such a conference if it is to be successful.

CONSIDERATIONS FOR CONFERENCE PLANNING

1. Identify specific areas of misconduct.
2. Provide documented evidence of chronic misconduct.
3. Establish concrete goals for improvement.
4. Identify specific consequences for failure to remedy misconduct.
5. Plan for concluding the conference.

EDUCATOR–LEARNER AGREEMENT

This agreement is entered into between:

Learner: _____

Educator: _____

Terms of the agreement:

_____

_____

_____

_____

_____

_____

_____

_____

Consequences of failure to comply with terms of the agreement:

_____

_____

_____

_____

_____

_____

_____

_____

_____

_____

Date for evaluation of the effectiveness of agreement:

_____

_____

Learner's Signature _____Date_____   Educator's Signature _____Date _____

Figure 8–2   Agreement between educator and learner.

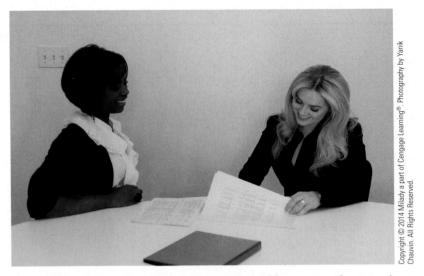

Figure 8–3   The conference environment should be as nonthreatening as possible.

The environment for the conference should be as nonthreatening as possible (Figure 8–3). The educator and learner should sit face-to-face with no barriers between them in a private area. The purpose of the conference is to bring about change, not to intimidate or control. The meeting should be focused on the violations of the rules rather than the character of the learner. The learner should understand how the conduct is a personal hindrance as well as a hindrance to other learners. The educator should ask sufficient questions to obtain the learner's view or perspective of the circumstances and practice effective listening skills during the meeting. Follow-up conferences are recommended to review progress and revise previously adopted plans and agreements if necessary. When progress or improvement has occurred, the educator has a wonderful opportunity to give recognition, approval, and positive reinforcement to the learner.

✓ Managing Difficult Learner Behavior

situational barrier
a situational barrier to learning occurs when a learner temporarily exhibits difficult behavior that is different than the personality or behavior usually exhibited.

chronic barrier
a chronic barrier to learning occurs when a learner behaves in a difficult manner consistently and creates a barrier to learning for other students.

We've discussed some *general* principles in managing learner behavior within the classroom. Now we will consider more detailed techniques that can be used for *specific* behaviors that create learning barriers. Anyone or anything that prevents students from achieving the learning objective is considered a learning barrier. When a learner temporarily exhibits "difficult" behavior that is different than the personality or behavior usually exhibited, that learner creates a **situational barrier**. On the other hand, when a learner behaves in a difficult manner consistently and affects other learners in an uncomfortable way, the barrier is *chronic*. The educator will need to be able to differentiate between situational and **chronic barriers** to learning.

If the behavior has occurred numerous times, it is likely that you are dealing with a chronic learning barrier or obstacle. If the behavior resulted from a particular incident, it is likely a situational barrier. The educator's role is to get the learner back on track without ridicule or embarrassment. Effective communication is critical in dealing with the various obstacles or barriers to learning. Relationships are mutual in that they are defined by both parties. The relationship will change when the communication between the parties changes. Changing relationships, however, takes time and patience. The more options you have, the better your odds of getting your desired results—in the classroom and in relationships with your learners.

Experienced educators and trainers have identified the types of difficult learner behaviors they have encountered throughout their careers. While some of the behaviors are rare, others are quite common. Each behavior causes potential learning barriers for either the learner exhibiting the behavior or others in the classroom. Master educators need to learn to identify the symptoms for each behavior in order to prevent the problems they create. We have already established that learners respond better to praise for positive behavior or performance than to criticism or punishment for their negative behavior. The principles of managing classroom behavior covered earlier suggest that strategies range from indirect or preventive (low-profile intervention) to more direct and corrective (high-profile intervention). Various levels of intervention are included in the strategies listed for each behavior that presents a barrier to learning.

Constant Attention-Seeking and Interruptions

Most of us have been in classrooms where we felt we were being held hostage by at least one of the learners. This is the student who sometimes has something to offer and sometimes does not, but talks anyway. Such learners are easily recognized because they interrupt throughout the presentation to share their personal experiences on the matter. They love to hear themselves talk and will take much longer to get a point across than most other students. The challenge with this behavior is that the leadership of the classroom can be sabotaged and the lesson steered off its charted course. An additional problem is that other learners may feel that "favoritism" exists in your classroom. Some strategies for dealing with this behavior are as follows:

- **The Unspoken Message.** Position yourself on the far side of the room from this learner to send a "quiet" message that the constant attention-seeking is not rewarded. Avoiding direct eye contact with this learner will send a similar message.
- **Pairs for Projects.** Assign learners to work in pairs, requiring the attention-seeker to work with another learner and acknowledge the partner's contribution.
- **Involve the Group.** Exhibit impartiality and fairness by deliberately calling on all learners in the classroom.
- **What Are the Rules?** Consider beginning class by drawing a vertical line down the center of a chalkboard or multipurpose board and putting the heading "Educator" at the top of the left one and the heading "Learner" at the top of the right one. Then ask the class if they have ever been in a class where the educator displayed annoying characteristics. Ask them to identify some of the behaviors of that educator and list them on the left side of the board. Answers might be some of

☑

IT'S WORTH REMEMBERING ✳

Master educators will minimize any negative impact that barriers have on learning in the classroom.

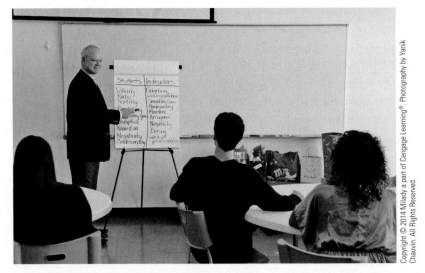

Figure 8–4   Identify distracting behaviors that can be displayed by both educators and learners.

the following: was monotonous and boring, didn't know the material, chewed gum, played with pocket change, and so on. Then ask them if they have ever been in a class where another student hindered the experience. Ask them to state the behaviors that were distracting and list them on the right side of the board (Figure 8–4). Answers might be constantly interrupted, carried on private conversations, argued every point, had an answer for everything, and so on. Once your lists are complete, you can make the commitment to your students that you will do everything in your power to avoid behaving in any of the ways listed on the left if they will avoid all of the behaviors listed on the right. The master educator will find a way to get all the characteristics or behaviors that she wishes to address on the right side of the board.

- **Let Groups Be the Guide.** Using small groups, rotating group leadership and members, and setting forth group questions are all effective measures for controlling the interrupter. We've talked about each of these solutions with other difficult learner behaviors, and those same principles apply here. This learner cannot control the entire activity if leadership is rotated and the entire group is required to participate in developing questions or finding solutions to questions that have been posed.

- **Play for Prizes.** Using incentives and token rewards encourages all learners to participate and therefore limits the opportunity for the troublesome learner to monopolize the entire class (Figure 8–5).

- **Chilly Chatter.** One method that works well in limiting each learner's response or contribution on any subject matter is to have them place their hand into a bucket of ice cubes. They are allowed to talk as long as they can hold their hand in the ice. When they remove their hand, they have to cease speaking. It brings humor to the classroom and also limits the showstopper from taking over the class. It's a great technique for fast-paced, brainstorming activities.

- **Help Is on the Way.** Solicit the help of the attention-seeking learners with special projects. They might be useful in designing and creating

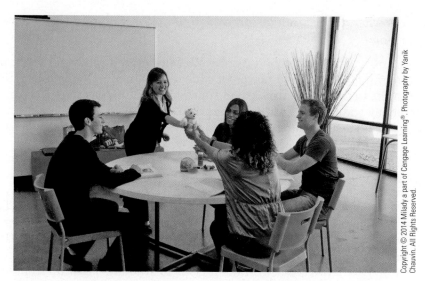

Figure 8–5 Use incentives or token rewards to encourage student participation.

flip charts for the topics of the day. Designate them as the official recorders of information on the wall charts. This keeps them physically busy and prevents the unnecessary interruptions that might otherwise occur.

- **Applause for Pauses.** Even these learners have to come up for air. When they pause to take a breath, you can simply thank them for their comments and redirect your body and your eye contact to another learner whom you ask to expand on the topic being discussed.
- **Pass the Baton.** This strategy allows you to compliment the learner and also redirect the attention of the class to another student. You might say, "Thank you for your responses; now let's hear from Maria."
- **The "Eyes" Have It.** When this learner raises his hand to ask a question, simply look at him directly and state that it is time for feedback from another learner and redirect your eye contact to a different student.
- **The Court Convenes.** As stated previously in the section on managing chronic misconduct, there comes a time when a personal conference or meeting with the student may be required. A one-on-one conversation with the learner will allow you to convey your appreciation for the learner's interest and commitment and your need to maintain impartiality in the classroom. Explain your need for the learner's help in accomplishing that goal. This addresses the learner's "real" need, which is tuned into station MMFI-AM (Make Me Feel Important About Myself)!

Chronic Tardiness

Every educator experiences learners who are consistently 5 to 10 minutes late for class. Such learners miss class frequently and usually turn in homework late. The challenge this behavior presents is a disruption of the flow of information, not only for the tardy learner but also for all the other learners when tardy students arrive late for class. Solutions for this behavior include:

- **Thank You and Thanks Again.** We have stated repeatedly that positive reinforcement is a powerful educational tactic. Giving a heartfelt thanks to those who arrived on time is rewarding positive performance. Convey your thanks at the beginning of each class, after breaks, and again at the end of the class. This ensures that your good students are tuned into MMFI-AM as well.

- **Rear Entrance Only.** It may not always be possible, but if the entrance to the classroom is opposite the main presentation area, the late arrival is less likely to disrupt the entire class.

- **Timely Beginnings.** Keep to the schedule. Beginning your class late to accommodate latecomers rewards the poor performers and penalizes the positive ones. By starting the class late, you are encouraging the remainder of the class to arrive late as well.

- **What Did You Expect?** Make it clear to students right up front what is expected of them during the training, including prompt attendance. As stated earlier in this chapter, get all learners involved in setting the guidelines for the classroom so they will take ownership of them and responsibility for complying with them.

- **What Did I Miss?** If tardy students arrive in the middle of a dynamic opening activity, they will either be unable to participate because they missed pertinent information or, if they join in, they may not be able to achieve the same results as other learners who were on time. If they miss the activity entirely, they will hear about it from other learners during the breaks or after class.

- **"Break" the Break Schedule.** Rather than providing one 15-minute break in the morning and another in the afternoon, consider a 5- to 10-minute break every hour. This helps retain learner interest because students can only focus for so long before their minds wander. It also allows only enough time to take care of necessities, such as use of the restroom and stretching. This prevents learners from engaging in other activities or conversations that may keep them from returning to class on time.

- **The Riddle Race.** Get the learners' attention by posing a riddle, asking a trivia question, or introducing a word puzzle. Give a token reward to the first learner who provides the solution or answer.

- **Ticklers and Teasers.** Try tactics such as placing a brightly colored gift bag at the front of the classroom (Figure 8–6). Your students, who are curious by nature, will eventually ask what's in the bag. Tell them that you will explain later and continue with your class. Just before a break or lunch, inform the students that you will open the bag and reveal the contents upon return and that those present will have the opportunity to receive or win a prize. The bag could contain nothing more than a handout relevant to your presentation, but it could also include small tokens or wrapped candy that is given to those who return to class on time.

- **Play for Prizes.** Offer more significant rewards for those who arrive on time or return from breaks on time. Create tokens that can be redeemed at the end of a day or week of classes. The tokens are awarded to students who are present on time. At the end of the designated period, the student with the most tokens gets to choose a reward from the

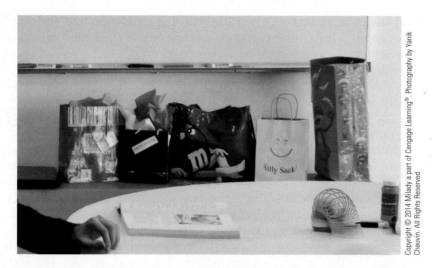

Figure 8–6   Arouse curiosity by placing a brightly colored gift bag in front of the classroom.

prize table. Your token could be stickers, buttons, poker chips, or dried beans. The prize table can be filled with both tangible and intangible items.

- **Group or Growl.** When classes are conducted in small groups, hold the group and group leader accountable for getting the entire bunch back to class on time. Announce that you will give a three-minute warning for the conclusion of the break. Give the group leader responsibility for ensuring that all learners are back to class on time. If group leaders have not already been assigned, use creative ways to delegate leadership. They could range from the person in the group who is the tallest, the oldest, the youngest, has the lightest hair, has been in school the longest, to the one who stands up last!

- **Time Will Tell.** At the beginning of the class, have all students synchronize their watches to an agreed-upon time. When it is time to take a break, designate an atypical amount of time, such as 7 minutes or 11 minutes. Announce, for example, that it is now 9:58 and class will resume at 10:07. This is consistent with taking shorter breaks more often. It causes learners to get physically and mentally involved in complying with the break "rules." You might even write the times for the beginning and ending of the break on the board as a reminder.

- **The Flat Tire.** Remember that all your learners will have legitimate reasons for being tardy from time to time, such as having a flat tire on the way to school. You should never prejudge any of your students. Doing so will only cause an adversarial relationship, which is detrimental to the educational process. Instead, apply all your strategies for dealing with tardy behavior in a positive manner and assume the best from all your learners. If they are, in fact, negligent, they will eventually get the message through the strategies you are employing. If their tardiness is unavoidable, they will appreciate your professionalism in handling them fairly.

- **The Flat Tire Welcome.** By assuming the best of your learners, it is appropriate that you warmly welcome all latecomers in a manner that expresses your sincere appreciation for their presence. Assure them that they will receive any materials already disseminated and you'll arrange for a brief review of material missed. If their reason for being late is legitimate or lazy, they will appreciate not being put on the spot or embarrassed in front of the other learners.

- **Tea for Two.** This is a simple approach of assigning teams of two to monitor each other's attendance and promptness in returning from breaks. It's logical in this instance to ensure teams are composed of at least one person who usually arrives on time.

- **You Pay, We All Pay.** Use the transfer technique and have learners create the "payback" for being late. Once the students have established the "fines" for being tardy, make certain that they are imposed without fail. Fines could include singing a song in front of the class, giving an impromptu speech in front of the class on today's topic, or paying a small fine into the student council fund.

- **No Interruptions, Please.** We've emphasized the need for not interrupting the flow of information delivered in the classroom. Depending upon your institution's tardy policy, latecomers may not even be allowed to enter class once the doors have been closed and class has begun. However, if policy allows them to enter, make sure that interruptions are avoided at all costs (Figure 8–7). When setting guidelines for the classroom, establish that handouts and other relevant materials will be made available to the learner at the break or end of class, whichever comes first. Let them know that they are to take a seat where you designate and that learning for other students is not to be interrupted.

- **Does Your Watch Work?** Involve chronic latecomers in the process of keeping time for the class. Assign them the task of making sure breaks begin on time and that breaks end on time as well. This requires them to be in the classroom as scheduled and helps ensure that all other learners are punctual as well.

- **The Court Convenes.** As with the learner who constantly seeks attention, there may be times when a personal conference or meeting

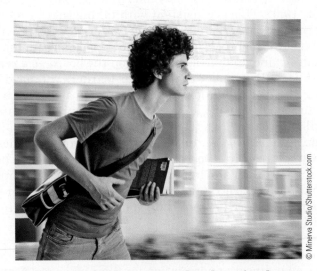

Figure 8–7　Make the chronic latecomer the class timekeeper.

with the student is required. It is important for you to understand the cause of the learner's tardiness. It may be something out of the control of the learner. It may be something that you or the resources available at the school could help eliminate. A conference may allow you to identify such personality characteristics as shyness or being an introvert that cause the student to be late in hopes of avoiding being called upon. Whatever is determined, the master educator will use creative skills to work with the student to find a suitable solution.

Too Shy to Participate

In almost every class, you will encounter a student who is quiet and shy. You will recognize such learners by their lack of outgoing energy and an apparently passive attitude. This behavior can be a challenge if the learner is entering a field that requires lots of energy and outgoing, expressive behavior. Some strategies for this behavior are as follows:

- **Ask the Group.** By employing group questioning, you allow everyone to participate in the answer even if they are too shy to respond individually. You might give small groups a couple of minutes to brainstorm about the answers to questions you pose and then have the group "reporter" state the answer (Figure 8–8). Conversely, you might allow the small group time to brainstorm the questions they would like to ask you, the educator. This ensures that even the most timid students can get their questions answered without having to publicly ask them.
- **Who's the Leader?** When utilizing small groups, make an effort to rotate the leadership role on a fairly frequent basis. This ensures that shy, introverted learners will eventually have the opportunity to serve in the role of leader. They will more likely be willing to lead a small group at first and might eventually become comfortable with taking on larger roles.

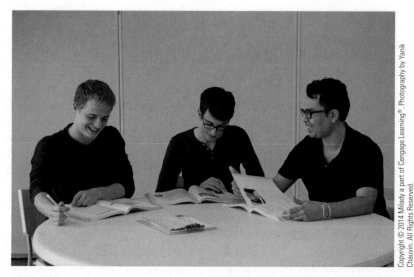

Figure 8–8   Many learners are more comfortable working in small groups.

- **Keep Groups Small.** Learners are more comfortable working with groups of five to seven people. Shy learners will generally be more willing to participate actively with a small group rather than with larger groups. They will want the group to succeed and will likely get involved and make a positive contribution.
- **The Group Writes.** Ask the groups to write their responses to specific, open-ended statements or questions and then read them to their group first. This is an effective tool for getting shy learners to share their thoughts and ideas. The questions should be related to the topic of the class. For example, if you were teaching a class on business management, you might designate the following statements for completion:

  a. The best ways to increase my client base are . . .
  b. The best way to deal with a dissatisfied client is . . .
  c. Coworkers will cooperate better with each other if . . .
  d. When fellow workers do not follow company policy, it makes me feel . . .

Give learners about three minutes to complete the statements and then have them share their responses with their small group. They will begin to observe the similarities and differences within the group responses. Eventually, all members will feel accepted and safe within the confines of their group.

- **Open the Network.** We've talked repeatedly about the importance of using powerful openings for the beginning of classes and presentations. Openers that incorporate networking among the learners are effective at bringing out bashful or shy students. Carefully select opening activities that will help learners get to know one another and will reduce the fear and anxiety felt by shy learners. The few extra minutes spent on such an activity will be rewarded with higher retention of the material by your learners.
- **Why Volunteer?** Shy, introverted behavior usually means these learners are the last to volunteer for anything within the class because they fear embarrassment or being put on the spot. As the facilitator, you can send the message that it is a good thing to volunteer because rewards accompany the risk. Make sure that the first volunteers you select are asked to do something extremely painless and even fun if possible. Make sure they are recognized to show that there need be no fear in volunteering in your classroom. Similarly, you can also ask shy learners to help you with nonverbal tasks such as distributing materials, taping flip chart paper to the walls, or gathering reports from groups. Involving them physically will soon result in better interaction with the whole group.
- **Participation at Will.** Occasionally, you will encounter shy learners who are just not comfortable with open participation. Never employ strategies that force learners to do something they really do not want to do. For example, when you are rotating leaders, if a learner is vehement about not assuming the leader role, by all means, do not force the issue. Usually, the learner will gain support and encouragement from the small-group partners and will eventually take the chance.
- **A Gift for You.** Incentives have been determined to be an effective tool in obtaining learner participation, even for the shyest students. You do not have to spend a great deal of money on rewards and incentives. Something as simple as individually wrapped candy makes learners excited about their accomplishments, however small. Most communities have "dollar stores" that are a great resource for inexpensive prizes. Stickers like those used in elementary school are effective,

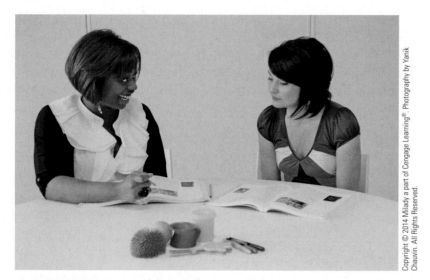

Figure 8–9   **Pair the shy learner with one who is more outgoing for more effective mentoring.**

especially if awarded by other class members. They come in stars and other shapes with brief expressions like "You're great," "Terrific," "Wonderful," "Outstanding," and so on. Have group members apply various stickers to the name tags of other learners during the class to recognize them for their contributions. This small symbolic act tells the learners how appreciated and important they are. Recognition will bring out the best in your shy learners.

- **Match with a Mentor.** When your activities involve pairs, make an effort to match the shy learner with one who is relatively outgoing (Figure 8–9). Take care to ensure that the other learner is not someone so domineering that the shy learner won't be able to participate or contribute. This can work well in career education by pairing more advanced, experienced students with newer students.

- **Link the Learners.** Consider approaching your shy learners privately and ask for specific feedback about what has been discussed in class. Very often, their comments will reflect thoughtful consideration and may be relevant to the small group or entire class. Ask shy learners if they are willing to share their thoughts with either group later. If the learner agrees, you might tell the group about your discussion and then have the learner give the details. This approach allows you to provide the link between this learner and the rest of the group or class, and the shy learner becomes involved. The shy learner may even need private coaching before speaking openly with the group or class. You might let such learners know ahead of time that you are going to call on them with a specific question, which gives them the opportunity to prepare their responses in advance and practice their delivery.

Sleeping in Class or Inattentiveness

Nothing can be more frustrating or disillusioning to an educator than to have a learner who sleeps through class. You may recognize this behavior by something as simple as closed eyes and head nodding off or audible snoring, which is found humorous by the rest of the class. In addition, we've all had students from time to time who appear to be floating about in outer space. They are fairly easy to recognize in that their eyes don't really seem to focus. They may even be preoccupied in other activities such as writing letters or making lists. The challenge for these situations is that absolutely no learning will occur for this student. The material will not even be heard, let alone retained. Some strategies for dealing with this behavior are as follows:

- **"Break" the Break Schedule.** The strategy that works well for tardy behavior is also suitable for inattentiveness. Rather than providing one 15-minute break in the morning and another in the afternoon, consider a 5- to 10-minute break every 45 to 50 minutes. This helps retain learner interest because some people can only focus for so long before their minds wander. Conduct an unplanned, brief break when you notice a learner is fighting to remain awake.

- **Engage the Energizer.** Stretch breaks and energizers can be used to vary the stimuli of the learners and keep learners from nodding off. These can be incorporated into your presentation without breaking the flow of your material. You might have students stand rather than raise their hands when they have a question or have completed an assignment. Allow them to stand until everyone is standing and then they can all take their seats again. This allows everyone the opportunity to stand and stretch during the class. Adding an energizer, such as a crossword puzzle relating to the topic, can capture your learners' interest and get them involved with the learning.

- **What's in It for Me?** These learners need to be constantly reminded of how they will benefit from the training provided. They must see how it will benefit their performance on the job in their new careers and their future success as well.

- **Guide in Groups.** All classes will be more learner-centered if group activities are utilized on a regular basis. Small-group involvement creates interest and usually physical activity that will keep your learners from entering into "dream" world. Have discussion topics or questions prepared in advance that can be assigned to small groups for brainstorming at any low or "sag" point in the presentation.

- **The Unspoken Message.** As stated in the principles of managing learner behavior, a powerful means of gaining a learner's attention is to move toward the learner. The closer you get, the more likely it is that the learner will focus attention on you due to your awareness of them and your presence close to them.

- **Involve the Learner.** If sitting quietly in the classroom is promoting sleep for certain learners, get them physically involved. Designate them as your "hand-out control officers" or use them to record information on flip charts or to post charts on the wall. Physical activity will restore alertness.

- **Vocal Variation.** Remember that *how* you say something represents a large percentage of what your learners hear and retain. By using your voice effectively, you will more effectively retain the interest of your students. Vary the pitch, tone, and pace of your voice and use emphasis for key terms.

- **The Biological Clock.** Most learners need more physical activity in the afternoon to retain the material presented. A master educator will plan mornings around theoretical information that requires more mental concentration. The afternoon can then be used for more practical, hands-on, skills-type training with group activities and physical assignments. Avoid scheduling reading or videos right after lunch. Involve the students in a physical activity immediately after lunch and make every effort to keep them energized for the remainder of the day.

- **What *Not* to Do.** These learners will be able to identify well with humor used to show how something should *not* be done as opposed to demonstrating the proper procedure. Humor will tend to lower the learner's resistance to the objectives of the lesson.

- **Park the Personal.** At the beginning of the class, have all students make a list of the pending activities that must be accomplished before they go to bed that evening. Once they are done, ask them to put the lists away until the class is over. They can now concentrate on the content of the presentation without being worried about all the tasks that await them after class.

- **Pairs for Projects.** Assign learners to work in pairs, which will intensify learner participation.

- **Diversity at Its Best.** The more diverse the format of your classroom, the more your learners will pay attention. We've talked about varying the stimuli, changing the pace, and incorporating numerous group activities and exercises (Figure 8–10). Even inattentive or uninterested learners want approval from their peers and have the opportunity to gain it in small-group activities.

- **From Ordinary to Extraordinary.** Take a few minutes to focus your presentation on any element of it that may be unusual or different. The unexpected can help regain the attention of the preoccupied.

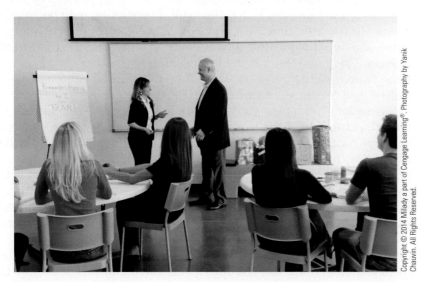

Figure 8–10 **A variety of teaching methods and activities must be employed to prevent boredom and dozing in class.**

- **The Court Convenes.** As with other behaviors, there may be times when a personal conference or meeting with the learner who constantly "nods off" or is totally preoccupied is required. It is important for you to understand the cause of the learner's inability to remain awake or attentive during class. It may be something out of the control of the learner. There may be something that is keeping the student from getting needed sleep or from focusing in class. Explore the possibilities for resolving the problem with the learner.

Distracting Side Conversations

Every class has at least one learner who is constantly engaged in side conversations. These learners also tend to try to monopolize discussions in the classroom. They love to socialize and find out what is going on in every other learner's life. The challenge with these learners is that they cause a major distraction to you, the facilitator, as well as to all other members of the class. Strategies that may be effective for this type of behavior follow.

- **The Unspoken Message.** As stated in the principles of managing learner behavior, a powerful means of controlling side conversations is to physically move toward the learners who are talking. The closer the educator gets, the more likely it is that they will cease the conversation because they will become alert to the educator's awareness and presence.
- **Let the Groups Grade.** As with other difficult behaviors, switching to small-group activities can be effective in curtailing the side conversations held by these learners. The group will usually apply enough peer pressure to eliminate the disruption and inattention. Rotation of group members may be required if the side conversations are between the same two learners.
- **Answer a Question, Ask a Question.** Ask the learners who are in conversation if they need an answer to a specific question or clarification of a point made in the presentation. If they do, you will be able to address it and move on. If not, the brief interruption may be enough to end the conversation. Also, you can address one of the offenders by name and direct a question at that learner regarding the topic of discussion. This requires that the learner focus attention on the matter at hand to answer the question. The side conversation will cease.
- **Pause and Whisper.** As we discussed in Chapter 7, "Effective Presentations", stopping your delivery for even a few seconds can really grab the attention of the learners in the room. During your pause, focus your eye contact on those engaged in the side conversation. Usually, when they find themselves the only ones speaking, they will quickly cease. When they do, thank them and continue. Another option is to greatly reduce your voice volume. Like the pause, this causes the voices of those in the side conversation to become louder and more noticeable. Other learners will usually try to quiet those socializing in the attempt to hear what you are saying.
- **The Court Convenes.** If your other strategies have failed in getting the learners to cease the disrupting side conversations, it may be time to announce a short break and initiate a private discussion with the learners about the behavior. They may not even be aware that the side conversations have been so disruptive to the other learners and to you. If the problem is of a chronic nature, it may be time for a scheduled

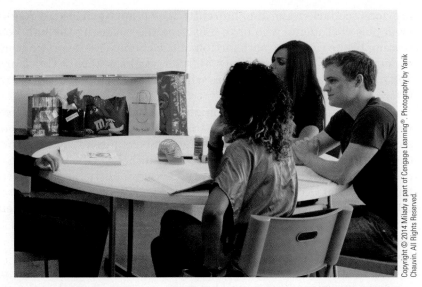

Figure 8–11 **Do not allow side conversations to distract other members of the class.**

private conference to really get to the bottom of the problem. You may have to show the learner you are human and explain how distracting it is for you to have learners not focused on the important material at hand. Explain that it would really be a great help to you if the side conversations were avoided (Figure 8–11). Many times, when learners see how much it matters to you, they feel they are contributing with their cooperation, and that makes them feel important and appreciated.

Doubt and Pessimism

Some individuals that find their way into your classroom are just eternal pessimists. You will be able to recognize them by their negative body language and their constant argument that what you are suggesting will never work. The problem arising from these learners is that you might be caught off guard by their challenges if you are not sufficiently prepared. Possible solutions for dealing with this behavior are as follows:

- **Just the Facts, Please.** Be prepared to present facts, figures, historical data, and other information that will give concrete support to the concepts or information you are presenting. This learner is not as interested in opinion as she is in hard factual data.
- **Ask Why.** When faced with the inevitable statement that your theories will never work, don't let the learner stop there. Ask the learner to explain why your concept, procedure, or principles will not work. Often, you learn that their doubt has little to do with the topic at hand. In fact, it may be nothing more than the learner's fear of change that causes the problems. The learner may be so uncomfortable with a change to an already-mastered procedure that the learner refuses to believe it will work. Communication is the key. Engage the learner in sufficient dialogue to determine what it will take to turn that opinion around.
- **For Example.** When you can offer real-world examples of how something works, the naysayer will begin to accept your ideas. Using the

previous scenario regarding haircutting, you might choose to give examples of students who have mastered the cut using the half-head parting to the complete satisfaction of the client. The reverse of the old elementary school activity, show and tell, works well with this learner. Tell *and* show and these learners will be more receptive to your information.

• **Stand Up and Testify.** Testimonials from prior learners are a great way to convince today's pessimist that something really works. Consider having more advanced students who have already taken your class return to share their experiences with the specific technique or procedure that you are covering in the lesson. This helps to show the naysayers that the concept really works.

• **Disarm and Diffuse.** When faced with a blatant negative comment from the learner, smile and say something like, "You may be right … this procedure may not work well for you. If you'll bear with me, though, I'd like to show you how I've made it work for me. In fact, I can even show you how lots of students before you have made it work using some minor modifications. Our main concern, after all, is the end result, isn't it?" This approach removes any atmosphere of confrontation and usually gets the learner to focus on what the class is really all about.

• **Convene the Court.** If you are faced with a chronic doubter who challenges every class or concept, it may be time to initiate a private conference to get to the bottom of the issue. This is a great opportunity to employ your active listening skills, which include the use of the words *feel, felt,* and *found.* It works like this: You might say, "I can certainly understand why you *feel* that way. Actually, other students have *felt* that way at this point in their training too. But they *found* that when they practiced long enough, these techniques ultimately produced the desired results." Notice that you have not told the student "you are wrong." You have not said "I am right." You have displayed empathy by stating your understanding of the learner's perspective. The learner now realizes that you are concerned about the opinions of your students and is no longer armed for battle. It might be appropriate to follow up with, "So, the issue is not whether the procedure will work, but whether you are willing to invest the time and effort to learn it. Why don't we get started?"

Having All the Answers

We have all been in classes with students who have the answer to everything, or at least think they do. They are fairly easy to identify because they have a comment for every single issue. It's important for the master educator to be able to discern whether these learners really have a great deal of knowledge or if they simply *think* they do. The challenge faced with this behavior is that the enthusiasm and overt participation can squelch the participation of the other learners. Some strategies for handling this behavior follow:

• **What Do You Really Know?** Master educators will learn to incorporate *pretesting* into their educational process. This technique can be helpful in many areas, including letting you identify those students who have a strong grasp of the material and those who simply act as if they do.

- **Match with a Mentor.** When your activities involve pairs, make an effort to match the overenthusiastic learner with a slower learner. Ask the one with all the answers to explain the procedure or coach the other student in the technique. This can work well in career education by pairing more advanced, experienced students with newer students.
- **Help Is on the Way.** If these learners do, in fact, know most of the answers or information, solicit their help with special projects. They might be useful in designing and creating flip charts for the topics of the day. Get them involved in reports, monitoring group activities, and helping other learners throughout the class. They will feel needed, appreciated, and important while helping other learners get the most from the class.
- **The Impossible Opening.** A simple technique for showing these learners that they, in fact, do not "know it all" is to open with an exercise for which they will not have all the answers. This could be something as simple as asking them to draw a touch-tone telephone keypad (with both numbers and letters) or completing a brain teaser or puzzle. Students will not be able to do either with 100 percent accuracy. This helps to put these learners into the correct frame of mind for learning more.
- **Questions, Questions, Who Has a Question?** Meet with this learner on break and ask him if he would be willing to take questions on the subject at hand from the entire group. If he is confident in his knowledge, he will be more than willing. If he is not, he will likely deny the opportunity and minimize his "know it all" attitude during the remainder of the presentation.

Conflict Management

In a classroom filled with adult learners from diverse backgrounds and cultures where choices exist, the potential for disagreement will always exist. When those differences are handled in a proper manner, effective interaction and creative solutions can be the result. The master educator's goal should be to turn the differences into opportunities for learning and opportunities for building relationships. If effective solutions are not reached, psychological distance between the parties may exist and create competition, disregard, alienation, or just simple dislike.

Students will definitely differ in their sensitivity or response to the actions and comments of others. Everyone needs to find a constructive outlet that will allow dissipation of the resulting stress. Practicing random acts of kindness, reading, exercise, or meditation may all be effective at channelling negative feelings and reducing the buildup of steam before it actually explodes. However, when any type of conflict exists between two individuals, the only viable solution is working through the difficulties together, even though yielding or avoiding the issue entirely may be the first choice. We should never assume there is no possible solution for a conflict or disagreement. Effective dialogue should not only resolve the challenge but also reduce stress and increase productivity. As human beings, we instinctively adopt a "position" when faced with a disagreement. Usually, that position is established around our personal concerns, needs, and fears. That means that the parties involved in the disagreement have likely adopted two very different positions, which create contention from the onset.

CONSIDER AND CONNECT

You will have far fewer difficult learners as compared to those who sincerely want to learn, but it is helpful to learn and practice effective strategies to ensure that every class you teach achieves the maximum potential for learning for all students present.

CONSIDER AND CONNECT

The master educator's goal regarding conflict management should be to turn differences into opportunities for learning and building relationships.

FOUR ENEMIES OF CONFLICT MANAGEMENT AND RELATIONSHIP BUILDING

1. I go first. We all think if we get a chance to explain our perspective first, the other party will totally understand and give up.
2. Ineffective listening. Hearing is not listening. We must all practice active, empathetic listening.
3. Fear. We are reluctant to enter negotiation because we are afraid we won't get the desired outcome. We are afraid that we may not "win" or that we might be made to look stupid. We may even fear that we are actually wrong.
4. No one wins. Perhaps the greatest enemy of effective conflict management is the assumption that if one of us wins, the other one loses. We may believe that the only way a solution can be reached is through out-and-out competition.

Conflict management
conflict management involves implementing strategies to limit and manage negative aspects of conflict and to enhance learning and group effectiveness or performance in an educational setting.

Conflict management could be reframed as "effective communication." Steven Covey offered one important concept in his book *Seven Habits of Highly Effective People*. This principle is "Seek first to understand, then to be understood." In other words, let the other person go first and they might be more likely to actually listen to your perspective on the situation. Another important principle has been identified by Roger Fisher and William Ury, who maintain that people in disagreement should focus on their "needs" rather than their "positions." If you think about it, when our focus is on our position, the entire dialogue is about why there is disagreement. If we focus on our mutual needs, we might actually find some common ground from which to move forward. Our ultimate goal should be a "win–win" situation. We need to learn to work through our disagreements and agree to disagree in an amicable manner.

While effective listening is critical in the conflict management process, we must not make the mistake of giving up on our needs entirely. For example, after listening thoroughly to the other person's point of view, we might follow up with, "I understand how you feel even though we look at this issue from different perspectives. I'm anxious to share my thoughts on this, but I want to focus on your needs and ideas first. So, help me understand why you feel the way you do." Of course, the real challenge may be the inability to really listen without interrupting with objections or arguments.

On occasion, it may be necessary to involve a third party in conflict management (Figure 8–12). Telling students to shake hands and get along will not create an acceptable solution even if it sends the problem into the shadows for a short while. It will likely resurface in the future. When selecting a third party, remember that the involved individuals should respect the third party's integrity, impartiality, and ability. Visual aids can often help in the conflict management process. Since our goal is to focus on needs rather than positions, creating a chart that helps clarify that process might be of assistance. Create a table on a flip chart or board with two headings: Participant

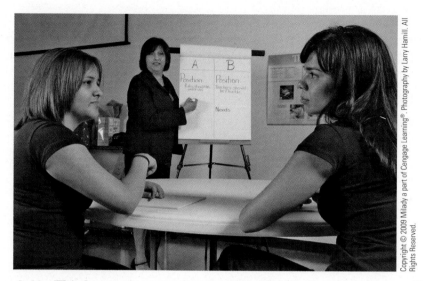

Figure 8–12 **Third-party intervention is often effective in managing conflict between learners.**

A and Participant B with subheadings "Position" and "Needs." They will then take turns and seek to understand and record the needs of the other person. They are free to restate, modify, and clarify the position. After both have completed the "position" portion of the exercise, have them move into the "needs" portion. They should take the time to ask effective questions of each other. They should brainstorm about how to fulfill the needs. Solutions that require no further interactions should be resisted. It is hoped that participants can develop tentative coauthored agreements and record them. Part of their plan should be to evaluate the results at predetermined time periods and then fine-tune the agreements as needed or as they encounter further challenges.

Wrapping It Up

The responsibility of creating a positive classroom environment challenges educators to use their skills as leaders, teachers, supervisors, managers, advisors, disciplinarians, and student advocates. The master educator who learns to balance each of these roles effectively will be rewarded with positive and stimulating learner experiences in the classroom. Educators need to skillfully integrate organizational and communication skills to effectively manage a classroom. Educators must ensure that their classrooms are safe environments in which their students can learn.

Master educators will inform students of what to expect and they will make themselves available for students to discuss issues of importance and relevance to learner progress through the course or program. They will address challenges consistently and uniformly as they arise in the classroom. The master educator will strive to develop and maintain high levels of student motivation and interest in an effort to minimize disciplinary challenges in the classroom.

In Retrospect

1. Explain low-profile and direct, high-profile control techniques that are used in dealing with learner misconduct.

2. Explain specific techniques used in remedying misconduct.

3. Explain the difference between a situational barrier to learning and a chronic barrier to learning.

4. Describe various difficult learner behaviors and explain methods for managing them.

5. List and explain four enemies of conflict management.

Objectives (Desired Performance Goals):

After reading and studying this chapter, you should be able to:

- List "major life activities."

- Define the term *learning disability*.

- Explain the four stages of information processing in learning.

- Use questions to help determine if a student is projecting symptoms of dyslexia and ADHD.

- List symptomatic chronic behaviors of students.

- List strategies for alleviating learner anxiety.

- State three strategies for fast-paced learners.

! CRITICAL CONCEPT

Master educators impact learners more by what they do and who they are than by what they say.

Special Learning Needs

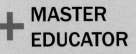

Americans with Disabilities Act in front of ADA
The Americans with Disabilities Act signed into law in 1990.

major life activities
human functions, including caring for self, performing manual tasks, walking, seeing, hearing, speaking, breathing, learning, and working.

THE ULTIMATE GOAL of this text is to help educators achieve successful learner results. Therefore, considerable time has been spent on the qualities and characteristics of different learner types as well as how to deal with various difficult behaviors exhibited by learners. In this chapter, we will attempt to explain techniques that can be employed with learners who have special needs and those with chronic behavior concerns (Figure 9–1). In addition, we will consider general barriers to learning and how they can be overcome.

The provisions of Title III of the Americans with Disabilities Act (ADA) of 1990 prohibit discrimination against people with disabilities. The protection is similar to that which has been provided to women, minorities, and others since the Civil Rights Act of 1964. Over 50 million Americans, 18 percent of the population, with physical or mental impairments that limit daily activities are protected under the ADA. According to the brochure published by the Office on the Americans with Disabilities Act, *Title III Highlights*, an individual with a disability is one who:

- has a physical or mental impairment that substantially limits one or more "major life activities," or
- has a history or record of such an impairment, or
- is regarded by others as having such an impairment.

"**Major life activities**" include functions such as caring for self, performing manual tasks, walking, seeing, hearing, speaking, breathing, learning, and working. Individuals who *currently* engage in the illegal use of drugs are not protected by the ADA when an action is taken on the basis of their current illegal use of drugs.

The document continues to provide examples of physical or mental impairments that include, but are not limited to, such contagious and noncontagious diseases and conditions as orthopedic, visual, speech, and hearing impairments; cerebral palsy; epilepsy; muscular dystrophy; multiple

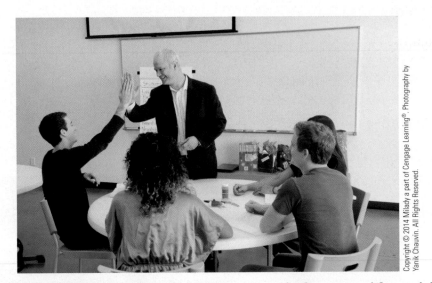

Figure 9–1   Employ a variety of techniques to assist learners with special needs.

sclerosis; cancer; heart diseases; diabetes; mental retardation; emotional illness; specific learning disabilities; HIV disease (whether symptomatic or asymptomatic); tuberculosis; drug addiction; and alcoholism. Homosexuality and bisexuality are not physical or mental impairments under the ADA.

The ADA prohibits discrimination on the basis of disability in both public- and private-sector employment, services rendered by state and local governments, places of public accommodation (including private career schools), and transportation and telecommunications services. The ADA sets forth parameters for removing barriers that deny individuals with disabilities equal opportunity to share in and contribute to the vitality of American life. The ADA means access to jobs, public accommodations, government services, public transportation, and telecommunication. The intention is that Americans with disabilities will have full participation in, and access to, all aspects of society.

Title III Highlights explains that places of public accommodation, including private career schools, have several specific requirements to meet:

* They must remove barriers to make their goods and services available and usable by people with disabilities to the extent that it is readily achievable to do so. "Readily achievable" means to the extent that needed changes can be easily accomplished and carried out without much difficulty or expense.
* Furnish auxiliary aids when necessary to ensure effective communication for those with sensory or cognitive disabilities, unless an undue burden or fundamental alteration would result.
* Make reasonable modifications in policies, practices, and procedures that deny equal access to individuals with disabilities, unless a fundamental alteration would result in the nature of the goods, services, or training provided.
* Eliminate unnecessary eligibility standards or rules that deny individuals with disabilities an equal opportunity to enjoy the goods and services of the place of accommodation.

The Americans with Disabilities Act Title III Technical Assistance Manual explains that some general requirements of the ADA with regard to courses offered by institutions include modifying the course to ensure that the place and manner in which the course is given are accessible. Examples of possible modifications that might be required include extending the time permitted for completion of the course, providing auxiliary aids or services, and offering the course in an accessible location or making alternative accessible arrangements. Alternative arrangements must provide comparable conditions to those provided to others, including similar lighting, room temperature, and the like. The institution must ensure that the course materials provided are available in alternate formats that individuals with disabilities can use.

If the course uses published materials that are available from other sources, the institution offering the course is not responsible for providing them in alternate formats. The institution should, however, inform students in advance of what materials will be used so that an individual with a disability can obtain them in a usable format.

In addition, an institution offering a variety of courses may not limit the selection or choice of courses available to individuals with disabilities.

CONSIDER AND CONNECT

One example of providing assistance might be class handouts in Braille or on audio cassettes for individuals with visual impairments.

Courses offered to fulfill a continuing education requirement for a profession, for example, are covered by the requirement that they be offered in an accessible place and manner, and an entity that offers such courses may not designate particular courses for individuals with disabilities and refuse to make other courses accessible.

Persons with disabilities who desire to enroll in a postsecondary institution have the responsibility of providing documentation of their disability and making a formal request for accommodations and access to classes. When students make such a report and request, it is the responsibility of the institution to provide an *individual accommodation plan* for that learner. The accommodation plan offered by the institution provides the necessary information for the learner regarding the steps the school is able to reasonably take to accommodate the individual's special needs (Figure 9–2). If the learner does not report a special need to the school, the school is not responsible by law to provide specific accommodations. However, the school may later determine that reasonable accommodations should be made for the student and can make those accommodations based on the school's desire to do so.

The accommodation plan might include implementing the use of auxiliary aids and services such as qualified interpreters, listening devices, note takers, and written materials for individuals with hearing impairments or qualified readers, taped texts, and Braille or large-print materials for individuals with vision impairments. Remember, however, that the ADA does not require the provision of any auxiliary aid that would result in an undue burden or in a fundamental alteration in the nature of the goods or services provided by the institution. Instead, the institution may provide alternative auxiliary aids, if available, that would not result in undue burden or alteration of services.

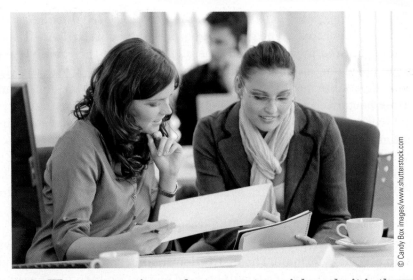

Figure 9–2   When prospective students report special needs, it is the responsibility of the school to provide an individual accommodation plan for each learner.

Learning Disabilities

In North America, the term *learning disability* refers to a group of disorders that affect a broad range of academic and functional skills, including the ability to read, speak, listen, spell, reason, and organize information. It must be made clear, however, that a learning disability is not necessarily indicative of low intelligence. It has been determined that people with learning disabilities may have difficulty achieving their potential because of a deficit in one or more ways the brain processes information.

The National Dissemination Center for Children with Disabilities (NICHY) states that learning disabilities fall into broad categories based on the four stages of information processing used in learning. The categories are input, integration, storage, and output.

- **Input.** This is the information perceived through the senses, such as visual and auditory perception. Difficulties with visual perception can cause problems with recognizing the shape, position, and size of items seen. Problems can occur with sequencing, which can relate to deficits with processing time intervals or temporal perception. Difficulties with auditory perception can make it difficult to screen out competing sounds in order to focus on one of them, such as the sound of the teacher's voice. Some students appear to be unable to process tactile input. For example, they may seem insensitive to pain or may dislike being touched.

- **Integration.** This is the stage during which perceived input is interpreted, categorized, placed in a sequence, or related to previous learning. Students with problems in these areas may be unable to tell a story in the correct sequence, be unable to memorize sequences of information such as the days of the week, be able to understand a new concept but be unable to generalize it to other areas of learning, or able to learn facts but be unable to put the facts together to see the "big picture." A poor vocabulary may contribute to problems with comprehension.

- **Storage.** Problems with memory can occur with short-term, or working, memory or with long-term memory. Most memory difficulties occur in the area of short-term memory, which can make it difficult to learn new material without many more repetitions than is usual. Difficulties with visual memory can impede learning to spell.

- **Output.** Information comes out of the brain either through words, that is, language output, or through muscle activity, such as gesturing, writing, or drawing. Difficulties with language output can create problems with spoken language, for example, answering a question on demand, in which one must retrieve information from storage, organize thoughts, and put the thoughts into words before speaking. It can also cause trouble with written language for the same reasons. Difficulties with motor abilities can cause problems with gross and fine motor skills. People with gross motor difficulties may be clumsy. They may be prone to stumbling, falling, or bumping into things. They may also have trouble running, climbing, or learning to ride a bicycle. People with small motor difficulties may have trouble buttoning shirts, tying shoelaces, or with handwriting.

learning disability
a group of disorders that affect a broad range of academic and functional skills, including the ability to read, speak, listen, spell, reason, and organize information; it does not necessarily indicate low intelligence.

input
one of four stages of information processing used in learning; the information perceived through the senses, such as visual and auditory perception.

integration
one of four stages of information processing used in learning; in this stage perceived input is interpreted, categorized, placed in a sequence, or related to previous learning.

storage
one of four stages of information processing used in learning.

output
one of four stages of information processing used in learning; in this stage, information comes out of the brain either through words (language output) or muscle activity (gesturing, writing, or drawing).

THE FOUR STAGES OF INFORMATION PROCESSING

1. Input: perceiving information through the senses.
2. Integration: Interpreting, categorizing, and placing in sequence; relating to previous learning.
3. Storage: Short-term and long-term memory.
4. Output: Information comes out of the brain through words or movement.

Some of the more common disabilities that affect learning are reviewed in this chapter in an effort to help educators recognize them and to provide techniques or strategies that may improve the educational process. Master educators will take every step possible to achieve learning results for all students, regardless of their abilities.

☑ Dyslexia

dyslexia
a neurologically based, specific learning disability that hinders the learning of literacy or reading skills and creates a problem with managing verbal codes in memory.

Dyslexia is a specific learning disability that is an impairment in the brain's ability to translate written images received from the eyes into meaningful language. The term *dyslexia* comes from an ancient Greek word meaning *difficulty with words*. It hinders the learning of literacy or reading skills. It creates a problem with managing verbal codes in memory. It is neurologically based and has now been firmly established as a congenital and developmental condition. Symbolic systems such as musical notes or mathematics may also be affected. It can occur at any level of intellectual ability. Sometimes dyslexia is accompanied by lack of motivation, emotional disturbance, or sensory impairment. The cause of dyslexia has not been confirmed. As an educator, you may find that 15 percent to 20 percent of your students experience language-based learning disabilities.

Symptoms of Dyslexia. An educator can ask a number of questions to determine whether learners who are age 12 to adult may have a potential problem. If the answer to the majority of the following questions is yes, the educator should refer the student to a specialist for advice:

- Does the student read slowly with many inaccuracies?
- Does the student have difficulty filling in forms?
- Is the student shy and holds back in discussions?
- Does the student avoid reading and writing tasks?
- Does the student spell incorrectly and frequently spell the same word differently in a single document?
- Does the student have trouble answering open-ended questions on tests?
- Does the student work slowly?
- Does the student have poor short-term memory skills?
- Does the student have an inadequate vocabulary?
- Is the student bright in some ways but experiences complete "blocks" in other ways?
- Does the student experience difficulty when taking notes or copying written work?

IT'S WORTH REMEMBERING ✳

Imagine how a young person with a learning disability must feel when no one can see or understand that there is anything wrong. Imagine the disappointment they feel when they appear to frustrate their parents, their peers, and their teachers. Imagine their own frustration knowing that they are actually intelligent, even though they may have some specific challenges.

- Does the student experience difficulty with planning and writing essay assignments or responding to test questions?
- Does another family member of the student experience similar difficulties?

A common problem with dyslexic learners is that they often appear to be displaying other characteristics to the educator. For example, it may appear to you that the learner is just not listening, is lazy, is careless and doesn't check the work, is not concentrating, or is being awkward or difficult on purpose. Very likely these perceptions are inaccurate. Educators will often find that dyslexic learners have a good "visual eye"; they are imaginative and skillful with their hands; they are practical; they often excel at individual sports; and they may have a wonderful imagination.

If a student is unsure whether she is subject to a learning disability such as dyslexia, she can ask herself a series of questions. In addition, you may refer the student to www.dyslexia-test.com for an inexpensive test or to a professional diagnostician to make a formal determination regarding learning disabilities. The self-questions are as follows:

- When writing checks, do you frequently find yourself making mistakes?
- When using the telephone, do you tend to get the numbers mixed up when you dial?
- Is your spelling poor?
- Do you mix up dates and times and miss appointments?
- Do you find forms difficult and confusing?
- Do you find it difficult to take messages on the telephone and pass them on correctly?
- Do you transpose numbers, such as 95 for 59?
- Do you find it difficult to say the months of the year in order in a fluent manner?
- Did you find it hard to learn your multiplication tables at school?
- Do you take longer than you should to read a page of a book?
- Do you have difficulty in telling left from right?
- When you have to say a long word, do you sometimes find it difficult to get all the sounds in the right order?

Teaching Dyslexic Learners. The goal of every master educator ✓ should be to teach every student to become an independent learner. The educator should review the learner's past academic file, if it is available, and gain a clear understanding of the student's specific difficulties and individual learning style. Only then can teaching strategies be employed that address the individual learner.

A master educator will attempt to make every required topic one of interest for the student and employ teaching strategies that engage and address the individual learning style for each student. Dyslexic learners have a great need for efficient time and task management, which will give them a sense of control and mastery over their own lives. This will help to overcome the many frustrations they experience daily. The educator should evaluate the student's learning and study environment and assist the student in keeping desk space arranged for easy location and access of materials. In addition, the educator should provide assistance with time management, whether it is having the student keep a daily log or journal or posting a month-by-month or program-at-a-glance wall

CONSIDER AND CONNECT

Dyslexic learners need to understand the "how and why" of what they are learning and be involved in the learning process.

planner. Also, having students color-code files or tabs of information helps them keep it organized and properly sequenced.

Some teaching tips for educators of dyslexic learners are as follows:

- Whenever possible, use highly focused teaching in groups of two or three students.
- Implement peer coaching and mentoring.
- Maintain a sense of humor and make learning fun.
- Work at a gradual pace and break information into small, manageable chunks.
- Give acknowledgment, recognition, and praise for good work.
- Use structured multisensory methods for teaching and have students use multisensory methods for practicing and learning (use visual, auditory, tactile, and kinesthetic methods, including games, activities, humor, and technology).
- Reassure learners that their difficulties are not their fault; be encouraging and find things they are good at.
- Encourage hobbies, interests, and extracurricular activities.
- Find something the learners are good at and focus on their strengths.
- Mark written work on content rather than spelling; check what is correct rather than what is incorrect.
- Leave notes on the board as long as possible if learners are being asked to copy them.
- Use written notes and lists rather than prose.
- Use color in visual aids; have students use colored pens and highlighters.
- Employ mind mapping and window paning (as discussed in Volume I).
- Teach learners good study skills.
- Before exams, have learners check to see that they have thorough notes and give them the opportunity to have their notes checked for omissions or errors.

Considerations for Handout Development

- Use clean, larger font such as Arial.
- Use left justification.
- Include diagrams and visual information such as mind maps.
- Do not start a sentence at the end of a line.
- Use boldface type to emphasize information rather than italics or underlining.
- Avoid using abbreviations.
- Use colored paper or colored film overlays with a matt finish; color effectiveness may vary by learner.

Some behaviors to avoid when teaching dyslexic learners are as follows:

- Do not ridicule or employ sarcasm (this should never be done with any learner).
- Do not make dyslexic learners read aloud in the classroom if they do not wish to.
- Do not compare the dyslexic learner's work with that of other students.
- Do not correct every single mistake made in written work; this will be too discouraging.

Some thoughts educators should remember about dyslexic learners are that they

* may not get the sense of a paragraph or chapter, even though they read it correctly.
* tire more quickly than learners who are not dyslexic; learning requires far greater concentration for people with dyslexia.
* may have difficulty with figures or musical notes.
* may omit words or write words twice.
* suffer from their own uncertainty in how to process words.
* have difficulty taking notes because they cannot listen and write simultaneously.
* feel constant time constraints because they read slowly.
* are often personally disorganized and may be clumsy or forgetful even when trying very hard.

Attention Deficit Disorder or Attention Deficit Hyperactivity Disorder (ADHD)

Attention deficit hyperactivity disorder (ADHD), is defined by the American Academy of Pediatrics as "a chronic neurological dysfunction within the central nervous system and is not related to gender, level of intelligence, or cultural environment." The cause of this disorder is still unknown, although some environmental factors, including diet and parenting techniques, appear to affect it. ADHD appears to run within families but the pattern of inheritance is not yet clear.

Some medications that are taken to treat other ailments or health concerns may also make ADHD symptoms worse. Statistically, between 3 percent and 8 percent of school-age children are diagnosed with ADHD; of those diagnosed, males outnumber females by a ratio of 3 or 4 to 1. More than half the children diagnosed continue to have problems into adulthood. It has been determined that most people known to have ADHD also have average or above-average intelligence and ability.

Symptoms of ADHD. Students with ADHD are natural multitaskers and pay attention to everything simultaneously. The educator can watch for a number of symptoms, as listed next, to determine if a student may have ADHD. If the symptoms are serious enough, the educator should refer the learner to a specialist for a complete analysis and diagnosis.

* Inattention. Learners with ADHD have problems staying on required tasks, especially if they are not interested in the subject matter.
* Hyperactivity. Learners with ADHD are always active, fidgeting, moving; doing one thing at a time is boring to them.
* Impulsiveness. Learners with ADHD often act before they think about what they are doing.
* Forgetfulness. Forgets things and loses needed items, such as books and pens.
* Social Ineptness. Learners with ADHD often have problems interacting with family or peers. They may talk excessively and interrupt frequently.

attention deficit hyperactivity disorder (ADHD) attention deficit hyperactivity disorder, a chronic neurological dysfunction within the central nervous system that is not related to gender, level of intelligence, or cultural environment.

IT'S WORTH REMEMBERING ✳

In some cases, diet, such as sensitivity to certain artificial flavors and certain types of foods, may make ADHD problems worse.

- Multiple Settings. Learners with ADHD usually display behavioral problems in at least two environments, such as school and home or school and work.
- Inconsistency and Continuity. The problems learners with ADHD experience usually continue over a long period of time, even though the behaviors are variable and inconsistent. In fact, the learners with ADHD may at times be the model student and at other times the educator's worst nightmare.

Research shows that many hyperactive youngsters do become less "hyper" as they grow older, but they continue to have problems with inattention, impulsiveness, and social interaction skills. You may notice this as fidgeting, twitching, or constantly moving in the classroom. If not treated effectively, ADHD can lead to chemical dependency, poor social outcomes, and even problems with the law. If appropriately treated and with appropriate family and social support, many individuals with ADHD develop effective coping strategies and achieve rewarding and creative careers. In addition to professional treatment, learners with ADHD should seek support from their family, school and work associates, and friends. Acceptance by others is critical to their success. Learners with ADHD need to work on both educational and social development and conduct self-monitoring on an ongoing basis. Building self-esteem and setting goals are essential for them to attain optimal living. Most of all, they must be encouraged to persevere—to never quit! The master educator can be highly beneficial in providing the encouragement that learners with ADHD need.

Teaching Learners with ADHD. Master educators will attempt to provide needed support to learners with ADHD while also encouraging growth. Specific strategies can be employed to foster independence and self-support. Educators should try lower-level accommodations first and move into higher-level accommodations only if necessary. Some strategies that have proven beneficial include:

- Seat learners in a quiet area without distractions, especially when they need to study or take tests.
- Whenever possible, give them room to move about and release excess energy.
- Tell students in advance what they can expect to learn (Figure 9–3).
- Prepare students in advance for changes in routine, such as theory to lab or theory to field trips.

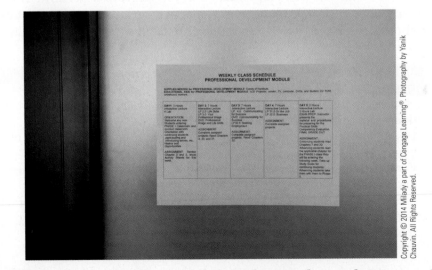

Figure 9–3   Posting a weekly schedule helps learners know what to expect.

- Provide assignments and instructions both in writing and orally.
- Follow a consistent schedule that is posted in the classroom or given to each student.
- Provide a printed outline to learners prior to the lesson or lecture.
- If possible, provide a note taker to record comments made during classroom discussions and lectures.
- Divide projects or assignments into shorter, sequential segments.
- Provide regular guidance and supervision to avoid procrastination and miscalculation by the learner.
- Allow sufficient time for the learner with ADHD to thoughtfully consider questions and prepare answers.
- Develop a system of discreet "cues" that will alert learners in advance that you are going to call on them for a response.
- Identify the learners with ADHD's strengths and present or teach to those strengths.
- Use high-impact audiovisual aids.
- As with learners with dyslexia (and all other learners), avoid sarcasm or criticism at all times.
- Allow learners to request the educator to review homework or written assignments after the first few items have been completed for confirmation that the assignment is being done correctly.
- Give practice quizzes prior to the official tests.
- Consider alternative testing methods that will also demonstrate what the student has learned.
- Never use hand-written tests or handouts. They should be typed, clear, and easy to read.
- Provide learners with training in study skills, test-taking skills, organizational skills, and time management skills.
- Train learners in alternative methods of note taking, such as mind mapping or window paning (Figure 9–4).
- Learn to recognize skill deficits on the part of learners with ADHD rather than assuming they are simply not complying with instructions.
- Provide immediate feedback to learners with ADHD every time desired behavior or performance has been achieved. Be positive.
- Never reprimand publicly; provide public recognition for learner accomplishments.
- Provide rules and consequences in a clearly stated manner and ensure that they are consistently carried out for all learners.

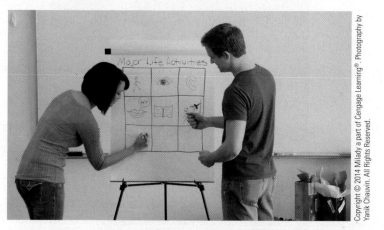

Figure 9–4 Window paning provides students with an alternative form of note taking as well as allows them to break the information into manageable chunks.

Master educators take personal steps to become knowledgeable about all learning disorders or disabilities in order to be better equipped to facilitate learning for those who experience them. Master educators accept the characteristics of learners with ADHD, especially their inconsistent performance. They recognize that learners with ADHD especially require an academically, emotionally, and socially safe environment in which to learn. We must also recognize that no two learners with ADHD are alike and that multiple approaches must be employed with each student. We must be flexible and learn to accept behavior or performance that may not meet the standards we have established for other learners. We must certainly recognize that the learners' poor performance is not due to laziness, poor motivation, or other internal characteristics.

Research indicates that a twitch or fidget is a sensory input, and to be effective, the second sensory-motor activity is one different than that needed for the primary activity (Figure 9–5). The effective second sensory-motor activity, such as tapping a pencil or foot, clicking a pen, twirling hair, clicking a pen, or listening to music, will help the learner stay alert and focused on the primary and important learning activity. A master educator will facilitate effective twitching for the learners with ADHD as long as the twitching or fidgeting is respectful of other learners and does not bother or distract them. We might think of it as "twitching to transformation." For example, the educator might facilitate the various sensory modalities, such as sight, sound, movement, taste, smell, and touch, by using color or computer games, music, or clicking timers; having students exercise, handout materials, or suck on hard candy; and giving students access to scented markers or candles, Koosh balls, or Slinkies. At each learning center, consider placing the following: colored sticky notes, scented markers, hard candy, a Koosh ball, a Slinky, a ruler, a worry stone, tape, and so forth.

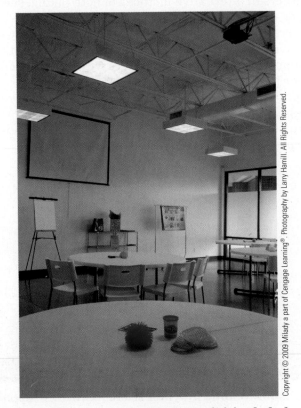

Figure 9–5   Effective second sensory-motor activities help learners stay alert and focused.

Educators should recognize that the goal of independence for these learners may be achieved only when:

- appropriate supports are consistently provided;
- learners have mastered time management and planning; and
- learners feel in control and comfortable.

Chronic Behaviors

According to the National Institute on Alcohol Abuse and Alcoholism (NIAAA), nearly 14 million Americans (1 in every 13 adults) abuse alcohol or are alcoholics. Several million more adults engage in risky drinking patterns. The costs to society in terms of lost productivity, health care costs, traffic accidents, and personal tragedies are overwhelming. According to the Alcohol Drug Abuse Help and Resource Center, the most recent estimate of the overall economic cost of alcohol abuse is over $185 billion annually. Absenteeism in the workforce is estimated to be four to eight times greater among alcoholics and alcohol abusers. The Substance Abuse and Mental Health Services Administration (SAMHSA) reports that approximately 16.5 million of the current users of illicit drugs in the United States hold full-time jobs.

These reports indicate that an extremely large percentage of America's workforce has some type of chronic negative behavior.

It is helpful for educators to learn to recognize symptomatic chronic behaviors, as discussed next.

> **CONSIDER AND CONNECT**
>
> Educators can expect to encounter chronic behaviors in their adult classrooms and must be prepared to deal with them.

Symptomatic Chronic Behaviors

Such symptomatic behaviors include, but are not limited to:

- Inattentiveness or memory lapses
- Poor attendance
- Improper diet
- Poor motivation and lack of interest
- Inability to reason or function adequately
- Physical weakness or debilitation
- Hallucinations or delusions
- Poor self-esteem
- Inappropriate responses to various circumstances or situations
- Inability to be productive

Coping with Chronic Behavior

Educators should not attempt to label learners or even diagnose chronic behavioral problems. If a learner exhibits any of the behaviors just listed, the learner should be referred to an appropriate professional source. It is likely that the learner can be helped with proper diagnosis and treatment. Remember that these individuals may be protected as "handicapped" or disabled persons who have the right to file discrimination complaints against educators and institutions if they are not carefully and appropriately handled. Should such a lawsuit be filed, the educator and/or institution must be able to show that the learner was given "reasonable accommodations."

A *written referral* to a professional source of help will be beneficial if such a lawsuit should arise. Legal counsel should be sought before taking action with anyone who you suspect may be mentally disturbed or have a substance abuse problem.

Accommodation Plan

accommodation plan
an accommodation plan provides the necessary information for the learner regarding the steps the school is able to reasonably take to accommodate the individual learner's needs.

As previously stated, accommodations that are reasonable should be made for learners with disorders and disabilities. In order to assist you in developing such a plan for learners, a sample plan is shown in (Figure 9–6). This type of plan could be adapted or modified as needed for your specific educational environment. The sample plan contains six key areas listing specific actions that may or may not be selected as part of the plan, depending upon the individual learner's needs.

Schools may also choose to provide proper notice to potential students with regard to their rights as pertaining to Section 504 of the Rehabilitation Act of 1973. A sample notice is provided in (Figure 9–7).

Barriers to Learning

Certain barriers or roadblocks to learning affect all learners, whether or not they have a learning disability. Master educators will make a concerted effort to remove any such barriers and provide an open, positive environment for learning by all students. An awareness of the various barriers to learning will make the teaching and learning process a more meaningful and rewarding experience. Following is a discussion of some of the barriers that may impact learning in your classrooms.

Learner Apprehension

empathetic
characterized by an understanding so intimate that the feelings, thoughts, and motives of one individual are readily comprehended and understood by another.

One of the most common barriers to learning your students bring with them is apprehension and fear, otherwise known as anxiety. Learners will be apprehensive about the changes they will be asked to make; they will be nervous about their performance in a classroom and how it will be evaluated. Previous learning experiences influence the attitudes of adult learners. They may feel threatened in a learning environment because they are worried about competing successfully with other learners. Some learners are simply uncomfortable talking in front of even a small group of other learners. They worry about how they will look and sound if they are called upon.

Some learners will have trouble answering questions because of their fear of making a mistake or looking foolish. Such anxiety is clearly a barrier to learning. As a master educator, you must learn specific ways to draw your learners into the class, reassure them, and make them active participants. Some steps you can take to help alleviate learner anxiety are as follows:

> ### IT'S WORTH REMEMBERING ✳
>
> Students will constantly compare themselves, their knowledge, and their responses to the way they perceive everyone else in the classroom.

• **Be empathetic.** Put yourself in the place of the learners. Find out as much about them and their prior experiences as possible. Asking questions of your learners and paying attention to their answers will immediately establish your rapport with them.

ACCOMMODATION PLAN

Name: _____ Course: _____ Entry Date: _____

It has been determined that this student meets the classification as a qualified handicapped individual under Section 504 of the Rehabilitation Act of 1973. In accordance with Section 504 guidelines, the school has agreed to make reasonable accommodations to address the student's individual needs by offering the following plan as marked.

PHYSICAL ENVIRONMENT

☐ Seat student in quiet, distraction-free area.
☐ Seat student near educator.
☐ Seat student near a positive role model.
☐ Prepare students for change in routine.

☐ Stand near student when giving directions or presenting lessons.
☐ Create a nonthreatening environment.
☐ Other: _____

LESSON PRESENTATION

☐ Pair student to check work.
☐ Write key points on board.
☐ Give written and verbal instructions.
☐ Allow learners to tape-record class.
☐ Incorporate a variety of activities.
☐ Use high-impact audio/visual aids.
☐ Use interactive audio/visual for review.
☐ Follow consistent, published schedule.

☐ Provide written outline before lesson.
☐ Use multisensory teaching.
☐ Provide note taker if possible.
☐ Conduct oral reviews.
☐ Provide peer coaching.
☐ Allow breaks during class.
☐ Provide a reader.
☐ Other: _____

ASSIGNMENTS/WORKSHEETS

☐ Allow extra time for task completion.
☐ Simplify complex directions.
☐ Handout worksheets one at a time.
☐ Allow tape recording of assignments.
☐ Provide study skills training.
☐ Avoid handwritten assignments.

☐ Divide work into shorter segments.
☐ Schedule shorter work periods.
☐ Provide review of assignments before completion.
☐ Reduce homework.
☐ Other: _____

TESTING AND EVALUATION

☐ Give practice quizzes before tests.
☐ Give written information on test content.
☐ Give oral exams whenever possible.
☐ Allow extra time to complete.

☐ Allow learner to take test in quiet place to reduce distractions.
☐ Use typewritten tests, not handwritten.
☐ Other: _____

ORGANIZATIONAL PLANNING

☐ Provide organizational-skill training.
☐ Provide time-management training.
☐ Provide daily assistance in use of planner.
☐ Give daily and weekly progress reports.
☐ Incorporate mnemonic strategies.
☐ Provide consistent coaching.

☐ Provide task-management assistance.
☐ Teach how to scan for key points.
☐ Assign volunteer homework partner.
☐ Support formation of study groups.
☐ Other: _____

EDUCATOR BEHAVIORS AND ATTITUDES

☐ Provide immediate praise for achievements publicly.
☐ Develop a set of cues for students to remain on task.
☐ Give needed reprimands privately.
☐ Accept the characteristics of the learner's disorder, disability, or handicap.
☐ Avoid sarcasm and criticism.

☐ Recognize *efforts* that learners make.
☐ Match teaching methods with student's learning style.
☐ Accept lesser-quality handwriting.
☐ Maintain flexibility.
☐ Contract with learner.
☐ Other: _____

Figure 9–6 A reasonable accommodation plan should be created for learners with disorders or disabilities.

Section 504 and the Americans with Disabilities Act

- You have the right to be informed by the school of your rights under Section 504 and the ADA.
- The student has the right to an appropriate education designed to meet his or her individual needs as adequately as the needs of nondisabled students are met.
- The student has the right to free educational services except for those fees that are imposed on nondisabled students or their parents.
- The student has a right to facilities, services, and activities that are comparable to those provided to nondisabled students.
- The student has a right to an evaluation prior to an initial Section 504/ADA placement and any subsequent significant change in placement.
- The school shall consider testing and evaluation information from a variety of sources, including teacher recommendations, physical condition, social or cultural background, and adaptive behavior.
- The student has the right to notice prior to any action by the school in regard to the identification, evaluation, or placement of the student.
- The student has the right to examine relevant records.
- The student has the right to an impartial hearing with respect to the school's actions regarding identification, evaluation, or educational placement.
- If the student wishes to challenge the actions of the 504 committee in regard to identification, evaluation, or educational placement, he or she may file a written request for due process with the school's Compliance Officer within 30 calendar days from the time the student received written notice of the committee's actions. A hearing will be scheduled before an impartial hearing officer and the student will be notified in writing of the date, time, and place for the hearing.
- On Section 504 matters other than identification, evaluation, and placement, the student has a right to file a complaint with the district's 504 Compliance Officer, who will investigate the allegations to the extent warranted by the nature of the complaint in an effort to reach a prompt and equitable resolution.

Figure 9–7   Notice of student rights.

- **Treat each learner as an individual.** The previous step started you in that direction. Don't assume that everyone will learn at the same rate or as fast as you think they should. Adult learners are especially sensitive to being treated as if it doesn't matter who they are or what they are thinking.
- **Establish strong and frequent eye contact.** Make sure your learners understand what you are saying before you move on to the next topic or step. Encourage them to ask questions and make sure they understand the answers.
- **Encourage self-confidence.** Being a facilitator means you are helping your students learn for themselves. You must encourage them and convince them that they have the ability to understand or do whatever it is you are teaching.

- **Never talk down to your learners.** Adult learners are sensitive and exceptionally quick to recognize condescending attitudes. If you act superior, as if you are smarter than they are, they will sense it immediately.
- **Use repetition and reinforcement.** Some learners need it more than others. If a learner doesn't understand something one way, explain it in a different manner.
- **Avoid being in competition with learners.** Occasionally, educators don't want their learners to grasp the new material too quickly or too well. They are afraid the students might be able to perform the task better than they do. A master educator will never want a learner to fail.
- **Limit evaluation of learning activities.** Many topics and tasks within the field of cosmetology require rigorous testing and evaluation. However, self-evaluation or peer assessment will often provide a valid measure of the learner's accomplishments as well as eliminate the anxiety often experienced during testing.

Learner Recall

You may often hear older learners comment that they don't remember things as well as they did when they were younger. Sometimes decreased memory or recall abilities are real and sometimes they are imagined. Master educators incorporate the use of cues to aid recall, reduce interference during the learning process, and allow sufficient time for learners to form a response. Cues such as mnemonics should be used to aid the learner in memory retrieval. For example, a student could use the mnemonic **M**y **V**ery **E**ducated **M**other **J**ust **S**aid **U**h-oh **N**o **P**luto to remember the planets in the order of their distance from earth (Mercury, Venus, Earth, Mars, Jupiter, Saturn, Uranus, Neptune, Pluto). Memory cues are any type of hint or signal that indicates the nature of something to be remembered. Cues can be verbal or physical, such as cue cards (like those used in acting). The master educator will develop a portfolio of cues that can be used in the educational process and keep it at hand for ready reference.

Interference during the learning process includes any type of activity occurring during a class that causes distractions for the learners. Distractions include music, workplace noise inside or outside the facility, other students talking during class, the telephone ringing, and so forth (Figure 9–8). The educator cannot always control the conditions that result in learner interference or barriers. However, master educators should take all steps possible to create a safe learning environment that is physically comfortable and conducive to the educational process.

Rapid Response

Another barrier to learning can be the requirement for learners to respond rapidly. We need to provide opportunities for self-pacing and eliminate, whenever possible, the requirement for learners to respond immediately. Training in the practical disciplines within the field of cosmetology, however, does eventually require learners to develop a competitive level of speed. Therefore, after training at their individual paces, learners must ultimately concentrate on timing of practical skills.

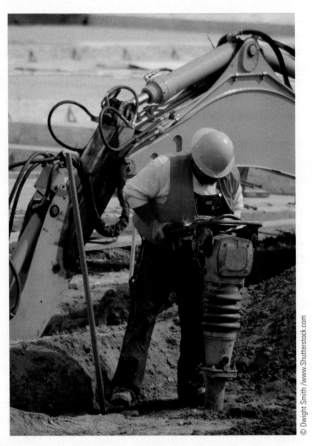

Figure 9–8   Construction noise inside or outside the facility can create a distraction and barrier to learning for all students.

Teaching Fast-Paced Learners

Although students who advance at a more rapid rate do not have the same issues as those with learning disabilities, they do present their own set of challenges to the educator. Research shows that in addition to the highly varied list of instructional methods used by master educators on a regular basis, a few other strategies have been effective. For fast-paced learners, educators found that less repetition in course content, advanced-level reading assignments, and higher-level questions worked more effectively. In addition, more independence for self-paced learning achieved better results. Moving beyond the core textbook for enrichment materials and individualized homework assignments has also proved beneficial. As stated in Chapters 2 and 4, "The Teaching Plan and Learning Environment" and "Basic Learning Styles and Principles," getting to know your learners and their learning styles will aid the educator in personalizing instruction for learners at all levels and learning abilities.

Lack of Learner Motivation

A serious barrier to learning occurs when learners simply do not want to be in the classroom. There is a limitless array of reasons why they may not want to be there, some of which are relevant and valid. Master educators will incorporate tactics to motivate learners and help them see the benefits they will enjoy by attending class. Educators can incorporate a variety of openers for classes that will allow learners to vent their frustrations about being there. These can be quite effective in getting the learners involved in the class while also serving as fun ice-breakers. A couple of ideas follow:

- **Assign learners to a two-member team.** Their responsibility is to face each other and, one at a time, "vent." Each person is to take two minutes to explain to the other learner all the reasons why they do not want to be in class. They are encouraged to show all the emotion they feel. The partner's role is to look the speaker in the eye and listen without interrupting. The educator calls time after two minutes and the learners exchange roles. The other one gets to "vent" while the first speaker listens. The educator simply wraps up with the explanation that now that they have gotten all that off their chests, they can get into the important lesson or material of the day. At that point, the educator should be prepared with a strong, motivational opener that clarifies for the learners why it's important for them to be in the class.
- **Handout cards entitled *Wow!* and *Yuk!*** Ask the learners to take out the "yuk" card first and write down all the reasons they did not want to come to class today. Have them list where they would rather be and why and so forth. Then have them take out the "wow" card and write all the reasons they wanted to come to class today. Have them list what they hope to gain from the instruction and what benefits they are seeking by being in the class. After all the cards have been completed, collect them and have a student helper tape them to the walls for all learners to read during breaks. The educator can wrap up this activity in much the same way as the first one.

Educator Behaviors

The greatest barriers to learning may be created by the behaviors and attitudes of the educator. We have already discussed various circumstances or situations that can be created by the educator to help learners become motivated. The opposite of those circumstances or behaviors can clearly create significant barriers to learning. For example, we suggested that the educator should establish strong personal contact with all learners. Failure to do so indicates that you are not interested in the learners or do not care about them. That will greatly inhibit the learning process. It has been suggested that learners should be put in an active mood by varying the stimuli and asking questions to keep the learners involved and make the class interesting. Conversely, if the educator does not allow questions, presents a boring lecture, avoids eye contact, or keeps the room at an uncomfortable temperature, learners probably will not learn! It was also suggested that master educators use examples and illustrations to support the content of our classes and show learners how the information will work for them. The opposite of that would be to simply assume our learners are going to apply what we have taught. After all, they are adult learners, and it's their responsibility to grasp the information and make it work for them, isn't it? That attitude will create a serious barrier to learning.

A significant barrier to learning would be to criticize learners in public or make them feel dumb for asking a question. Another earlier suggestion

CONSIDER AND CONNECT

Praise, recognition, and approval should be used regularly and frequently to reach every learner regardless of learning styles and ability.

was to encourage interpersonal relationships among learners and allow them to expand their network of support. A barrier to learning could be created by not allowing learners the opportunity to network. After all, by encouraging learners to interact with others and experience peer support, the educator may be relieved of the pressure to be available for each and every student at all times.

Wrapping It Up

Master educators learn to recognize behaviors and signs of learning disorders and disabilities and refer those learners to the appropriate professionals for diagnosis and treatment. They will also continue to improve their own knowledge of learning disorders so that they can more effectively serve every learner. They will accept the characteristics of learners with disabilities and those that advance at a much faster pace. They will ensure that all learners have an academically, emotionally, and socially safe environment in which to learn.

In Retrospect

1. List "major life activities."

2. Define the term *learning disability*.

3. Explain the four stages of information processing in learning.

4. List questions that can be used to help determine if a student is showing symptoms of dyslexia and ADHD.

5. List symptomatic chronic behaviors of students.

6. List strategies for alleviating learner anxiety.

7. State three strategies for fast-paced learners.

10 Program Development and Lesson Planning

Objectives (Desired Performance Goals):

After reading and studying this chapter, you should be able to:

- List the steps in the curriculum development process.

- Explain the purpose of the use of an advisory council in the curriculum-development process.

- Define the three domains for instructional outcomes and write learning objectives for each.

- Conduct a sound orientation program for new students.

- Explain the value and advantages of lesson planning.

- Describe each component of a lesson plan.

! CRITICAL CONCEPT

Experience has proven that the time spent in planning significantly reduces the time spent in execution. Plan your educational programs carefully.

Planning Concepts and Preliminary Analysis

FOR MOST SCHOOLS THAT OFFER career education, the courses or programs will also encompass cognate areas that serve to supplement the practical, scientific, and business skills of the professional. In some cases a state regulatory agency will prescribe the core content required in each of the programs. Schools are also required by accrediting agencies to offer programs of study that are appropriate in content and length to meet the stated mission of the institution.

A properly developed program of study will result in an orderly and systematic process of education that ensures students will progress satisfactorily through the program and achieve all the established objectives for the program.

Curriculum Development

The institution's curriculum includes a set of courses constituting an area of specialization. So, regardless of the programs offered at your institution, effort must be put into the development process, includes completing a thorough review of program content and identifying units of instruction prescribed by any applicable oversight agency; defining and allocating learning outcomes for students; organizing and sequencing material; allocating appropriate time for subjects and units of instruction; developing a program outline and schedule for classes; developing lesson plans; and creating a systematic method of student evaluation.

Steps for Developing a Program of Study

Following is a sequential procedure for developing a program of study.

1. **Determine Resources for Program Content.** This step will be somewhat directed by applicable state regulatory agencies and will lead you to existing literature, documents, and textbooks that are available for review and consideration.
2. **Review Information Obtained.** This begins the development process. The materials gathered will be reviewed and a determination made regarding the extent to which the information will be included in the curriculum. Likewise, a determination will be made as to whether any additional information will be needed to supplement the content.
3. **List Essential Tasks and Topics.** The occupational knowledge, skills, and competencies that are needed by professionals within the career field must be identified in order to be included in the curriculum.
4. **Sort the Topics and Tasks.** You will need to logically organize the various topics and tasks into related groups. These groups will eventually become the specific subjects or categories of study.
5. **Sequence the Subject Categories.** A logical order for subjects or categories might be the order in which tasks are performed within the occupation. It might also be organized in steps, so that learning begins with basic skills and builds to more complex skills. Another option

---

MASTER EDUCATOR

1. Use lesson plans as a guide, but make them their own.
2. Bring their own talents, experiences, and personal characteristics to each classroom.
3. Follow the program outline and ensure all educational objectives are met.

CONSIDER AND CONNECT

Preliminary analysis of the programs, educational objectives and goals, lesson plans, and scheduling must occur before teaching can begin.

might be to schedule from general to more specific subject matter. Ultimately, you must ensure that topics are not scheduled before prerequisite topics have been covered.

6. **Allocate Time for Each Subject Category.** The overall time allotment established for each category may be prescribed by the regulatory oversight agencies. Keep any such standards in mind as time is planned for each category.

7. **Identify Units of Instruction.** Units are subsections or topics within each of the subject categories. The general subject includes all topics to be covered, but a unit concentrates on only one or a few of the topics within that subject area.

8. **Allocate Time for Each Unit of Instruction.** The overall time allotment for each unit of instruction may or may not be established by the state regulatory agency. Therefore, the school must make a determination as to how many hours will be spent in the various units of study for the designated program.

9. **Develop a Program Outline or Syllabus.** A program outline is a comprehensive and organized written plan of instruction that usually includes a general description of the program, topics to be taught, learning goals and objectives, resources, instructional methods, grading procedures, materials, and supplies and facilities needed to deliver the program. A properly prepared program outline is the result of considerable study and careful planning. The major pieces of the overall program are outlined in a clear and logical manner.

10. **Develop Lesson Plans.** An important step in the curriculum development process is the creation of daily lesson plans. Lesson plans serve as the road map for each class session and will ensure that students receive the detailed information needed for each unit of study. There will be more in-depth information on lesson-plan preparation later in this chapter.

11. **Develop a Systematic Method of Student Evaluation.** Evaluation is the collection and analysis of information that leads to a judgment concerning the learner's knowledge and performance. A systematic approach should be used that assists the learner in achieving satisfactory results. Assessment and evaluation should be considered when developing learner outcomes or objectives.

12. **Develop a Comprehensive Schedule.** After the content has been identified and the sequencing of the various subjects has been determined, a detailed schedule of learning should be created. The schedule should cover the entire program of study and coordinate with the lesson plan. It will help ensure that program and institutional objectives are met and that all required lessons can be completed in the time allocated within the program outline. The schedule will also enable the educator to appropriately integrate academic learning with practical skills development. A well-planned schedule is essential to the learning process and will outline how each day will be spent for both the educators and the students.

13. **Develop an Orientation Program.** The orientation program should provide information about the educational program. It should cover the detailed program syllabus and all its elements, school policies and procedures, and any other general information pertinent to the student's success in the program.

The first eight steps discussed are considered to be level-one steps in the curriculum development process (Figure 10–1). Level-one steps include the selection and organization of curriculum content. Steps 9 through 13 represent the second level of the process and include development of the instructional program itself. The educator will generally be more involved with the second level than with the first.

Advisory Council

As previously stated, the minimum requirements for the program of study are often set forth by a state regulatory agency. The eight steps contained in the first level of curriculum development can be more effective and expeditious if the use of an institutional advisory council is employed. The **advisory council** is generally composed of school owners and directors, educators, and employers within the applicable field of study; graduates of the institution; representatives from local or state professional trade organizations; and even, perhaps, representatives from the regulatory oversight agencies. The council can be helpful in identifying and prioritizing subject matter and skills that need to be taught as well as assigning relative importance to each category of study. The council members will bring to the table their own experiences and education as well as additional resources from which they can draw to satisfactorily address the current needs of the industry with respect to the ability of those students graduating from your institution.

advisory council
a committee composed of school owners and directors, educators, and employers within the applicable field of study; graduates of the institution; representatives from local or state professional trade organizations; and even, perhaps, representatives from the regulatory oversight agencies. The focus of the council should be curriculum, facilities, equipment, and institutional outcomes, at a minimum.

Organizing Material

Once the search and review steps have been completed and the subjects and tasks have been identified for the course or program of study, those subjects must be organized and sequenced in a logical manner to ensure maximum learning and retention by the students. For proper sequencing to occur, you must determine whether specific subjects, topics, or tasks must be preceded by others. Allotment of time for each subject and unit of study should be considered during the sequencing of the information. Time allotments may be driven somewhat by the oversight agency's prescribed curriculum. Hours allotted to each area of study will also be driven by the relative difficulty and relative importance of each subject and unit. In addition, consideration should be given to how well the components of the program blend together. It is important to avoid major gaps in or overlaps of subject matter.

Instructional Outcomes

The key elements of program development revolve around intended learner outcomes that are reflected in various goals and objectives. Questions applicable at this stage include "What knowledge should students have and what skills should students be able to perform as a result of completing the program of study?" Since there may be much more that could be taught in

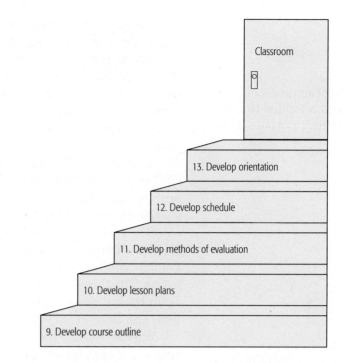

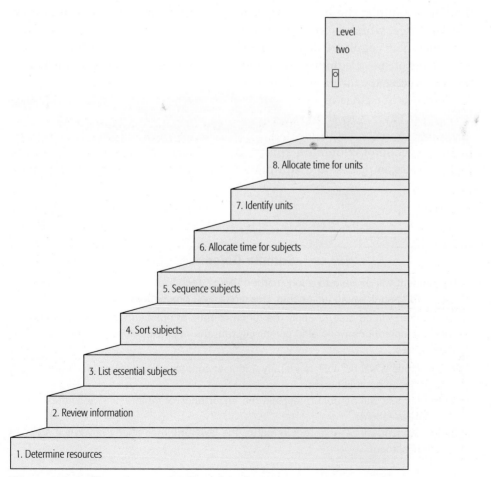

Figure 10–1 Step in curriculum development.

objectives
something that one's efforts or actions are intended to attain or accomplish; purpose; goal.

cognitive domain
the cognitive domain includes those performances that require knowledge of specific information, such as principles, concepts, and generalizations necessary for problem solving.

psychomotor domain
Objectives in the psychomotor domain relate to skill performance, which requires tools, objects, supplies, and equipment.

the program than time or resources will permit, it is essential that the most important goals and objectives are identified as to what can be acquired in the time available.

The terms *goals, aims, objectives*, and *outcomes* are often used interchangeably in the context of education. For the purposes of this text, the terms *goals* and *objectives* will be used to address the outcomes expected for the program of study. Goals or objectives are established for various levels within the program-development process. First, they are defined for the overall program of study. Second, goals or objectives are established for each subject or category of study. Third, instructional goals or objectives are set forth for each lesson plan found in a unit of study. Program goals generally specify the learning outcomes of the program of study. Subject or category objectives will more specifically address the objectives or outcomes for the general subject area. Instructional objectives address specifically what the student will know or be able to accomplish upon the conclusion of a daily lesson. The three different types of objectives are similar and differ primarily in their degree of generality. Refer to the accompanying chart of objectives and their examples.

You can see the natural progression from a general program goal, to a subject goal or objective, to a specific instructional objective within a unit of study. When defining goals and objectives, it is helpful for the educator to relate the goals to the different types of performances that need to be specified. For example, the intended learning objective may be the acquisition of *knowledge*, which is known as the **cognitive domain** of instructional outcomes. The cognitive domain includes those performances that require knowledge of specific information, such as principles, concepts, and generalizations necessary for problem solving.

For another class or unit, the outcome desired could be *skill development* as it relates to the performance of a specific task or activity. This would be the **psychomotor domain** of instructional outcomes. Objectives in the psychomotor domain relate to skill performance, which requires tools, objects, supplies, and equipment. A primary goal of training in most

OBJECTIVES AND EXAMPLES

Type of Objective	Sample Objective
BUSINESS 101 - PROGRAM GOAL OR OBJECTIVE (general outcome)	The student will be able to apply learned theory, technical information, and related matter to ensure sound judgments, decisions, and procedures.
SUBJECT OR CATEGORY OBJECTIVE – BUSINESS ADMINISTRATION	The student will be able to apply the fundamentals of business management and business operations while also complying with the applicable local, state, and federal laws.
INSTRUCTIONAL OR LESSON OBJECTIVE (specific to daily lesson): BUSINESS FINANCE AND LAWS	1. The student will be able to identify financial considerations involved in operating a business establishment. 2. The student will be able to explain the importance of maintaining accurate business records. 3. The student will be able to summarize the laws and regulations governing an establishment.

career education is to enable students to acquire the mastery of those skills needed to become professionals. To become proficient, the students will perform physical or psychomotor tasks under the supervision of an educator. Repeated use of the skills required will eventually transfer to routine practice in the workplace.

There are fewer occasions where the objective would reflect a desire for the development of an *attitude* or *value* related to the subject matter. This is known as the **affective domain** of instructional outcomes. In the affective domain, the desired performance includes the demonstration of feelings, attitudes, or sensitivities toward other people, ideas, or things. Surveys of employers consistently reveal their interests in hiring people who have positive attitudes, get along well with fellow workers, possess a good work ethic, and are happy in their profession. All of these qualities are indicative of positive attitudes, values, and feelings. In addition to having knowledge and quality technical skills, new professionals must also possess the affective factors that influence how they will perform in the workplace. Refer to Figure 10–4 for an example of objectives in each domain.

Objectives serve little purpose unless they are measurable and unless efforts are made to assess their achievement. The sample objectives contained in this chapter indicate the desired behavior or outcome to be demonstrated by the student (Figure 10–2). This allows the educator to decide on the conditions of the learning activity, the desired performance for the student's class level, and the measurement procedures that will be used in determining whether the learner's performance meets desired standards. The master educator will recognize that treating all students or groups of students exactly alike in the assessment process is as inappropriate as teaching everyone the same way, regardless of their learner type or abilities. By defining outcomes-based objectives, the educator can make decisions that are in the best interest of the students with regard to assessment and evaluation.

If the goal is for graduates to think critically and creatively, to be able to analyze situations and draw conclusions about what they observe, they must be given the opportunity for such learning in school. The committed educator will ensure that learning goes beyond the mere acquisition of knowledge (the ability to recall factual information) and incorporate higher-level objectives into daily lessons.

affective domain
In the affective domain, the desired performance objective includes the demonstration of feelings, attitudes, or sensitivities toward other people, ideas, or things.

Domain	Sample Objective
Cognitive Domain	The student will be able to identify from a list of chemicals those that should be stored in a locked room or cabinet.
Psychomotor Domain	The student will demonstrate how towels are to be folded and placed in a closed cabinet.
Affective Domain	The student will demonstrate responsibility by following school policies and procedures at all times.

Figure 10–2 Sample objectives for instructional outcome domains.

✓ The Program Outline

When the preliminary analysis and research have been completed, the subjects selected, and the material organized and sequenced, a program outline or program syllabus should be developed. Step 9 in the curriculum development process lists the various components generally found in an outline for a program of study. Program outlines will vary in design, style, and content, but generally include the following:

a. The name of the program
b. A brief description of the program
c. Learning goals and objectives
d. Subjects and topics of instruction integrating academic learning and practical skills training
e. Hours or competencies applied to each subject and/or unit of instruction
f. Instructional methods, including materials, equipment, and facilities used
g. Grading procedures
h. Other pertinent information such as references, learner prerequisites, and so on

Chapter 12, "Assessing Progress and Advising Students," will discuss the foundation and purpose of grading as well as the development of practical skills competency evaluation criteria that can be used in collecting and analyzing information that can lead to a judgment by you, the educator, with respect to a learner's performance or progress through the program of study.

Orientation Program

When all other steps in the curriculum development process are completed, it is time to introduce new students to the program of study. The master educator will work with administration to prepare and implement a comprehensive **orientation program** that provides information about the instructional program, the goals for the program, any policies affecting students, and any student services available during their training. Orientation should be scheduled on or before the first day of class. A well-prepared and well-planned orientation program can be the first step in creating a successful program graduate. New-student orientation is also an opportunity to review many of the policies and procedures that were discussed with the applicant during the registration process. It is an appropriate time to review the "consumer information," which is required by various accrediting and federal agencies as well.

The purpose of a sound orientation program is to ensure that the new students are able to:

• Understand the general objectives of the program of study.
• Identify the various career opportunities within the field of the program in which they are enrolled.
• Recognize the lifestyle changes that may be needed as a result of becoming a full-time student.
• Understand the various rules and policies affecting students enrolled in the program of study.

orientation program
A program or class that occurs on or before the first day of class that provides information about the educational program. It should cover the detailed program course outline and all its elements, school policies and procedures, and any other general information pertinent to the student's success in the program.

COSMETOLOGY PROGRAM OUTLINE EXAMPLE

DESCRIPTION 1500 Hours

The primary purpose of the Cosmetology Program is to train the student in the basic manipulative skills, safety judgments, proper work habits, and desirable attitudes necessary to obtain licensure and for competency in entry-level positions in cosmetology or a related career field.

PROGRAM GOALS OR OBJECTIVES

Upon completion of the program requirements, the determined graduate will:

1. Project a positive attitude and a sense of personal integrity and self-confidence.
2. Practice effective communications skills, visual poise, and proper grooming.
3. Respect the need to deliver worthy service for value received in an employer-employee relationship.
4. Develop effective work habits in the interest of safety and infection control.
5. Perform the basic manipulative skills in the areas of hair styling, hair shaping, haircoloring, texture services, scalp and hair conditioning, skin care and makeup, and nail care.
6. Perform the basic analytical skills to determine proper makeup, hairstyle, and color application for the client's overall image.
7. Apply learned theory, technical information, and related matter to ensure sound judgments, decisions, and procedures within the scope of the job.

To ensure continued career success, the graduate will continue to learn new and current information related to skills, trends, and methods for career development in cosmetology and related fields.

REFERENCES

A comprehensive library of references, periodicals, books, texts, and audio/videotapes are available to support the program of study and supplement student training. Students should utilize these extensive materials at every possible opportunity. Students will receive *Milady Standard: Cosmetology* textbook and *The Essential Companion Study Guide*.

INSTRUCTIONAL METHODS

The clock-hour education is provided through a sequential set of learning units that address both theoretical knowledge and the specific practical skills necessary for certification or licensure, graduation, and entry-level job skills. Student salon equipment, implements, and products are comparable to those used in the industry. Each student will receive instruction that relates to the performance of useful, creative, and productive career-oriented activities. The program is presented through comprehensive lesson plans that reflect effective educational methods and follow *Milady Standard: Cosmetology*. Subjects are presented by means of interactive lecture, demonstration, student participation, and student activities. Audiovisual aids, guest speakers, field trips, projects, activities, and other related learning methods are used throughout the program.

GRADING PROCEDURES

Students are assigned theory study and a minimum number of practical experiences in each category of study. Specific academic learning and practical assignments are designated as requirements for graduation from the program. Theoretical knowledge is evaluated after each unit of study. Practical assignments are evaluated as completed and counted toward program completion only when rated as satisfactory or better. Practical skills are evaluated according to text procedures and the published competency criteria. Students must maintain a written grade average of 75% and pass a final written and practical exam prior to graduation. Students must make up failed or missed tests and incomplete assignments. Numerical grades are considered according to the following scale:

WRITTEN:			PRACTICAL:		
	93–100	EXCELLENT		4	EXCELLENT
	85–92	VERY GOOD		3	VERY GOOD
	75–84	SATISFACTORY		2	SATISFACTORY
	70–74	NEEDS IMPROVEMENT		0–1	UNSATISFACTORY

(continued)

SUBJECT HOURS	UNIT HOURS	SUBJECT/UNITS
75		THEORY—CLASSROOM INSTRUCTION—Limited to:
	5	Orientation
	5	Career Information
	10	State Laws and Regulations
	8	Professional Image
	2	First Aid
	10	Chemistry
	10	Electricity
	15	Job Seeking
	10	Professional Ethics
75		BACTERIOLOGY, DECONTAMINATION, INFECTION CONTROL
	10	Types and Classifications of Bacteria, Growth and Reproduction, AIDS
	10	Biology, Health and Public Sanitation
	10	Disinfection, Sterilization, Sanitation, Chemical Agents and Products
	5	OSHA
	40	Tools, Equipment Use and Safety, Practical Application of Procedures
75		SHAMPOO, RINSES, SCALP TREATMENTS, AND RELATED THEORY
	5	Properties of Hair and Scalp, Hair Growth
	20	Hair Analysis and Scalp Care and Practical Application of Procedures
	5	Hair Loss, Disorders of the Hair and Scalp
	15	Draping for all Services, Practical Application of Procedures
	30	Shampooing and Related Theory, Practical Application of Procedures. The Chemistry and Use of Shampoo and Conditioning Products
150		HAIRSTYLING AND RELATED THEORY
	10	Tools and their use
	50	Wet Hairstyling, Finger Waving, Pin Curls, Roller Curls, Comb-out Techniques, Braiding- and Practical Application of Procedures
	75	Thermal Hairstyling and Pressing, Curling Irons, Blow Dry Styling, Air Waving, and Practical Application of Procedures
	15	Artistry of Artificial Hair
200		HAIRCUTTING AND RELATED THEORY
	5	Basics of Haircutting, Tools and Their Use and Safety
	20	Sectioning and Practical Application of Procedures, Guides, Elevations
	125	Cutting High Elevation, Reverse Elevation, Blended Elevation, and Practical Application of Procedures
	50	Razor, Clipper, and Scissor-over-Comb Techniques, Special Effects, and Practical Application of Procedures
125		HAIRCOLORING AND RELATED THEORY
	10	Introduction, Nature's Color, Client Communication, Color Theory
	10	Types of Haircolor: Temporary, Demipermanent, Oxidative Deposit-Only, Nonoxidative Permanent, Oxidative/Lift-Deposit, Hydrogen Peroxide Developers, Chemistry of Haircoloring
	50	Color-Application Techniques and Practical Application of Procedures
	50	Hair Lightening, Special Effects Highlighting, and Practical Application of Procedures
	5	Special Problems in Haircolor/Corrective Coloring, Safety
200		CHEMICAL REARRANGING (TEXTURE SERVICES) AND RELATED THEORY
	5	Introduction and History, Modern Chemistry, Perm and Relaxing Products, Chemistry of Products

SUBJECT HOURS	UNIT HOURS	SUBJECT/UNITS
	10	Hair Structure and Chemical Reformation, Rod Selection, Sectioning and Wrapping Techniques
	100	Perming Techniques and Practical Application of Procedures
	10	Steps in Chemical Relaxing, Hair Analysis
	75	Chemical Hair Relaxing Processes, Chemical Blow-out, Soft-Curl Permanent, Safety Precautions, and Practical Application of Procedures
175		MANICURING AND PEDICURING AND RELATED THEORY
	10	The Nail and Its Disorders
	5	Introduction, Shapes of Nails, Equipment, Implements, Cosmetics, and Materials
	90	Preparation of Manicuring Table, Plain Manicure, Safety Rules, Individual Nail Styling, Theory of Massage, Hand and Arm Massage, Other Types of Manicures, and Practical Application Procedures
	50	Advanced Nail Techniques, Nail Wrapping, Sculptured Nails, Dipped Nails, Nail Tipping, and Practical Application of Procedures
	20	Pedicuring, Foot Massage, and Practical Application of Procedures
175		FACIALS AND RELATED THEORY
	10	The Skin and Its Disorders
	5	Introduction, Facial Treatments, Facial Massage, Facial Manipulations, and Practical Application Procedures
	75	Facials for Dry Skin, Oily Skin, Comedones, Milia, and Acne; Packs and Masks; Light Therapy, and Safety
	65	Preparation for Makeup Application and Cosmetics for Facial Makeup, Chemistry of Cosmetics, Makeup Application Techniques, and Practical Application of Procedures
	10	Lash and Brow Tinting, Artificial Eyelashes, and Practical Application of Procedures
	10	Removing Unwanted Hair and Practical Application of Procedures
50		SALON BUSINESS, RETAIL SALES
	5	Introduction, Fundamentals of Business Management, Opening a Salon, Business Plan, Written Agreements
	10	Licensing Requirements and Regulations, Laws, Safety
	5	Compensation Packages, Payroll Deductions, Insurance
	10	Salon Operations, Policies, Practices, Telephone Use, Advertising
	10	Sales, Communications, Public/Human Relations
	10	Securing Employment
200		MISCELLANEOUS
		To be applied by the instructor to strengthen student performance: supervised field trips, topics identified by Institutional Advisory Council as relevant to current trends within the industry, or other related training.
1500		TOTAL HOURS

The training hours specified in the above table must be met by each student in each category in order for the earned hours to be accepted by the state licensing board for examination. The generous portion of miscellaneous hours is to be applied as needed in curriculum-related areas or if the student requires additional time in a given category or desires to specialize in a specific area.

- Know the most recent performance outcomes achieved by the institution with respect to completion, licensure, and employment.
- Understand the importance of consumer safety and general safety procedures followed in the chosen field.
- Understand OSHA requirements, as applicable.
- Understand any other applicable policies or standards that are applicable to the student's course completion.

A comprehensive orientation program can best be accomplished with the use of prepared lesson plans that cover all the requisite information. It is recommended that a three-ring binder be used to organize the materials presented in the orientation program. The binder should include the orientation lesson plans as well as the forms, policies, and handouts that will be used to deliver the information. Orientation is a great opportunity to have students acknowledge the receipt of certain information required by state regulatory and accrediting agencies. Some typical topics to be covered in a new student orientation program are as follows:

- Staff and student introductions
- An ice-breaker or opening activity that will allow new students to bond with continuing students
- An explanation of the importance of developing people skills as well as technical skills for career success and the qualities needed
- An explanation of the importance of student desire, personal commitment, and drive to succeed
- A history of the applicable field as a profession
- The job outlook for careers in program-related fields
- Program length and licensure requirements for the jurisdiction
- Tips to students for behavior modification and time-management strategies to help with the addition of 20 to 40 student hours weekly to their existing schedule of responsibilities
- Obstacles the students may encounter to program completion and possible solutions to them
- The rules or standards of conduct required for students within the institution
- The various policies affecting students, such as clocking procedures, hours of attendance, class schedules, leaves of absence, reference library procedures, satisfactory academic progress requirements, grievance procedures for students, the school's suggestion box policy, advisement procedures, disciplinary policies, privacy policy, the Campus Crime and Security Report, and so on
- Emergency evacuation procedures, use of fire extinguishers, first aid stations, and so on
- OSHA regulations and basic requirements for a safe workplace
- Financial aid programs if applicable

All staff members should participate to some degree in the orientation program, at least to the extent that all are introduced to students. It would be appropriate for the educator to cover most of the material while an admissions representative could review the consumer information that was provided during the registration process. The financial aid officer might review how financial assistance will be affected by student progress and attendance in the program of training.

Use your own creativity in developing ice-breakers and bonding activities for the beginning of the orientation program (Figure 10–3).

Remember, a professional orientation program that conveys to new students all the critical information about what they can expect during their program of study will prevent many potential future problems. Consider referring to your new students as *graduates* the minute they enter your orientation class. A master educator will ensure that all *critical firsts* for students, including their first day of orientation and/or school, are memorable ones.

Lesson Plan Development

We have learned all the elements required for developing an overall program of study. We also learned that the detailed program outline and class schedule will serve as the blueprint for charting what is to be taught, when it is to be taught, and how it is to be taught. When the program subjects and units have been defined and the program outline completed, it is time to begin the most detailed step in the process of program development: creation of lesson plans. All the research, review, and planning activities that have taken place prior to this point will only have value when all that effort has the opportunity to come to life in the classroom.

Teaching without a lesson plan can be compared to driving across an unfamiliar country without a map. Comprehensive lesson plans will serve as the road map to be followed for each day's classes. The lesson plan should be a clearly written, flexible, and individualized guide for conducting a lesson. Each lesson should be based on the needs, interests, and abilities

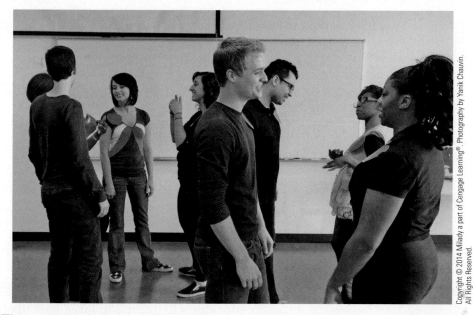

Figure 10–3   An ice-breaker or opening activity during the new-student orientation allows new students to bond with each other.

LEARNING REINFORCEMENT IDEAS AND ACTIVITIES FOR ORIENTATION

- Have existing or continuing students attend orientation and introduce themselves and state briefly something special they have learned or enjoyed since enrolling. Then have new students introduce themselves and give a one- to two-minute personal history and personal accomplishment of which they are proud.
- The "personality name badges" activity reinforces the definition of personality as the outward reflection of inner feelings, thoughts, attitudes, and values. It is also a good way for new students to bond with other new students and/or students already enrolled in the school. Stick-on name badges and colorful markers are required. After orientation is completed, the school's standard name badges can be issued.
  a. Issue a stick-on name badge for all participants.
  b. Instruct participants to write their first name in large letters centered near the top of the badge.
  c. Using each letter in their name, ask participants to create words that describe their inner feelings, thoughts, attitudes, and/or values (personality).

  Example:

S	**A**	**R**	**A**	**H**
W	C	E	T	O
E	T	B	H	N
E	I	E	L	E
T	V	L	E	S
	E	L	T	T
		I	I	
		O	C	
		U		
		S		

  d. Ask participants to use their colorful markers and create a border for their name badge that reflects their personality.
  When everyone has completed their name badges, discuss the fact that personalities are all different and use the wide variety of words chosen by students to describe themselves as evidence.

- Develop a "Just for Laughs" quiz on your school policies and other information covered during orientation. It will not be graded but can be used by the instructor to determine what, if any, policies or procedures need further clarification. Remember, you are covering a lot of information for new students. The "quiz" could help with their retention of the important information. Develop handouts for any information not already contained in the student catalog or contract.

of students and should address the goals, needs, and style of the individual educator. Your success as a master educator will depend in large part upon your ability to effectively plan and present your subject matter. You must know exactly what you are going to teach and how you are going to teach it.

Advantages of Lesson Planning

A master educator must take advantage of the many tools and resources available for improving the quality of education offered in the classroom. A well-prepared lesson plan is one of those tools. It requires the educator to carefully consider the selection of the subject matter, procedures, and the preparation of tests to check student progress. As the profile of today's learner changes, lesson plans will have to be changed and updated frequently to ensure educators are delivering the most current information to their students. Some of the advantages achieved through daily lesson plans are as follows:

- Owners and educators can maintain confidence that program and lesson objectives will be met.
- Learners receive the benefit of effective teaching principles, such as connecting new material that was learned previously and having information presented logically and sequentially.
- Educators are prepared with appropriate review questions and answers.
- Learners receive the benefit of appropriate summarization and review.
- Learners know exactly what is expected of them and have follow-up assignments to ensure they achieve the needed level of competence.
- Educators have the opportunity to consider a variety of learning styles when developing each lesson plan, which ensures that more students benefit from the training.
- Educators will supply the needed teaching materials and aids to provide a quality presentation.
- The confidence level of the educator will soar due to prior preparation and knowledge that the material will be presented in an organized manner.

The Lesson Plan: Pieces, Parts, and Points

While a well-designed lesson will consist of three main parts—the introduction, the main body, and the conclusion—the plan used to deliver that lesson will contain many more components. Lesson plans will vary in form and content based on the subject matter and the style of the educator. There is no single best model, but all good lesson plans will contain the following minimum components:

- Program title
- Subject and topic (also known as unit and lesson title)
- Lesson objectives (also known as behavioral performance objectives)
- Implements, equipment, and supplies required for both students and the instructor
- Teaching aids (also known as educator materials, instructional aids, and educational aids)
- Facility
- Time allotment
- Prior student assignments (also known as prerequisites of the learner)
- Educator references (might include supplemental materials used)
- Notes to educator
- Learning motivation (also known as lesson introduction)

- Subject matter and in-depth notes (content presentation)
- Activities for lesson (also known as instructional activities or learning reinforcement ideas and activities)
- Summary and review
- Follow-up assignments, if applicable
- Evaluation procedures (also known as testing or practical projects)
- Other pertinent components (some forms identify a separate component for safety guidelines; others incorporate that information into the presentation outline)

Though some of the components of a lesson plan are self-explanatory, others require clarification, and these are discussed next.

Lesson Objectives. The objectives should indicate measurable knowledge, skills, and attitudes students should possess upon completion of the lesson. Some lessons lend themselves to the acquisition of knowledge while others are geared more toward skill development. Other lessons, such as those dealing with people skills, may focus more on the development of attitudes. Each lesson objective will have a focus on a particular domain—the cognitive, the psychomotor, or the affective. However, some lessons may contain multiple lesson objectives and involve more than one instructional domain. The master educator will keep lesson objectives clear, concise, and simple whenever possible. The learner should be able to have a clear understanding of what she will be able to accomplish or know upon completion of the lesson and assigned practice.

Implements, Equipment, Supplies. This part of lesson planning requires the educator to list the implements, materials, and equipment needed to deliver the lesson. It also addresses what materials students will need during the lesson. By preparing lesson plans ahead of time that contain this component, the educator can notify the students in advance of what will be needed so that the class can begin on time and progress in an orderly and organized manner.

Educational Aids. In addition to materials, equipment, and supplies, the educator must determine in advance which instructional aids are needed to deliver the scheduled lesson. The school resource center, for example, may have available a video that shows techniques that are to be covered in the lesson. Therefore, the educator needs to ensure that the LCD projector is operational and that the TV and VCR or DVD player are available for the class. The educator may have other charts or visual aids that will help the students understand the procedure covered in the lesson. By having all required teaching aids listed in the lesson plan, the educator can ensure that the entire class can be presented in a well-planned, orderly fashion. Further in-depth information on the creation and use of educational aids can be found in Chapter 11, "Educational Aids and Technology in the Classroom."

Facility. The educator will want to identify for students where the presentation will take place. If the lesson is strictly a theory class presentation, the theory classroom would be listed. If it is a practical class with a demonstration, the practical classroom or lab space should be designated. There may be times where a special model is going to be used for a specific practical skills presentation, and the laboratory may be the most appropriate location for the class. Again, this is just one more step in ensuring that everyone knows where they need to be at the time of the scheduled class.

Time Allotment. The time allocated for the lesson should be listed. A master educator will bear in mind that the amount of time required for a lesson will vary depending on how many students are in attendance and how many activities are incorporated into the lesson. The existing knowledge and skills abilities of a certain group of students could also affect the length of the class. The educator should maintain flexibility to accommodate these elements when planning the time to be spent on each lesson.

Prior Student Assignments. This component ensures that all students are prepared for the class. For example, if you are going to be teaching the practical application on a given topic, students must have read and received training in the prerequisite information.

Educator References. This component requires the educator to list a variety of references that are available for research and additional preparation. The educator may also want to identify these references for the students as well if those resources are also available to individual students for independent study.

Notes to Educator. This component is generally used when lesson plans are being developed that will be used by other educators within the institution. Notes to the educator would include reminders regarding any applicable research that should be completed prior to delivery of the lesson. They might suggest reviewing the variety of learning reinforcement ideas and student activities found within the lesson so that a determination can be made ahead of time with regard to which ones will be included in the actual lesson. This ensures that the educator has gathered all the appropriate props and materials prior to class.

Learning Motivation or Introduction. Some educators consider the introduction or learning motivation to be the most critical component of any lesson plan. This orientation to the lesson prepares the students for the upcoming instructional tasks and the purpose of the lesson. Students enrolled in any program of study are usually tuned in to the radio station WII-FM: "What's in it for me?" In this element of the lesson, the master educator will convey to learners why the information they are about to receive is important to them. The introduction or learning motivation may also consist of a review of prior learning, a statement of the lesson objectives, and a statement of what is expected of students during and after the class.

One common thread for every classroom is that students do not enter the classroom in the same mind-set. Students' minds will be on different matters; they may be removed from the world of education; they may be thinking about what they did the evening before or how they are going to reconcile (or not) with their significant other; or they may be concerned with a variety of other things that are distracting to the educational process. Therefore, the master educator will learn to introduce the lesson in such a manner that it will gain the attention of the learners and motivate them so that their attention will be maintained

EXAMPLE OF A LESSON PLAN COVER SHEET FOR TEACHING COMMUNICATION SKILLS

COURSE MANAGEMENT GUIDE

INSTRUCTOR NAME: _____   **DATE TAUGHT:** _____

SUBJECT: Orientation
TOPIC: Communicating for Success

LESSON OBJECTIVES:

Upon completion of the lesson, the student will be able to:

1. List the "golden rules" of human relations.
2. Explain the definition of effective communications.
3. Conduct a successful client consultation/needs assessment.
4. Handle delicate communications with your clients.
5. Build open lines of communication with coworkers.

IMPLEMENTS, EQUIPMENT, SUPPLIES REQUIRED:

STUDENT	INSTRUCTOR	ITEMS
X	X	Standard Textbook
X	X	Standard Workbooks and Study Guide
X		Student notebook
X		Pens, pencils

TEACHING AIDS (Audio/visual equipment, handouts, etc., used by instructor):

1. Electronic whiteboard
2. LCD projector and instructor-support slides
3. *Standard DVD Series* and DVD player

FACILITY: Theory classroom

TIME ALLOTMENT: 1 to 2 hours (adjust based on school schedule and student activities/participation)

PRIOR STUDENT ASSIGNMENT:

1. Read Chapter XXX, *Standard Textbook*

EDUCATOR REFERENCES:

1. *Standard Textbook*
2. *Standard Workbooks and Study Guide*

NOTES TO EDUCATOR:

1. Review chapter, entire lesson plan, and instructor-support slides prior to lesson.
2. Review Learning Reinforcement ideas/activities and predetermine which are to be used.
3. Check projector to ensure it is working properly.
4. Gather all materials and supplies needed for demonstrations prior to starting class.
5. Have students sign in for class and document attendance based on school's procedure.
6. During the instructor-preparation time and while students are entering and getting settled for the class, have the first instructor-support slide containing the inspirational quote projected (or write it on the board or flip chart). This will help get instructors and students into the appropriate mind-set for learning and for the day.

during the entire lesson. This introductory process is referred to as the *anticipatory set*.

The anticipatory set is a process. It begins before students enter the classroom and continues during the activity that occurs when learners are arriving physically and then mentally adapting to what is about to occur in the classroom. It is the process of getting students ready to learn. The master educator will become comfortable with several different approaches to establish the mood or "set" for the classroom. She might ask a provocative question or make a startling statement, or share a story relating to the topic of the day. The master educator will learn early in her career to maintain a journal of events and activities that can be shared in the classroom environment. The learning motivation or introduction should be carefully planned to capture the attention of the learners and stimulate their interest in the class or lesson that is about to occur.

Presentation Outline and Notes. This is the most substantive part of the lesson plan. It actually represents the formal part of the class presentation. The instructor should outline the topic to be presented in an organized and properly sequenced format. In addition, she should record detailed notes to supplement the outline during the presentation. A lesson plan should be comprehensive enough that a substitute instructor could readily present the class with a brief review of the material. In many disciplines, well-prepared, commercially published lesson plans are available that follow the content in the core textbook used for a program of study.

Activities for Lesson. Activities are experiences, participatory exercises, projects, and assignments that will enable the learners to achieve the objectives of the lesson. It has been determined that the educator must vary the stimuli for students at least every eight minutes during a lesson to maintain interest. This can be done through a variety of methods that are covered elsewhere in this text. Use of student activities during a lesson is an excellent way to ensure maximum retention of the material. Therefore, the master educator will include learner-centered activities in each lesson as well as learner-centered projects and assignments after the lesson that will ensure that learning objectives are achieved. Activities could include games or competitions during the lesson, a research assignment after the lesson, a group field trip, a video presentation, or a group activity with requirements to report back to the entire class. The master educator will consider prior knowledge and skills necessary for completing activities. She will also consider the opportunities for students to practice the behavior specified in the objective and the opportunity for providing prompt feedback to students with regard to the activity.

Summary and Review. The lesson summary brings closure to the class and provides an opportunity for the educator to summarize the main points or provide an overview of the lesson. An effective ending is just as important as an effective beginning. The master educator will condense the lesson into a few basic points that can be delivered quickly and concisely. She will prepare in advance review questions and answers or group activities that can be used to reinforce key points in the lesson. To ensure that

anticipatory set

a process that begins before students enter the classroom and continues during the activity that occurs when learners are arriving physically and then mentally adapting to what is about to occur in the classroom. Essentially, it is the process of getting students ready to learn.

IT'S WORTH REMEMBERING ✳

Educators must remember that adult learners must make school a priority; however, they must recognize that it will never be their first priority. Their other responsibilities as an adult prevent school from being their absolute top priority.

CONSIDER AND CONNECT

It has also been determined that the amount of information learned in an adult classroom is directly proportional to the amount of fun the learner has.

the summary is more than just a review and achieves maximum results, follow these tips:

– List major points or headings on the board or slide.
– Distribute a handout to the students that covers the major points of the lesson.
– Ask students to review their notes and then present one key point to the class.
– Conduct an informal oral review by asking students questions regarding the lesson and allowing them to answer them individually or in teams.
– Have students work in teams to write review questions and conduct an activity of them questioning each other. Use a beach ball or other item toss to determine which team asks the next question, and so forth

CONSIDER AND CONNECT

Involving learners in developing the review questions and activities will ensure their ultimate ownership of the information.

Follow-up Assignment. Without a doubt, meaningful and interesting work can be done outside the framework of the supervised laboratory or classroom, which will enhance learning. Clearly, homework or outside assignments should only be given when students have achieved sufficient knowledge or skills to proceed successfully in an independent environment. Follow-up assignments may:

– lengthen the amount of time students spend in learning activities;
– foster initiative, independence, and responsibility;
– reinforce classroom and practical skills learning;
– promote self-discipline for learners; and
– enable the educator to allow for individual differences in learners.

The master educator will make certain that assignments are clear and comprehensible and that they are meaningful and of interest to the students.

Evaluation Procedures. No lesson plan would be complete without including a component that can be used to measure the learners' successes in achieving lesson objectives and assess the effectiveness of the educational activities and procedures used to deliver the material contained in the lesson. When planning every lesson, the master educator will take into consideration a number of methods that can be used to determine the level of knowledge or skills achieved by the learners. This evaluation will enable the educator to proceed with subsequent learning or to engage in remedial or relearning activities.

☑ Wrapping It Up

Quality instruction is a result of thoughtful planning and many different activities by many different contributors. The educator's involvement in the planning of daily lessons is crucial to the success of any institution. Master educators do more than simply mimic or parrot plans that are prepared by others. They may use those plans as their guide, but they make those plans their own by personalizing them and individualizing them to reflect their individual uniqueness. They bring their own talents, experiences, and personality characteristics to each classroom. They use that history and experience to bring life and excitement into each class. They shape their instructional programs in ways that will reflect their own personal strengths and preferences but also address the needs of the students they teach. This cannot be accomplished unless educators take an active role in the development of the daily lesson plans.

Planning and developing a program of study is an individualized project that includes input from a wide range of participants, including school personnel and advisory council members. Planning will take into consideration the prescribed state curriculum, the school's facilities, the school's mission statement, the program objectives, the resources available for program development, and much more. The program of study must be flexible enough to meet the educational requirements set forth by the state regulatory agency as well as the demands made by the current industry trends. It must present a planned and organized approach to a well-rounded educational program.

The master educator will follow the program outline exactly. She will prepare her teaching activities well in advance. She will establish measurable performance outcomes or objectives for each unit of study. She will respect and follow the **curriculum** and program of study established by the school without fail. As she progresses through a program of study, she will make regular notes regarding what works and what doesn't work so that information can be incorporated into future curriculum revision projects. A master educator will recognize her role in applying assessment and evaluation criteria to students on an individual basis to ensure that each student is receiving maximum benefit from the program of study. A master educator will also recognize that a proper and complete program outline and class schedule will become the blueprint that will enable educators to know:

curriculum
a set of courses constituting an area of specialization.

- what is to be taught;
- when it is to be taught; and
- how it is to be taught.

The same program outline and class schedule will also advise educators and students of:

- where they are going;
- how they are going to get there; and
- why the program objectives are relevant.

Organization and careful planning make it possible for an institution to provide ultimate educational and training effort with maximum efficiency and maximum results.

In Retrospect

1. List the steps in the curriculum development process.
2. Explain the purpose of the use of an advisory council in the curriculum development process.
3. Define the three domains for instructional outcomes.
4. State the purpose of a sound orientation program for new students.
5. Explain the value and advantages of lesson planning.
6. List each component of a lesson plan.

CHAPTER

11

Educational Aids and Technology in the Classroom

Objectives (Desired Performance Goals):

After reading and studying this chapter, you should be able to:

- List the 10 advantages for using educational aids.

- List the eight important concepts to consider when preparing and selecting visual aids.

- Explain the guidelines for effective use of multipurpose boards and flip charts.

- Explain the basic rules for preparing and using slides.

- List key tips for using electronic whiteboards.

- Employ the general guidelines that should be considered when using projected materials.

! CRITICAL CONCEPT

Effective use of educational aids and technology will enhance any class and ensure greater opportunity for the learner to retain the information.

The Master Educator's Role

THE MASTER EDUCATOR PLAYS an important role in the identification, selection, and development of instructional materials and teaching aids. Research in adult learning shows that lecture-only teaching is essentially obsolete. Classes need to be learner-centered, use a variety of teaching methods that appeal to the various senses of the learner, and involve learners in the educational process. **Educational aids** can boost student success in the classroom. These aids reinforce what a teacher says and help ensure the main points are understood. Educational teaching aids highlight important information, engage students' other senses in the learning process, and allow for different learning styles.

Why Use Educational Aids and Technology?

Learning resources, technology, and instructional aids support creative and innovative teaching methods. Varying instructional materials and teaching aids encourages student interest in the material being presented. Instructional aids provide for a change of pace and help to clarify important information. Visual instructional tools are effective across cultures and languages because they act as a natural bridge between intellectual understanding of and the ability to perform complex tasks. Infusing technology into the learning environment has become a national priority. Memorable teachers will master the use of instructional media in ways that best augment their teaching styles and learning objectives.

Advantages of Using Instructional Aids and Technology

There are a number of advantages to using effective instructional media, including minimizing or eliminating barriers caused by language, space, or time. These advantages are discussed next.

Reinforcement of Key Ideas. Learners often place more emphasis on what they see as opposed to what they only hear. Students tend to take more detailed notes regarding material projected or displayed through a visual aid than on information that is presented orally with no visual-aid support.

Create Attention and Interest. It has been determined that the average learner thinks at a rate of approximately 400 to 500 words per minute. The average educator speaks at the rate of 110 to 160 words per minute. The use of interesting **visual aids** can go a long way in filling in the gap between the rates of speaking and thinking. Creative visual aids can help focus the learner's attention on the topic being presented to avoid the inevitable mind-wandering that might otherwise occur.

Develop Understanding and Increase Retention. The more senses the presentation can address, the greater the opportunity for understanding by the learner. The greater the learner's understanding of the matter at hand, the longer he will retain the information. This can best be summed up by the words of Confucius, who said in 451 B.C., "What I hear, I forget; what

---

+ MASTER EDUCATOR

1. Use a variety of instructional media within each classroom.
2. Incorporate educational aids that help students understand, process, encode, and recall new information.
3. Are change masters and embrace growth and learning.

educational aids
aids that boost student success in the classroom and reinforce what a teacher says while helping to ensure that main points are understood. Educational teaching aids highlight important information, engage students' other senses in the learning process, and allow for different learning styles.

visual aids
an instructional tool, such as a video, poster, model, chart, graph, or slide, that presents information visually.

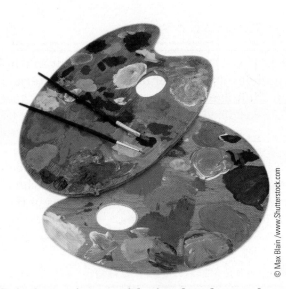

Figure 11–1   Painting a picture with visuals enhances learning.

I see, I remember; what I do, I understand." Hearing, seeing, and doing all appeal to different senses and increase retention for the learner.

Paint a Picture of Information. A picture is three times more effective than words alone, and words and pictures together can be six times more effective. This gives new meaning to the old adage that "a picture is worth a thousand words (Figure 11–1)."

Increase Comprehension. A well-prepared visual aid can give clearer meaning to words or directions that may otherwise be confusing. For example, when teaching cardiopulmonary resuscitation (CPR), the instructor can explain the steps by stating that the victim should be lying flat, his airway open with head tilted back with his nose pinched while giving two full breaths. However, if the educator makes that statement and while projecting on the screen or smart board a nine-pane matrix depicting the nine steps of administering CPR. (For an example of such a window pane, refer to Chapter 5, "Basic Methods of Teaching and Learning.") Use of the visual aid strengthens and supports the verbal and/or written instructions. Consider how today's Global Positioning Systems work in helping you to find your destination. The system projects a moving map on the screen, which is supplemented by voice support telling you when to turn and which direction to go. The system goes on to display how far you are from your destination and what time you will arrive.

Add Value to Time and Resources. For most students, 75 percent of what they learn is obtained visually, another 13 percent is gained through hearing, and a total of only 12 percent is accomplished through the other senses of smell, taste, and touch. Therefore, by adding visual aids to the spoken message, learners will gain the information more quickly and reduce required presentation time significantly. We have all heard that "time is money." Therefore, by saving time, overall costs will be reduced.

Add "Real-World" Perspective. When teaching the underlying theories, judgments, and skills required in career education, it is helpful to illustrate them with real-life examples. For instance, when teaching anatomy and the phases of cell mitosis, the educator could simply state that

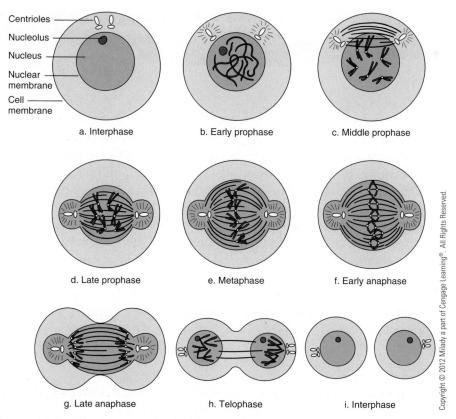

Centrioles
Nucleolus
Nucleus
Nuclear membrane
Cell membrane

a. Interphase   b. Early prophase   c. Middle prophase

d. Late prophase   e. Metaphase   f. Early anaphase

g. Late anaphase   h. Telophase   i. Interphase

Figure 11–2   The phases of mitosis.

there are nine phases in mitosis including: interphase, early prophase, middle prophase, late prophase, metaphase, early anaphase, late anaphase, telophase, and finally back to interphase (Figure 11–2). The statement alone would leave the learner with a huge gray fog in their brain. However, if the educator projected a slide depicting a real-life example of those nine phases, the learner would have a much clearer understanding of the process.

Organize and Cover Presentation Points. Visual aids can be a tremendously helpful tool when the educator is attempting to clarify his thinking and develop a logical sequence of the material to be presented. By arranging the visual aids in order prior to the presentation, the educator can also ensure that every key point in the lesson is covered during the class. In fact, slides that contain detailed notes can be printed and used as the lesson plan to ensure that all key presentation points are covered in proper sequence.

Ensure Consistency. The more visual aids used in the classroom, the more confidence the educator can have that all students are seeing and hearing the same thing. By using descriptive, clarifying instructional media, there is less chance of the learner misunderstanding the spoken words.

Create Educator Confidence. A master educator, regardless of his years of experience, will be remiss if he relies solely on his memory or experience for ensuring that all key elements of a lesson are presented. Even the sharpest of practitioners or educators can experience the mind going "blank." At the same time, a younger educator may be fearful or less confident that he will remember everything he needs to present in a given class. By having well-organized instructional media, educators, both new and experienced, can approach the classroom with more confidence in their ability to deliver a powerful and informative lesson.

☑ What to Consider

Teaching situations vary greatly and the need for and use of teaching materials will be adapted accordingly. The objectives established for each lesson will determine, to some extent, what types of teaching aids will be used. The instruction must be adapted to both the individual and collective needs of the learners in the classroom as well. This is a major responsibility and takes a good deal of planning on the part of the educator. By using a variety of teaching materials, there is greater opportunity that learners of different ability levels will ultimately absorb the information. For example, if the student has difficulty with reading or with the English language, visual aids should not be primarily of the print variety. It would be more beneficial to incorporate other aids such as photos, graphs, charts, maps, or models into the presentation.

Important Concepts

When selecting and preparing visual aids for use in the classroom, the master educator considers a number of important concepts.

Visibility. A visual aid is hardly effective if it cannot be seen clearly by all learners.

Clarification. An effective visual aid will explain a *single* concept or technique; it will show a relationship or present a procedure in a clear, concise manner; it will be relevant.

Color. Bright colors have aesthetic appeal for learners; colors create interest and have been proven to enhance retention of information.

Proportion. In depicting any physical technique or procedure, all parts should be in proper proportion to each other to avoid misleading or confusing the learner.

Construction. When preparing visual aids, the educator should employ good workmanship as well as quality materials.

Mobility. When preparing large instructional aids, the educator should take measures to ensure that they are portable enough to move from one classroom to another and can be properly stored and protected.

Terminology. Words used in visual aids must be clear and understandable for all learners. The terms used should be current and consistent with industry trends.

Protection. When preparing instructional aids, consideration should be given to how they will be protected for future use. This could be something as simple as maintaining overhead transparencies in sheet protectors or something as sophisticated as making a cover for a life-size model of the human skeleton that might be used when studying anatomy and physiology, or backing up electronic files on a CD-ROM or on portable storage devices such as flash or jump drives.

CONSIDER AND CONNECT

Visuals communicate messages more powerfully than just written or spoken words. Learners may miss written or spoken words, but they can encode visual information in an instant.

CONSIDER AND CONNECT

The master educator carefully chooses and prepares teaching materials and aids that will strongly influence the degree of success achieved by the learners.

Educational Materials

Every institution should maintain learning resources appropriate and essential for the achievement of the objectives established for each program offered. Learning resources include relevant educational materials, such as reference books, periodicals, business manuals, technical references, textbooks, workbooks, audiovisual materials, audiovisual equipment, and any other materials that support the educational programs.

Standard Print Materials

Print materials rely primarily on reading for comprehension. They are used more for reference, independent study, or as handouts, rather than as visual aids during a presentation. Some of the most common printed materials used in adult education are discussed next.

Textbooks. These are the fundamental sources of essential information (Figure 11–3). They generally include all the basics required for licensure in a given discipline. Though they play a major role in education, they should not be overused by educators. Other aids and resources should be used to supplement the basic textbook. Institutions should also not overlook the opportunity to use eBooks. Cengage Learning publishes electronic versions of textbooks within certain disciplines for instant online access by students. The use of such tools requires an Internet connection and enables highlighting, note taking, and bookmarking. Students can even use the search capability and benefit from the audio glossary. Further, students usually have the ability to print pages one at a time while connected to the Internet. In this age of computer technology, this is a great way for students to have access to the full content without having to carry the textbook at all times.

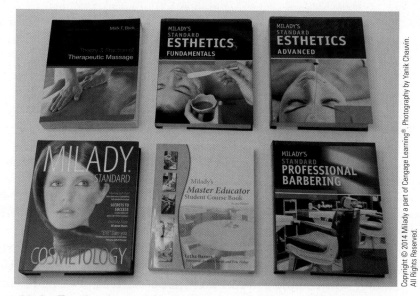

Figure 11–3 **Textbooks are the fundamental source of information for every program of study.**

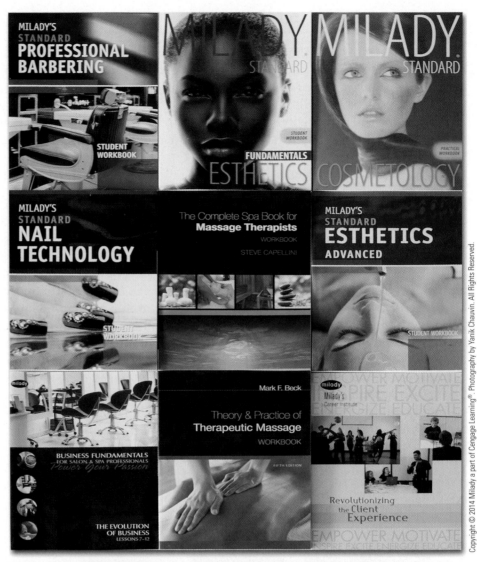

Figure 11–4 **Workbooks are used to complement and support basic text material. Cengage Learning also publishes Study Guides to accompany some of their core textbooks. These products are developed with all learning styles in mind and help students recognize, understand, and retain key concepts while minimizing the need for assistance from the educator. Many activities allow the students freedom to work in pairs and small teams, which appeals to the interactive, social learners.**

Workbooks. Workbooks are usually written to complement and support the basic text material. They contain exercises, tests, projects, and other activities that correlate with the textbook chapters. A major advantage is that they can be used independently and at the pace set by the learner (Figure 11–4).

Newspapers, Articles, and Clippings. Newspaper items or articles from trade journals or industry periodicals can be useful in the classroom because they will usually contain information that is even more current than that contained in the basic textbook. They can also be used to give credibility and strength to text materials or information presented by the educator (Figure 11–5).

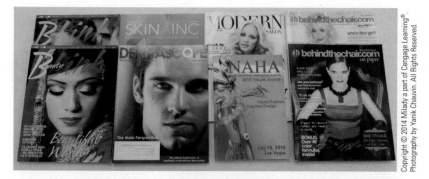

Figure 11–5   Trade journals or newsletters contain current information that adds credibility.

Brochures and Pamphlets. Inexpensive but useful information can be obtained from a variety of resources that support the education offered in the classroom. Sources for educational pamphlets are professional trade associations, industrial and commercial firms, and state and federal government agencies (Figure 11–6). For example, the U.S. Department of Labor publishes annually an *Occupational Outlook Handbook* that contains information about career opportunities in the United States. This could be beneficial for anyone pondering a career choice. A company by the name of Channing Bete Company, Inc. publishes a variety of booklets with such titles as *About Time Management, About College and Stress, How to Improve Your Listening Skills, How to Improve Your Reading Skills,* and more. All these booklets could be useful for the educator in any career-education classroom.

Reference Books and Exam Review Tools. Learning resources in any institution should include a well-equipped library of reference materials for use by both the educators and the students (Figure 11–7). They can be used for research when preparing for a presentation, by students

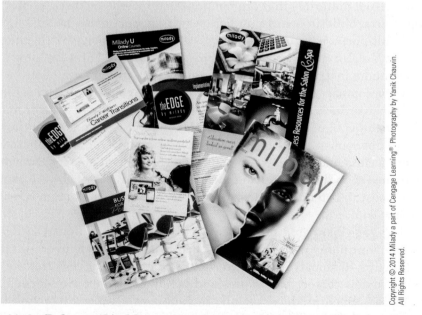

Figure 11–6   Relevant booklets are an inexpensive source of information that supports education.

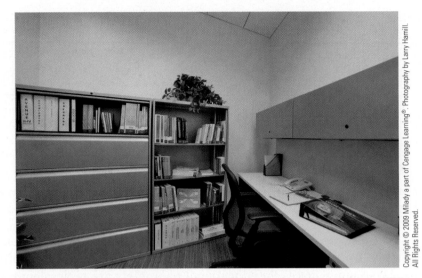

Figure 11–7   A well-equipped media or resource center can be used by students and educators.

to research materials for a special report or project, or just to increase general knowledge in a given subject matter. Cengage Learning publishes exam-review booklets for many disciplines in both hard copy and through a mobile application (app). The "on-the-go" app is designed to help students prepare for written exams. It is available for use with iPhone, iPod touch, and iPad devices. Features often include a "question of the day," randomized multiple-choice questions for each chapter, immediate feedback with rationales, and progress reporting for all chapter tests.

Nonprojected Audiovisual Materials

Audiovisual materials that are nonprojected include pictures, photographs, flip charts, bulletin boards, audiotapes or compact discs, posters, exhibits, and multipurpose boards. Following is a brief discussion of each category.

Audio Downloads or Compact Discs. As we enter the new millennium, audio instruction is presented primarily in the form of audio downloads, or compact discs. Audio files or discs are convenient and reasonably inexpensive. Such audio tools are useful to support the instructor and have long been popular tools in the educational process. In addition, they are a key component in self-study or self-instructional systems. Educators can record a class and then have the audio download available for students who were absent to listen to during independent study. The slower learner can also choose to listen to the class repeatedly to ensure maximum retention of the material.

Cengage Learning publishes highly effective student CD-ROMs to supplement many of their core textbooks. They include over 100 helpful video clips, demonstrating proper practice and procedures that help students review correct techniques and behaviors they have learned in the classroom. Such products usually include a randomized testbank unique to the tool to help the student review for key examinations. Often there is a game section included to create an entertaining form of education with word and image scrambles, Hangman, and other games. To reinforce terminology and pronunciation, an audio glossary is often included, with hundreds of terms from each textbook. Some products include games patterned after popular television game shows. Educators use these products as both a self-study tool for students as well as a way to facilitate interactive education and competitions right in the classroom. These tools have also been found to be very effective for students who need to "catch up" after having missed class due to an illness, for example. Some educators are using podcasts which are a type of digital media consisting of an episodic series of audio files subscribed to and downloaded through Web syndication or streamed online to a computer or mobile device for student use. The word is a neologism derived from "broadcast" and "pod" as a result of the success of the iPod. Podcasts are often listened to on portable media players by students in many different venues.

Pictures, Photographs, Charts, Bulletin Boards, and Posters. Visual representations made through pictures, photographs, charts, graphs, posters, or bulletin boards can be useful in presenting many types of information in interesting ways that enhance and motivate learning. These types of visual aids can increase retention, develop continuity of thought, provide variety in learning, and make effective use of instructional time. They can also provide experiences for the student that may not be available through other sources.

Exhibits. There will be times when it is appropriate for educators to display a group of objects that are used to form an integrated whole for instructional purposes. Such exhibits can be used in much the same way as the individual components are used in the educational process. Simple exhibits can be set up in many places, such as on a table, shelf, or desk. More complex exhibits may require considerable floor space and special construction. Students can participate in assembly of a more complex

---

GUIDELINES FOR USING PICTURES, PHOTOS, CHARTS, BULLETIN BOARDS, AND POSTERS

- Keep them current. An old, obsolete bulletin board is worse than useless. Properly attach the material. If using pictures, photos, diagrams, or charts on a bulletin board, make sure they are tacked down securely and do not hang askew.
- Keep it simple. Remember that "less is more." Focus on the key point or message and don't clutter the display with unnecessary information.
- Encourage creativity. Have learners prepare educational bulletin boards. Inspire their creative juices and let them exhibit their creativity about a given subject while also learning more about it.
- Use instant or digital cameras. The ability to take instantly developed or electronically printed pictures adds reinforcement to the classroom by allowing learners to capture certain looks or techniques they have created. Having photos of certain steps or experiences also increases learner retention.
- Practice and encourage humor. The master educator will use humor and cartoons whenever possible to emphasize learning points.

multipurpose board
a white magnetic marker board that functions in much the same way as a chalkboard but with many more uses.

exhibit. Such participation can foster teamwork and increase retention of the subject matter as well. An exhibit might be a display of the student's lab kit and educational materials during the new-student orientation class.

Multipurpose Boards. Although chalkboards may still be used in some classrooms, the more modern version is a white magnetic marker board, also commonly called a **multipurpose board**. Each type can be effective in communicating information to learners. As the name indicates, the multipurpose board may be used for several purposes.

Multipurpose boards have a smooth white surface that is magnetized. Special marking pens that come in a variety of colors are used with multipurpose boards. They are cleaned with a damp cloth. Because of their steel backing, other visuals can be attached to the board with the use of magnets. This is especially beneficial when the educator is building upon concepts within a given subject matter. The white, nonglare surface has other uses—it can be used for a projection background and materials, such as figures or letters that are cut from plastic, will adhere to the surface when rubbed in place.

There are a number of advantages of using a multipurpose board. Boards are flexible in that the educator can develop or prepare material in advance or use it during the presentation to provide direction in the learning process. It can then be erased for re use in the next part of the class. Another advantage is that these boards available in most classrooms. The use of colored markers can add variety (Figure 11–8). As with any teaching tool, there are also disadvantages. Boards are so common that their frequent use could fail to attract and retain the attention of the learner. Once the material placed on the board has been erased, it is difficult and time-consuming to refer back to it. Also, constant use of the board can result in the educator talking "to" the board rather than to the class. In addition, the chalk or markers may not always be easily read by everyone in the class.

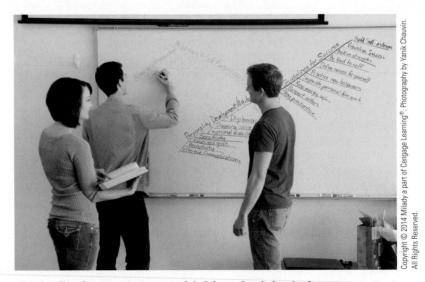

Figure 11–8   Students can create highly colorful mind maps on a multipurpose board.

TOP 10 USES FOR BOARDS

- List the objectives for the lesson.

- Outline the material contained in the lesson.

- Sketch items such as cross sections, diagrams, tools, and equipment.

- List quiz questions ahead of time.

- List new vocabulary.

- Notify learners of important announcements.

- Provide solutions of sample problems or challenges.

- Allow students to work through problems or make drawings under close supervision with easy opportunity for corrections.

- List assignments for the day or week.

- Use as the background for slide projection.

TOP 10 TIPS FOR EFFECTIVE BOARD USE

1. Always begin with a clean board. The chalkboard and chalk rail should be washed before each class. Make sure that chalk, a clean eraser, and other necessary supplies are available.

2. If writing a lot of material on the board, prepare a layout to ensure you have sufficient space, and do so ahead of time to avoid using too much class time for the task.

3. Use printed letters rather than script and make them at least 2 inches tall.

4. When presenting, remember to speak to the learners, not the board.

5. Take care not to use grease- or wax-based chalks or permanent markers that will not come off the board.

(Continued)

TOP 10 TIPS FOR EFFECTIVE BOARD USE

6. Use the board to supplement other instructional material, such as the key points of a video before showing it to the class.

7. Use a laser pointer to reference material on the board. In the absence of a laser pointer, an inexpensive quarter-inch dowel about 2 feet long will suffice.

8. Practice using simple sketching techniques, such as stick figures, which can be used in presentations.

9. Write material on the top half of the board as much as possible for greater visibility. If possible, the bottom of the board should be 36 to 42 inches from the floor.

10. If other educators share the same classroom area, use courtesy in maintaining the board. Clean it after each class. Do *not* write "save" on the board. Material that needs to be saved should be written on flip charts or paper panels on the walls.

Flip Charts. Flip charts are large pads of bound paper approximately 30 inches wide and 36 inches tall. They contain a large number of white or blank newsprint pages on which the educator can present visual information. Often the pages are perforated at the top for ease of removal from the padded chart. Commercial flip charts are available to accompany some instructional units, but educators can create their own in the classroom using the blank ones. Generally, they are suitable for a relatively small class of no more than 40 learners, depending upon the physical layout of the classroom. It is essential, as with all visual aids, that the charts are clearly visible to all learners. Flips charts are useful in teaching sequential steps in a process. Each major point can be illustrated on a single sheet for discussion before moving on to the next page. Almost any type of nonprojected visual may be used with a flip chart display, such as photographs, pictures, diagrams, or figures. Flip charts are portable, adaptable, and allow easy reference back to previous points. They provide an effective tool for review and can be stored for reuse as needed. They are not inexpensive to use, as the pads of paper can be used up quickly. A sturdy stand is essential to avoid awkwardness when writing on the pad. The pages can become worn if overused. Some key points for effective use of flip charts should be considered, as discussed in the accompanying box.

Projected Audiovisual Materials

We have discussed at length the various uses, advantages, and disadvantages of nonprojected audiovisual aids. Another category of effective instructional aids is projected visual aids. The most common projected visual aids include

TOP 10 KEY POINTS FOR FLIP CHART USE

1. Determine key points of the presentation in advance and pencil them in lightly at the top or side margin of the flip chart pages. During the actual presentation, the penciled notes will serve as your outline for using brightly colored markers to record the important information.

2. Prepare some of the pages in advance as appropriate (Figure 11–9). Prevent them from early review by learners by taping a couple of blank sheets over them until the time you wish to display the prepared material. This technique can be used for full or partial pages of the chart.

3. Use a variety of colored markers that are not commonly used. Design art markers are available in colors such as blue-green and red-violet. Such colors are unusual, attract the attention of the learner, and can be easily seen.

4. Unless the flip chart can be placed at least 36 to 42 inches off the floor, write on the top two-thirds of the chart to ensure that everyone in the class can see the material. If you are presenting from a platform it may be possible for everyone to see the entire chart, in which case you can use the entire page.

5. Enhance the visual appeal of each page by using techniques such as underlining, boxing, and geometric shapes to add visual interest for the learner.

6. Use flip charts for brainstorming sessions. This is a terrific tool in learner-centered education. Assign students to record key ideas on flip charts as they come up. This allows you to get the learners involved while also maintaining control of the class. You can clarify the ideas or concepts while the student does the recording.

7. Remember to stand to the side of the flip chart as you discuss the information recorded there.

8. Point to the item on the chart that you are referencing. A laser pointer can be used, or use a moveable keynote that you can place next to the item under discussion and move as needed.

9. For certain discussions, you will want to remove each flip chart page and tape it to the wall (unless using the very expensive charts that already have the "stick-on" feature) so the information can easily be referenced and reviewed during the remainder of the class.

10. Use masking tape to attach charts to the wall because it can be taped to most surfaces without causing any damage. Very fine straight pins may also be used on many surfaces.

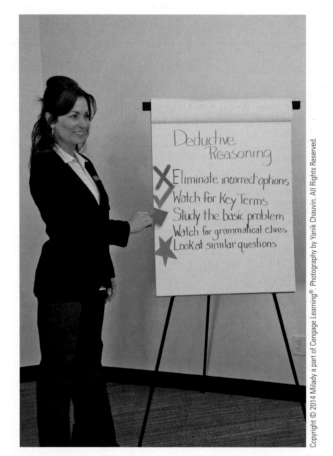

Figure 11–9   Prepare flip chart pages in advance and use color and keynotes for emphasis.

overhead transparencies, liquid crystal display (LCD), videotapes and DVDs, computer software, and electronic delivery. In the twenty-first century, technology is changing dramatically and millions of dollars will be spent to equip our nation's schools with technologies that facilitate the generation and dissemination of knowledge. Today's students have been raised in a media-oriented environment. As educators, we must use that same technology to enhance our teaching methods and the student's ability to learn. We will first discuss overhead projection, which is rapidly being replaced by improved technology.

Overhead Projectors and Transparencies. Although overhead projection using transparencies is rapidly being replaced with LCD projection, it is an economic and convenient alternative to using a board. It is a tremendously flexible instructional tool. It can project any material that is written, drawn, or printed on transparent film. Write-on transparencies can be used in the same manner as the chalkboard, but allow the educator to face the class even while writing the material on the film. Another advantage is the ability to use this type of projection in a fairly well-lit room, which facilitates note taking and interaction with learners. The educator can also build on concepts by adding overlays to base transparencies. Brightly colored markers can be used on transparency film to create interest and gain attention. Markers are available in either permanent ink or wet/dry-erase felt-tip pens.

One advantage of using overhead projection and transparencies is that they are extremely versatile. Educators can use commercially prepared transparencies or can make their own. In addition to writing on blank transparencies, the educator can produce fairly sophisticated film using a good word-processing program or publishing software. The laser-printed hard copy of the material can be converted to a transparency simply by running the appropriate type of transparency film through the copier. Take care to ensure that the film is appropriate for the copier. Incompatible film could result in the melting of the film inside the copier, which is an expensive error. Another advantage is that the equipment and tools are close to the front of the room near the educator and only a small amount of space is needed. One disadvantage is the fact that light bulbs for the projector invariably burn out in the middle of a presentation. It is recommended that a spare bulb be taped inside the projector so that the problem can easily be remedied if it occurs. Another disadvantage is that there is no audio to support the overhead. That, however, is where the educator comes in. You provide the audio to go along with these useful visual aids. Remember, classroom size and arrangement may not always be suitable for use of an overhead projector.

Computers and Computer Software. Due to improved technologies, computers are playing a much larger role in education. Visuals can be displayed on a computer monitor in a sequence much like slides and filmstrips, but also have the advantage of providing some video-like effects such as wipes, dissolves, fades, animation, and more. Graphics can be output from the computer into other forms of presentation media such as handouts or transparencies. Information can be projected on television monitors, video projectors, and projection screens. CD-ROM discs serve as a great source for independent study and/or classroom presentations. Computer software programs have made test creation, test-bank storage, and indexing of information much easier.

It is essential that today's learners have access to the use of computers and the accompanying technology for effective learning. Most schools are installing and upgrading computer labs, depending on the size of the school and the programs offered. Most will have at least a couple of computer stations available for students and others will have entire labs with numerous stations available for student use. In addition, many schools are using tablet technology and downloading relevant applications and allowing students access to the tablets. For example, at Dermalogica Academy in Manhattan, iPads play multiple roles throughout the academy, from acting as the reference library to being a personal tutor. With so many great apps available, the academy uses iPads to engage the learner individually and in groups. They use a number of apps for preparing student exams and playing review games that are fun and collaborative. They are also used to help students learn to build a client base, fill clinic hours with services, and establish ongoing relationships with clients using social media. They use the Facemapping® app as a tool to become a successful retailer and build a personalized product prescription for each client. With today's technology, a master educator is limited only by his imagination with respect to using technology in the classroom.

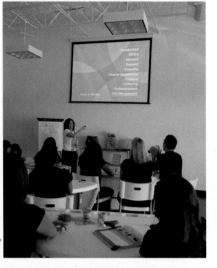

Figure 11–10   LCD projection eliminates the need for bulky televisions, and images may be projected on a much larger screen.

Liquid Crystal Display (LCD)

an LCD projector is a device that is used to display video images or data. Light from a halogen lamp passes through glass panels and produces an image that can be projected onto any flat surface.

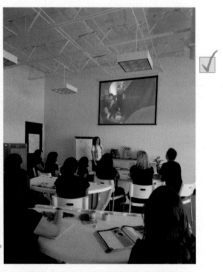

Figure 11–11   One advantage of using DVDs is that they can be viewed in a fully-lit classroom.

Liquid Crystal Display (LCD). Numerous features and benefits of the use of LCD projection warrant discussion. An LCD projector is a device that is used to display video images or data. It is the modern equivalent of the slide projector or filmstrip projector of the past. Light from a halogen lamp passes through glass panels and produces an image that can be projected onto any flat surface. Use of an LCD projector eliminates the need for bulky televisions. Images may be projected on a much larger screen than a typical television screen, providing for greater visibility for all students (Figure 11–10). LCD projectors are smaller and less expensive than ever and are a viable and affordable tool for today's classrooms. When considering the purchase of an LCD projector, various features should be considered, including resolution, brightness, contrast, weight, connectivity, and lamp life.

Slides, typically created in PowerPoint™, may be developed to present a complete lesson. Such instructor-support slides are available from Cengage Learning to support textbooks in a wide variety of career education disciplines. Slides may be developed using actual photographs that, when projected, appear more real than printed pictures because the colors are more brilliant and appealing to the learner. Slides may also be created from word-processing programs or publishing software on a computer. Again, clarity and vivid colors add interest to the presentation. LCD projection of PowerPoint™ slides can typically be accomplished in a fully lit room, provided there is not a significant wash on the screen from bulbs positioned directly overhead. A few hints to remember when using PowerPoint™ slides include printing out a handout so learners can take notes, having a backup plan in case of technology failure, and using a remote or having someone advance slides for you so that you can focus on your students. Cengage Learning provides a chapter-by-chapter outline of important discussion topics in Microsoft PowerPoint™ to support many of its core textbooks. The products usually include hundreds of slides featuring images from the text to capture the interest of the visual learner. Sides are easy to use and easy to edit. Additional visuals and photos can easily be dropped and the notes sections can be edited with each educators personal notes.

DVDs. "Digital Versatile Disc" or "Digital Video Disc" (DVD) is an optical disc storage format that can be used for storing data, including movies with high video and sound quality. DVDs resemble compact discs, as their diameter is the same (120 mm [4.72 inches] or occasionally 80 mm [3.15 inches] in diameter), but they are encoded in a different format and at a much higher density.

For the most part, films and filmstrips have been replaced with video and DVD technologies. One advantage of DVD/video use is that they can be viewed in a fully lit room (Figure 11–11). Video gives the educator the advantage of showing motion, which is important for certain kinds of learning, especially with respect to mastering technical skills. For example, many quality technical DVDs are available from Cengage Learning that show step-by-step procedures for learning a wide variety of technical skills. DVDs and CD-ROMs can also be used to present an example of behavior being discussed as it relates to the training program. DVD technology is used with this text to show interaction between an educator and students, or students and clients,

BASIC GUIDELINES FOR CREATING SLIDES

- Remember, less is more. Keep each slide simple and uncluttered. Limit the information to no more than eight lines per slide and no more than eight words on a line whenever possible.
- Use at least 18-point, bold, simple typefaces or fonts in both upper- and lowercase lettering.
- Vary the font size to emphasize relative importance of material.
- Provide ample space between letters, words, and lines. Leave a space equal to the height of an uppercase letter between each line.
- Be creative. Use cartoons, graphs, charts, and illustrations instead of relying solely on words to convey your meaning. Use tinted film and/or colored ink for emphasis and interest.
- Use horizontal visuals to allow maximum visibility.
- Avoid vertical lettering, which is hard to read and distracting.
- Use a maximum of two font styles on any single slide. If you use more, the type tends to compete with the content.
- Think in key points or bullets. Choose active words and short phrases.
- If items are nonsequential, don't number them. Use bullets, characters, arrows, boxes, and so on to delineate them.
- Use copyright-free illustrations found in clip-art books, which provide an inexpensive source of professional art.
- Prepare presentations well ahead of the scheduled class and support with detailed notes.
- Check the projector bulb, visibility and glare, position of the screen in relation to seating, and focus of the screen prior to the class.
- Go to a black screen whenever students will be coming to the front of the room for activities as the projector light can be very harsh.
- Point to specific items on the screen with a laser pointer, which is usually included with a remote control used to advance bullets and slides within a presentation.

and so forth. A video presentation of specific subject matter can often carry the bulk of the classroom presentation. Videotapes are economical, flexible, and easily stored. These are all reasons why video education is one of the most commonly used instructional materials in today's classrooms. In order to ensure that maximum learning is derived from the classroom presentation, the educator should consider a number of key guidelines. Remember, whenever the term *video* is used, it is referring to either video or DVD technology.

Television. Open-circuit television is the type that comes into our homes through broadcasts by networks and local stations. Closed-circuit television is a system through which the number of receiving units can be selectively controlled, usually accomplished through cable connections. Closed-circuit television is generally associated with the educational field. Modern videotaping techniques combined with closed-circuit television offers tremendous potential for the field of education. The hardware used with videotaping is generally a television monitor. When determining the size of a television monitor for a classroom, plan for one diagonal inch

CONSIDER AND CONNECT

Many teachers today are taking advantage of the wide array of free videos available from YouTube. They simply search a specific topic, review the clips, and share those that are the most applicable to the topic and bring the most interest and humor to subject matter.

TIPS FOR VIDEO/DVD EDUCATION

- Consider the objectives of the lesson. Does the video address those learning objectives?
- Be familiar with the content of the video. Make sure it deals with your subject in a manner consistent with your presentation.
- Prepare discussion questions for use before and after the viewing of the video.
- Make certain that learners know what they are expected to learn from the video. Explain the value of the knowledge they are about to receive.
- Introduce the key points of the video prior to the viewing. This encourages learners to pay attention to those points during the presentation.
- Discourage note taking during the video because it can cause learners to miss important points. Hand out an information sheet after the video instead.
- Eliminate all possible distractions (noise, glare, interruptions) and be sure the room is well ventilated.
- Ensure that the video is in focus and the volume and tone are appropriate for room size.
- Show only relevant parts of the video. Cue the video to the appropriate point ahead of time. To maintain learner interest and retention of the material, stop during long videos and lead a relevant discussion.
- Reinforce major points of the material either during the video or immediately afterward if the video does not already do so through repetition.
- After reviewing major points, discuss the principles and practical application of the information.
- Show the video a second time whenever possible, either immediately after the discussion or as a review at the beginning of the next class session.
- If the video presents a technical procedure, students should demonstrate the actual skills involved, rather than convey their learning through a written or oral examination.
- When reviewing, correct wrong responses from learners immediately to prevent learning of incorrect information or habit patterns.

of viewing screen for each student in the class. For example, if there are 25 students, you would want a 25-inch monitor. If that size of monitor is unavailable, the option is two 19-inch screens. For classes over 75, it becomes more effective to use a video projector on a much larger screen. When using a front-screen projector, a darkened room is necessary for clear viewing. Video education may be the most popular today, and a broad spectrum of subjects and titles is available at very affordable prices. When using television and DVD education, it is critical that the educator remains in the classroom, facilitates the use of the effective medium, and ensures interaction among the learners.

Electronic Whiteboards

Another term for an electronic whiteboard is a SMART board. It is a digital whiteboard that allows the use of touchscreen capabilities to manipulate information due to the connection to a computer. The screen works much like a computer in that there is a menu button, floating toolbar, notebook, keyboard, and write button. There are three main features: touch recognition that allows you to use a pen to write, your finger to navigate, and your palm to erase; a pen tray that works much like a chalkboard; and SMART software that is used for delivery of lessons.

- Use your finger or stylus to write notes and information, which can then be saved to a file or CD-ROM, printed out, or emailed to others.
- Have students use the highlighter tool to highlight key terms and definitions.
- Allow students to use fingers to point and interact with images, text, and other objects on the screen; this benefits students with limited motor skills.
- Use comic book software to create humorous stories about important program content or allow students to write and develop their own comic books.
- Use interactive Web sites with the whiteboard to research and report on key topics.
- Allow students to interact with software on the electronic whiteboard while you use an attached computer to manipulate features in the program.

Use of an electronic whiteboard has resulted in more motivation and interest on the part of the learner because the subject comes alive and captures the learner's attention. This technology encourages the involvement of learners while giving the instructor instant access to a vast array of electronic resources. In addition, it enables seamless links to be made between the technology and the subject material (Figure 11–12).

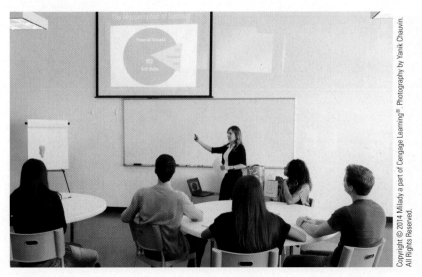

Figure 11–12 **Once an educator becomes trained in the use of the electronic whiteboard, the flexibility and scope for imaginative lesson planning is huge.**

distance learning
any mode of instruction in which there is a separation, in time or place, between the instructor and the student.

Electronic Delivery Systems (Distance Learning). Another technological innovation that has had a tremendous impact on education is that of electronic systems for the delivery of instruction. This impact has grown dramatically in the new millennium. In the not-too-distant past, the individual classroom educator was practically the sole facilitator of learning. Schools now use distance education to respond to students' needs for alternatives to the schedules and locations at which courses traditionally have been offered. More and more courses and programs are available online by way of the Internet. In addition to being a great resource for educators to research materials in education preparation, the Internet has already made its mark in the area of distance learning (Figure 11–13). The U.S. Department of Education defines **distance learning** as any mode of instruction in which there is a separation, in time or place, between the instructor and the student.

Cengage Learning publishes online courses for many disciplines that are designed to be used with core textbooks and to support the practical portion of some courses. The online courses focus on delivering the theory portions of the curriculum online while also addressing all types of learners. Features include interactive lectures with audio, video support, interactive learning reinforcement activities, including situational problems, games, automatically graded quizzes and tests as well as audio flashcards with glossary terms and definitions. Cengage Learning also offers many online learning programs for licensure examination preparation and teacher-training programs. Online testing preparation programs offer students a fast and convenient way to prepare for important examinations. Tens of thousands of students have successfully used these products, which offer review and chapter tests plus comprehensive tests. Extensive reports help students determine areas of study to focus on. A key advantage of online learning is that the student can set the pace and the schedule based on his or her own personal needs.

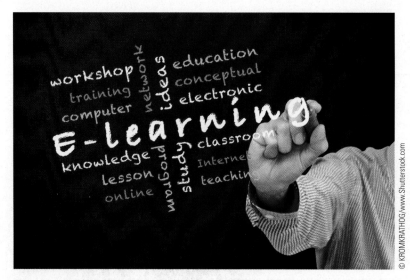

Figure 11–13 The Internet has made its mark in the area of distance learning.

Telecommunications courses are offered principally through the use of one or more technologies to deliver instruction to students who are separated from the instructor and to support regular and substantive interaction between students and the instructors. These technologies include television, audio, or computer transmission through open broadcast, closed circuit, cable, microwave, or satellite, and audio and computer conferencing.

Students should consider certain personal traits, however, to predict their success with a distance-learning program. Encourage students to answer some key questions prior to enrolling in a distance education program, such as:

- Do I enjoy, and am I good, at reading and writing?
- How do I handle project deadlines?
- How important to me is face-to-face interaction with my teachers and fellow students?
- How good are my computer skills?
- How much time can I devote to my coursework on a weekly basis?
- How good am I at organizing and managing my time?
- Am I willing to actively contribute in online discussions?
- What are my expectations from completion of the online course?

Instructors need to recognize that though distance learning is here to stay, due to the hands-on nature of technical skills training within many career-education disciplines, the educator will never be replaced by technology.

Social Media

In the twenty-first century, a master educator will not ignore the impact of social media on our adult learners and education. Facebook, Twitter, LinkedIn, and other means have revolutionized how the world communicates. Social media are used by young people, adults, grandparents, celebrities, and world leaders. The younger world leaders become, the more likely the methods for communication between nations will change and become more and more digital.

There is a variety of studies that show blogging can improve educational outcomes. One university reported that when they changed individual chemistry labs to groups of students doing their experiments and posting the results to a blog and receiving feedback from other students, the pass rate in the class was increased by 14.4 points.

By nature, we are all more attentive to the quality of our work when we know it will be public and viewed by many. In addition, blogging facilitates a learner-centered discussion, which promotes a stronger personal investment by students. Students are simply more engaged with the material. The focus is more on the process of constructing and evaluating knowledge, discussed in Chapter 10, "Program Development and Lesson Planning." One suggestion is to create a single class blog for any given course and/or program and post case studies, topics for commentary, and articles and new information and allow students to respond. Students can also be assigned to post notes on each class along with the three most important lessons they learned on the assigned material. Other students can comment on all

telecommunications courses
courses offered principally through the use of one or more technologies to deliver instruction to students who are separated from the instructor and to support regular and substantive interaction between students and the instructors. These technologies include television, audio, or computer transmission through open broadcast, closed circuit, cable, microwave, or satellite, and audio and computer conferencing.

postings. Blogs are a simple way to engage learners and create an environment that will appeal to many of today's learners who were literally raised on technology.

General Guidelines for Projected Materials

Some general guidelines should be considered when using projected materials:

- The bottom of any viewing screen or board should be at least 42 inches from the floor, which will allow most learners to see the full screen clearly.
- For best viewing, the screen should be placed in a front corner at an angle facing the center of the room.
- The projector should not obstruct the learners' view of the screen.
- Tilt the top of the screen forward so that the projector beam meets the center of the screen at a 90-degree angle. This will help eliminate image distortion and fading at the top.
- A matte-surface screen should be used for greatest image visibility and seating breadth in the classroom.
- The distance from the screen to the first row of seats should equal no more than twice the width of the screen (e.g., if the screen is 6 feet wide, it should be no more than 12 feet to the first row).
- The distance from the screen to the last row of seats should equal no more than six times the width of the screen (e.g., if the screen is 6 feet wide, it should be no more than 36 feet to the last row).
- No row of seats should be wider than its distance to the screen (e.g., the first row in the previous example given should be no wider than 12 feet, while the last row should be no wider than 36 feet).
- The projected image should fill the screen completely.
- Whenever possible, seat learners in a fan-shaped area of about 70 degrees with the center perpendicular to the screen. This will facilitate viewing for all participants.

✓ Equipment

Career education is heavily dependent upon educational equipment, including the tools and implements used within the various fields. Many of the educational aids already discussed in this chapter require the operation of specific equipment or hardware. The equipment and tools are generally provided by the institution, but it is necessary for the educator to know how to operate and maintain the equipment effectively and safely. In today's classrooms, the master educator can plan for regular use of a television and DVD player; an overhead projector with transparencies; a computer with PowerPoint™, CD-ROM, and DVD capability; mannequins and models, if applicable; and, of course, all the tools and implements appropriate for the program of study. In addition to these instructional aids, the educator must be knowledgeable and skilled in the use of the tools and implements that will be used by the students. The instructor will also need to be able to teach student instructors how to make intelligent decisions concerning purchase and maintenance of such equipment.

Much of the equipment or hardware used by the educator is subject to the issue of safety. Those items that are electrically powered must be handled with care and according to the manufacturer's directions. The durability or maintenance record of the equipment should be considered in the selection process. The quality of the warranty or manufacturer service should also be a consideration when selecting types and brands of equipment to be used in the classroom as well. Of primary importance when dealing with instructional equipment is that it is inspected and prepared prior to the beginning of any class to ensure that it is operational and functioning according to needed standards for quality education.

Wrapping It Up

In this chapter, we have learned the importance of using instructional media within the classroom. They are effective means for involving the learners in the educational process while at the same time increasing students' ability to retain the material presented. There are several types of educational aids, all of which play an important role in career education. While instructional media are a critical part of the educational process, they are not the message itself. They supplement and support the message of the educator. As with all other elements of teaching, the educator must prepare in advance for the use of instructional media. He must be comfortable with the equipment and confident about the presentation.

In Retrospect

1. List the 10 advantages of using educational aids.

2. List the eight important concepts to consider when preparing and selecting visual aids.

3. List the tips for effective use of multipurpose boards.

4. State tips for using flip charts.

5. List the general guidelines that should be considered when using projected materials.

6. List key tips for using electronic whiteboards.

IT'S WORTH REMEMBERING

The master educator knows that properly selected and effectively presented instructional media can add *power* and *impact* to every presentation.

Objectives (Desired Performance Goals):

After reading and studying this chapter, you should be able to:

- Explain the purpose of grading.

- Explain what categories should be graded and when grading should occur.

- List the characteristics of eight different types of grading styles.

- Establish a test plan.

- List advantages and disadvantages of various types of questioning used in evaluation.

- Explain the purpose and use of Likert scales, rating scales, checklists, performance checklists, multiple-category grading, rubrics, and point grading.

- Explain the basic principles and steps involved with academic advising of students.

! CRITICAL CONCEPT

Master educators know that students can always do better and will inspire them to compete with themselves for better performance.

What's in a Grade?

AS EDUCATORS it is essential that we become proficient in measuring the knowledge acquired by our learners. *Merriam Webster's Dictionary* defines **grade** in the noun form as "a step or stage in a course or process." In the verb form, it is defined as "to assign a number or letter that shows how well one has done." So, the purpose of grading is to evaluate learner achievement and build learner confidence. Learners get excited and feel good about enrolling in school when they get a good grade and positive feedback from their educator. The small "wins" achieved by our students through good grades provide positive reinforcement from the educator and build students' self-confidence. The good grade gives them the encouragement to try even harder the next time and to continue in the course of study.

Another purpose of grading is to identify educational progress and measure the knowledge, skills, and even attitude of the learners. As educators we must measure how far the learners have come in order to plan their future training. Effective grading procedures also establish fair and understandable methods for assessing performance. In other words, by establishing predetermined criteria to measure learner performance, all students will receive equitable evaluation. For example, performance of a skill in exactly the same manner by two students should not result in an A for one and a C for the other. Accrediting bodies set standards that require institutions and all educators to follow established grading procedures and criteria in a fair and equitable manner. Those standards suggest that every instructor should interpret and apply the grading procedures in the same manner. Performance of a given practical skill by a student should not result in an A from Ms. Easy Educator and a C from Mr. Hardnose Educator.

Master educators will use grading to challenge learners and assess their progress rather than to trick them. Learners of today must be constantly challenged so they will continue to study and learn. Students as well as educators need to know how they are progressing through their course of study. If learners believe the grading procedures to be fair, they will be motivated to improve their performance.

What to Grade

Grading must correlate with educational objectives that determine what the student is expected to know, feel, or be able to explain or do. Only when **educational objectives** are established and then evaluated can the master educator determine whether or not an outcome or change in behavior has occurred. To review the purpose and development of educational outcomes, refer to Chapter 10, "Program Review, Development, and Lesson Planning."

Usually three main categories are assessed and graded in schools of cosmetology and related career fields:

- Theoretical knowledge
- Practical skills development
- Attitude and professionalism

grading
the process of evaluating a student's performance or knowledge and assigning a letter or number that shows the student's level of achievement.

➕ MASTER EDUCATOR

1. Incorporates a variety of testing and evaluation methods to ensure learners reach the desired degree of competency.
2. Develops test plans to ensure educational objectives are appropriately evaluated.
3. Provides regular and thorough feedback to learners regarding achievement.

educational objective
a clear goal indicating what the student should be able to know or do as a result of the training.

IT'S WORTH ✳ REMEMBERING

Effective evaluation includes a multiplicity of strategies and options.

These areas are generally evaluated using a typical grading chart such as the one found here or in the sample grading procedures that follow. Scales and ratings may change from course to course or school to school. The concept, however, remains the same. Following is an example of a grading chart.

Grading Chart

A	100%–93%	5
B	92%–83%	4
C	82%–75%	3
D	74%–68%	2
F	Below 68%	1
Incomplete		0

Sample Grading Procedures

Students are assigned theory study and a minimum number of practical experiences in each category of study. Specific written and practical assignments are designated as requirements for graduation from the course. Written tests are administered after each unit of study. Practical assignments are evaluated as completed and counted toward course completion only when rated as satisfactory or better. Practical skills are evaluated according to text procedures and requirements set forth in established skills performance criteria. Students must maintain a minimum written grade average of 75 percent and pass a final written and practical exam prior to graduation. Students must make up failed or missed tests and incomplete assignments. Numerical grades are considered according to the following scale:

	Written		**Practical**
93–100	Excellent	4	Excellent
85–92	Very Good	3	Very Good
75–84	Satisfactory	2	Satisfactory
70–74	Needs Improvement	0–1	Unsatisfactory

This example shows how the former grading chart can be adapted to reflect a different scale and how numerical percentages might be used for written tests or grades while numerical ratings are assigned for practical skills evaluation.

The learner's theoretical knowledge is usually assessed through written testing consisting of one or more of the following categories:

- True-or-false questions
- Completion (fill-in-the-blank) questions
- Multiple-choice questions
- Matching exercises
- Essay questions

Practical skills and attitude, on the other hand, are generally assessed using performance evaluation methods, such as:

- Likert scales
- Rating scales

- Checklists
- Performance checklists
- Rubrics

These are considered teacher-centered methods because they do not involve cooperation of the learner. The educator merely observes and assesses learner behavior or performance of a skill and documents the observations. Later in this chapter, these methods of evaluation will be discussed more fully.

When to Grade

Master educators must have a plan for appropriate times in the course of instruction to assign grades. For evaluation to be thorough, it must occur before, during, and after instruction. It is important for all learners to understand the criteria with which they are being graded and to know how they are progressing throughout the course of study.

Outcome evaluation determines what the student knows after having been taught certain material or skills. This is often accomplished through pretesting, which occurs prior to teaching and learning, and posttesting, which occurs after teaching and learning. The grading system should allow learners to see how they are doing before the "final grade." Grades that are given to individual topics or performance areas *on the way* through the course of study result in outcome evaluation.

Summative evaluation is the process of assigning grades after testing has occurred. Educators generally give tests at the end of each chapter or unit of study. In developing a course of study, educators establish certain checkpoints or gates at which summative evaluation will occur. For example, in a 1,200-hour barber course, it may be determined that summative evaluation occurs upon completion of the first phase of study or 250 clock hours, upon completion of 600 clock hours, upon completion of 900 clock hours, and upon completion of 1,200 clock hours. The summative evaluations might include both written testing and practical skills evaluation.

Master educators learn to incorporate both outcome evaluation and summative evaluation into the courses of study they teach.

outcome evaluation
grading that determines what the student knows after having been taught certain material or skills.

summative evaluation
the process of assigning grades after testing has occurred.

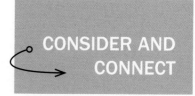

Evaluation occurs over time and tracks a learner's development and competencies over weeks or months.

Grading Styles

Master educators understand why consistency is important to both the educator and the learner. When grades are assigned to students in any given area, the educator must be prepared to explain the criteria used or the reasoning that resulted in the grade. Personal feelings about a learner or a learner's habits should never enter into a grading situation. Justice remains critical in our adult classrooms. Educators must be fair, honest, and just when determining grades. The following examples of grading styles depict numerous examples of how grading should *not* occur.

Grading by Disposition

Grading by disposition occurs when the educator gives grades according to his mood or disposition at the time of grading. If he has had an argument with his significant other on the way out the door that morning or had a flat tire on the way to work, he may be in a bad mood. If he has not taken control of his own attitude and has let his circumstances control him, his bad mood could be taken out on his students. In such a situation, he will ignore the predetermined performance criteria established for grading and automatically give all students a lower grade. By the same token, the educator may be in an outstanding mood due to some unexpected windfall, and just feels so good that he gives every student a better grade than deserved. Either approach is incorrect and harmful to the students.

Grading by Personal Fetish

This type of grading occurs when the educator always targets one detail or skill behavior that is his personal fetish or pet peeve and grades learners down in that particular area. For example, the educator may feel there is only one acceptable method for holding a particular implement or instrument. If a student doesn't complete the procedure using the exact technique that the educator feels is required, he automatically grades the learner down even if the end result was satisfactory.

Grading without Risk

In this type of grading, the educator wants to remain on safe ground so he always gives average grades, nothing too high and nothing too low. This is often caused by the educator not fully understanding the grading criteria and how they are applied. Unfortunately, the learners never have a clear understanding of how they are performing.

Grading with Spite

When the educator always gives low grades to a particular learner just because he doesn't like the student, he is grading with spite. This may result from one particular past event with the student that the educator has never forgotten. Clearly, this is prejudicial and unfair behavior on the part of the educator (Figure 12–1). It is harmful to the student's progress and self-esteem.

Grading by Assumption

Grading by assumption, also called the *halo effect*, takes place when the educator unconsciously gives certain learners higher scores, especially on essay-question tests, simply because he has had previously positive learning experiences with those particular learners. In other words, just because these students have performed well in other testing situations, the educator automatically assumes that they will do well in this situation and grades according to his expectations rather than the students' actual performance or ability. Similarly, this type of grading also occurs when the educator tends to approach learners who have done poor work in the past with an expectation of seeing poor work currently. He then automatically assigns

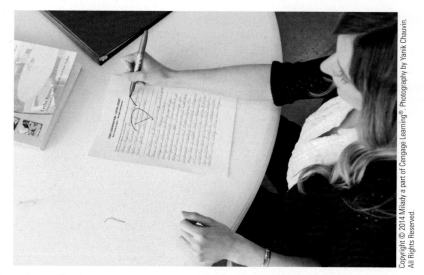

Figure 12–1 **Prejudicial grading is unfair and ineffective.**

a lower grade based on his assumptions or expectations. Both assumptions are inconsistent and unfair to the learners.

Grading *in Absentia*

Grading *in absentia* is performed by those infamous educators who give grades for work or skills they didn't actually see performed. For example, the institution requires that every skill performed in the practical lab be given a practical grade. The educator gets distracted and doesn't follow step three in his zone teaching assignment and fails to see the end results of all skill performances. He then sits down at the end of the day and simply writes out a bunch of grades for the students. This results in a catastrophic situation. It has removed any credibility from the grading and evaluation process. It more than likely has resulted in the loss of respect for the educator, and it has failed to provide the students with fair evaluations of their work.

Grading Improvement Only

This may be the least negative type of grading, in that the educator tends to offer higher scores simply for improvement the learner has made. In other words, the effort and better ability achieved by the learner results in a higher-than-deserved score. At least this educator is rewarding the student for positive performance, even if the grade is not based exactly on the published grading criteria. One benefit may be that the learner will become encouraged and continue to do well. The downfall occurs when the learner has progressed to expected levels and the grading is now adjusted according to the grading criteria. This could be somewhat disillusioning after having previously received the higher grades.

Grading with Warm Fuzzies

When grading with "warm fuzzies," everything looks "great" to the educator so every learner receives top scores. This educator does not want to deal with any questions and wants all learners to feel *great*. This type of grading

IT'S WORTH REMEMBERING ✳

Master educators know that what you evaluate is just as important as how you evaluate.

is more common with new instructors. They either lack confidence in their own skills ability or lack understanding of the grading procedures and criteria, or they simply fear rejection by the students if they assign a bad grade. They don't want to hurt anyone's feelings, so they give great grades to everybody. Here again, the credibility of the grading process has been challenged and the students have been harmed.

Master educators will not only avoid all of these grading styles, they will take tactful steps to ensure that their fellow educators will do the same. Fairness and consistency have been established as critical qualities and characteristics of a master educator. There is no area in which fairness and consistency are more important than in grading learners.

✓ Grading Methods: The Test Plan

test plan
consists of an outline of the content that will be covered by each test, applying weights to particular test questions based on lesson objectives.

weighting
the process of determining the importance of each content area that has   been selected to test.

Educators must identify the skills and knowledge to be learned and describe them in behavioral terms. Educators within an institution must agree that the content of their course or program tests is important and relevant to the educational objectives. Because testing is the most proficient method for measuring knowledge, educators must prepare a test plan. The *test plan* consists of an outline of the content that will be covered by each test. Educators will then determine the importance of each content area that has been selected to test. This process is referred to as *weighting*. Application of appropriate weighting requires careful decisions on the part of the educators. One of the worst criticisms in education is of educators who teach certain material and then test on something else. You may notice that chapter review questions have been added to this edition of *Master Educator*. Look more closely and you will see that the review questions at the end of the chapter tie directly to the performance goals stated at the beginning of the chapter. Similarly, the test plan must tie to the objectives of the lesson(s) taught, and it is logical that the amount of class time devoted to topic areas should be relevant to the weighting given to each topic on the test. An example of lesson objectives and a test plan for the study of Life Skills if found below. The plan is followed by an actual test that has been developed based on the plan (Figure 12–2).

OBJECTIVES	CURRICULUM AREA	WEIGHTS	NUMBER OF TEST QUESTIONS	QUESTION NUMBER(S)	QUESTION TYPE
List the guidelines for personal and professional success.	Orientation	10%	1	1	Multiple Choice
Create a mission statement.	Orientation	10%	1	4	Multiple Choice
Explain how to set short-term and long-term goals.	Orientation	20%	2	5, 10	Multiple Choice
Explain effective ways to manage time.	Orientation	20%	2	2, 3	Multiple Choice
Describe good study habits.	Orientation	20%	2	6, 7	Multiple Choice
Define ethics.	Orientation	10%	1	8	Multiple Choice
List the characteristics of a healthy, positive attitude.	Orientation	10%	1	9	Multiple Choice

Figure 12–2   The Life Skills test plan.

TEST: LIFE SKILLS

1. _____ is based on inner strength and begins with trusting your ability to reach your goals.

   a. Loyalty   b. Integrity
   c. Self-esteem   d. Honesty

2. In order to manage your time effectively, you must tap into your _____.

   a. inner organizer   b. inner spirit
   c. external skills   d. external resources

3. Three bad habits that can keep you from maintaining peak performance are procrastination, lacking a game plan, and _____.

   a. persistence   b. prevarication
   c. preparation   d. perfectionism

4. Your sense of purpose can be validated in a _____.

   a. trade magazine
   b. personal mission statement
   c. legal contract
   d. executive business plan

5. Long-term goals are usually those you expect to take more than a _____ to complete.

   a. day   b. week
   c. year   d. month

6. _____techniques will save you time by uncovering needed solutions.

7. If you find studying overwhelming, focus on _____.

   a. the big picture   b. your long-term goals
   c. improving habits   d. individual small tasks

8. Some ethical characteristics that you should aspire to include respect, courtesy, honesty, and _____.

   a. sincerity   b. abruptness
   c. aggressiveness   d. curtness

9. A combination of understanding, empathy, and acceptance is known as _____.

   a. attitude   b. personality
   c. mission   d. sensitivity

10. When you have goals, it is essential to have _____ for attaining them.

    a. a task list   b. a dream board
    c. an action plan   d. time log

The example depicts how the test plan identifies the number of test items to include in the test. The ultimate goal is to design a *power test* with an *objective* format. Power tests are those that can be completed by at least 80 percent of the students within one hour. An objective format is one in which most, if not all, of the educators agree on the correctness of a specific answer.

☑ Question Types in Test Development

A variety of question types can be used to develop testing tools that are appropriate for every type of learner and for various learning situations.

True or False. True-or-false questions have two distinct advantages. The educator can write a test that covers a large number of statements or items in a short period of time. Accordingly, students can read and respond to a large number of statements or items in a short period of time.

The use of true/false questions in testing is not as widely accepted as other forms of test development due to the disadvantages encountered. The first disadvantage is that a student who has no prior knowledge of a subject area has a 50 percent opportunity to choose a correct answer. The second, and probably more damaging, disadvantage is that the student may place into long-term memory the incorrect information or statement for recall at a future time. When true/false testing is incorporated into the curriculum, the educator should follow some well-established guidelines during test development:

- Initially, all test items should be written as true statements.
- Second, review all test items and convert at least half of them to false statements.
- Avoid the use of the word *not* in statement development.
- Keep the statement brief and ensure that it is clearly *true* or *false*.
- Whenever a test statement is attributed to an opinion, quote the source. For example, "according to the *Occupational Outlook Handbook* …"
- Do not use words such as *usually, always,* or *never*.
- Avoid direct quotes from textbooks, which require the student to rely too heavily on memory recall.
- Always avoid use of petty, trick statements.

Matching Items. Matching items are used to test the students' precise recall of associations and discriminations within their memory. One of the disadvantages of this type of testing is that unless there are more options listed in the definition or description column than there are in the terms or items listed in the first column, one incorrect answer will automatically result in another incorrect answer. Another disadvantage is that as the students progress through the test, there are fewer remaining choices, and thus previous answers tend to cue the correct answer to other items. Matching test questions also have certain advantages. They provide for the *chunking* of important knowledge or information needed by the student. Chunking of information allows the student to store it in memory for future use.

When writing matching test questions, the educator should consider the following guidelines:

- Items used in a set should be common to each other.
- The number of possible matches should exceed the problems or items listed.

CONSIDER AND CONNECT

The master educator will limit the use of True/False evaluation to avoid placing incorrect information into the learner's memory.

- Keep the sets to 15 items or less.
- Keep all items and possible matches on one page.
- Ensure that directions are clear for all students.

Essay Questions. Essay questions are those that require an answer in a sentence, paragraph, or short-composition format. They are used to determine the learner's knowledge and comprehension level as well as to determine whether the learner can analyze the information sufficiently to properly apply it in a practical situation. Essay questions allow the learner to provide an analysis or interpretation of a given subject or topic. The difficulty arises when varying educators score the same response differently. In other words, because the essay question response usually represents the learner's personal point of view or understanding of an issue, the responses become somewhat subjective. It follows, then, that the review of those responses may become subjective as well. Another disadvantage of using essay-type questions is that they often result in *halo effect* grading. Remember, this occurs when the educator unconsciously gives higher scores because of previous positive experience with a learner. The educator's impressions of a learner's competence or ability may affect his judgment regarding the learner's responses. Additionally, essay tests limit the educator to only a few questions per examination, which greatly restricts his ability to assess a larger sample of learner behavior and knowledge.

When preparing essay question tests, educators must carefully focus on the learning objectives of the lesson. The use of specific verbs, the meanings of which have been taught to students, is recommended. In fact, master educators will give their learners examples of how to answer essay test questions using specific verbs. This should be part of the lesson process whereby students are taught how to take an essay examination. Educators should consider use of verbs such as:

- Explain
- Describe
- Discuss
- Summarize
- List
- Cite
- Compare
- Contrast

In order to eliminate some of the subjectivity involved in scoring essay test questions, educators should first write a response to each question. Second, they should review the response and note each important point. When scoring of the test occurs, the educator can then mark or count the number of previously noted elements included in the learner's answer. If the learner includes additional points or comments that are also correct, extra credit or further points can be awarded. Whenever possible, educators should score essay questions without knowledge of the student's identity. This will help prevent the situation of grading by assumption. Assigning learners a number that can later be matched to their names will allow a degree of anonymity that could result in more objective scoring.

CONSIDER AND CONNECT

Rather than using matching questions for formal evaluation, the master educator will use matching exercises for partner competitions within the classroom, which facilitates fun while learning.

Completion Items. Completion questions are also known as *fill-in-the-blank* questions. These test items include statements wherein key phrases or words are left blank and provided by the learners. These are often a favorite among educators because a large amount of material or information can be covered in a relatively short period of time. These questions or statements must be prepared in such a manner that there is only one correct answer. However, this results in a disadvantage, because the stem of the question or statement may give hints about the correct answer in order to ensure that multiple responses are not possible. Some tips that should be considered by the master educator in development of completion questions are:

- Keep the questions as short as possible.
- Incorporate sufficient cues to ensure learners can correctly complete the items.
- Avoid leading questions that give learners the answer.
- Structure questions to ensure that there is only one correct answer.
- Keep the language and reading level appropriate for the level of the learners.
- Avoid long, rambling paragraphs, which can be confusing to learners.
- Ensure that all completion questions begin and end on the same page of the test.

Educators should remember that completion test questions are quite time consuming to create and score if not written correctly. Master educators will learn to incorporate a moderate degree of completion questions in testing or determining a learner's progress in a given subject or topic.

Multiple-Choice Questions. Multiple-choice questions present several answers from which the correct one (or most correct one) is chosen by the learners. The questions contain a stem or statement usually followed by a series of at least three or four possible answers. The possible answers that are incorrect are known as *foils* or *distractors*. Foils may be less correct than the answer with the greatest degree of correctness. They may also be only partially incorrect or totally incorrect. Multiple-choice questions offer many advantages in testing. They tend to reduce the amount of guessing done by students due to the foils or incorrect answers.

In addition, they are objective in scoring, which increases agreement among educators as to the correct answer. The difficulty of each question can be controlled by how similar the possible answers are. This form of questioning also allows educators to construct test questions that exceed simple recall of knowledge on the part of the learners.

When writing multiple-choice test questions, the master educator will take steps to:

- Ensure that the stem of the question is the largest portion of the question.
- Vary the location of the correct answer so that a pattern of correct answers cannot be identified by learners.
- Ensure that the length of the correct answer and the foils are equal or near equal.
- Ensure that foils have a potential for correctness; they shouldn't be totally ridiculous.

- State the stem or question in an affirmative rather than negative manner.
- Avoid writing stems (questions or statements) that give the learners answers to other questions on the test.
- Avoid using the terms *always* or *never* in the possible answers.

Again, master educators will learn to effectively incorporate the use of a variety of test-question types into the examination process. This will ensure that they can determine to a greater degree the level of learning and comprehension on the part of the learners in the classroom.

Project-Oriented Evaluation

Project assignments and assessments can be highly effective with adult learners who are independent and can work well alone or with partners or small groups. Based on the course objectives, a list of curriculum topics can be posted, allowing adult learners to choose one among several. All sorts of materials and supplies are made available, allowing students to use their creativity to design or devise a project that illustrates their understanding of a specific principle or concept. Evaluation of the project occurs over a period of time. Project-oriented evaluation is a true form of learner-centered, discovery-oriented learning that will stay with the student long term.

Descriptive Performance Evaluations

Because training in various career education disciplines requires practical, "hands-on" skills training, it is reasonable to assume that the practical skills abilities of learners must also be evaluated. This form of evaluation allows students the opportunity to demonstrate their understanding or mastery of important concepts through the manipulation of objects, concepts, and tools. Therefore, the master educator will ensure that all students are appropriately evaluated in their practical skills as well as their communication skills and ability to interact with others. The best way to accomplish this type of evaluation is through a teacher-centered activity that allows the educator to observe learners' behaviors. Many methods can be used to accomplish this type of evaluation. In this text, we will focus on five types of descriptive scales: *Likert scales, rating scales, checklists, performance checklists,* and *rubrics.* Master educators will establish the content of such scales to include the material knowledge, skills, and behaviors desired in the learners.

Likert Scales

Likert scales are simple to use and encourage educators to observe student behaviors in a natural environment using a systematic approach. A Likert scale uses a five-point rating scale ranging from "strongly agree" to "strongly disagree" or from "poor" to "excellent." Refer to the two examples of Likert Scales (Figures 12–3 and 12–4).

> **CONSIDER AND CONNECT**
>
> Educators can cover large amounts of subject matter in a reasonably short period of time using multiple-choice questioning.

> **Likert scale**
> a measurement that uses a five-point rating scale ranging from "strongly agree" to "strongly disagree" or from "poor" to "excellent."

Likert Scale 1

CLIENT/PATIENT COMMUNICATION	STRONGLY AGREE	AGREE	NO COMMENT	DISAGREE	STRONGLY DISAGREE
Greeted client/patient warmly with a smile.					
Introduced self.					
Called client/patient by name.					
Extended arm for handshake.					
Escorted client/patient to chair.					
Ensured client/patient was seated comfortably.					
Performed pre-service consultation.					
Listened attentively to client/patient.					
Asked intelligent, relevant questions.					
Was open to client/patient suggestions.					
Put client/patient at ease during consultation.					
Accurately recorded comments on card.					

Figure 12–3   Likert scales facilitate observation of student behaviors using a systematic approach.

Likert Scale 2

DISPENSARY DUTY	POOR	FAIR	NO OPINION	GOOD	EXCELLENT
Kept supply area replenished.					
Changed disinfectant soak solution as applicable.					
Conducted inventory of dispensary and stockroom.					
Reported inventory needs.					
Restocked dispensary as needed.					
Checked-in product deliveries as applicable.					
Stored all implements appropriately.					
Laundered linens and stored appropriately.					
Cleaned dryer filter after each use.					
Cleaned lint around dryer area daily.					

Figure 12–4   Likert scales use a five-point rating system, such as from "poor" to "excellent."

Rating Scales

Rating scales are similar to Likert scales but usually contain fewer rating categories. The rating scale can be used to compare a student's performance or behavior with specific standards or criteria established for a designated learning category, such as work habits and skills. They can also be used to compare a student's performance or behavior with that of other students (Figure 12–5). The ratings may range from "below average" to "exceptional," or the educator may choose to use ratings of "never" to "always." When comparing behavior with that of other students or coworkers, ratings might range from "unsatisfactory" to "better than average." For example, the educator can use the same performance criteria to evaluate a student's work habits and skills on an individual basis and on a comparison basis with other students as follows:

rating scale
a grading chart similar to Likert scales but usually containing fewer rating categories; it can be used to compare a student's performance or behavior with specific standards established for a designated learning category.

Individual Rating	Optional Individual Rating	Comparison Rating
A = Always	4 = Exceptional performance	4 = Better than average student
U = Usually	3 = above-average performance	3 = Competitive with average students
S = Seldom	2 = Average performance	2 = Requires more attention than average student
N = Never	1 = Below-average performance	1 = Lacks ability even after special training

N/A = Not Applicable (could be applied to any of the specific criteria in any rating scale).

Refer to the example of a rating scale for work habits and skills.

Rating Scale

WORK HABITS AND SKILLS	INDIVIDUAL RATING	COMPARISON RATING
Is prompt and dependable in attendance.		
Portrays a positive attitude, shows interest, and pride in work.		
Is neat, clean, and professional in appearance.		
Is cooperative; gets along well with others.		
Exercises initiative in starting and following through on assignments.		
Accepts constructive criticism; works toward improvement.		
Solves problems effectively and makes appropriate decisions on assigned work.		
Sets high standards and consistently achieves quality results.		
Meets industry standards with regard to the time element for delivering professional services.		
Pays close attention to instructions and details.		
Interacts appropriately with clients/patients, coworkers, and supervisors.		
Follows rules, regulations, and policies.		
Uses and cares for equipment and implements properly.		
Works independently without close supervision.		

Figure 12–5   Rating scales allow the educator to evaluate a student's skills on an individual basis as well as on a comparison basis with other students.

The Checklist

PERFORMANCE CRITERIA INFECTION CONTROL	ADEQUATE/ SATISFACTORY	INADEQUATE/ UNSATISFACTORY
Cleans implements thoroughly with warm, soapy water.		
Rinses implements thoroughly.		
Completely immerses implements in EPA-registered disinfectant for designated time.		
Stores implements in enclosed container or ultraviolet cabinet.		
Disinfects work station and work area.		
Washes own hands using antibacterial soap before and after contact with each client/patient.		

Figure 12–6   **Checklists are another variation of the rating scale.**

Checklists

checklist
a variation of the rating scale that contains fewer rating categories; generally, a specific performance is rated as *adequate* or *inadequate* or *satisfactory* or *unsatisfactory*.

performance checklist
a factual and objective form of grading that uses specific performance criteria that help to remove educator bias from the rating process, resulting in more consistency.

One variation of the rating scale is known as the **checklist**. Checklists are used in the same manner as rating scales but contain fewer rating categories. Generally, the educator would rate the specific performance criteria as either "adequate" or "inadequate" or "satisfactory" or "unsatisfactory (Figure 12–6)."

Performance Checklists

Master educators will find the **performance checklist** more factual and objective as compared to the Likert, rating, and checklist scales. Performance checklists require a great deal of time to prepare. However, they are highly rated among various professions because of the consistency in scoring reached among educators. The use of specific performance criteria that remove the opinions of the educator from the rating process results in a higher frequency of similar ratings on identical criteria among educators. This type of evaluation is useful when determining if certain competency levels have been reached before moving into the next category of training. In addition, performance checklists are effective in preparing students for the state licensing examination, which will probably follow a similar format in the practical skills categories. A performance checklist will usually consist of from one to seven subsets of behaviors with specific criteria that are rated for competency.

There are two schools of thought on how ratings are applied when using the performance checklist. National testing agencies tend to use "yes" or "no" ratings as to whether specific criteria have been met. Some educators choose to use a rating of from 0 to 3, with 0 meaning that performance was inadequate, 1 meaning that the step was completed with minimal educator acceptance, 2 meaning the performance was merely adequate, and with 3 representing a perfect score. Because educators differ in age, ability, knowledge, skills, attitude, personality, perception, and philosophy, it is important that the checklist be constructed in a way that minimizes educator subjectivity and focuses on whether or not the specific skill or task was

PERFORMING LASER OR IPL HAIR REMOVAL TREATMENTS	WORKMANSHIP/PROFESSIONALISM
____ Unlocked laser device.	____ Obtained and replaced key in a secure location.
____ Put on safety goggles and gloves.	____ Goggles were clean and gloves were properly placed.
____ Applied gel if recommended by manufacturer.	____ Properly removed and safely applied gel.
____ Set treatment parameters per guidelines or previous treatment.	____ Carefully checked previous treatment record for guidance and according to the response at the test site.
____ Performed treatment at highest fluence skin can tolerate.	____ Adjusted the time based on the spot size of the beam and the scanning pattern of the handpiece.
____ Compressed skin firmly with handpiece to disperse the oxyhemoglobin chromophore.	____ Held the handpiece properly.
____ Selected a starting spot and performed a test pulse.	____ Ensured that client could tolerate fluence.
____ Followed a well-defined pattern and worked across area where hair was to be removed.	____ Demonstrated accuracy in a well-planned pattern of procedure.
____ Administered a single pulse per area.	____ Worked only in areas where hair was to be removed.
____ Periodically cleaned handpiece to free it of carbonized hair.	____ Used ultrasonic gel on the skin to prevent accumulation of burned hair on the laser lens per manufacturer's recommendations.
____ Read the skin.	____ Made adjustments if cooling remedies did not reduce client's discomfort.
____ Removed any gel used with the device.	____ Operated in a clean and safe manner.
____ After treatment was complete, wiped down skin with soothing antiseptic lotion.	____ Consideration was given to client's comfort.

Figure 12–7   Multiple category grading: performing Laser or IPL hair removal treatments.

performed as written. This method of evaluation removes the requirement for the educator to make judgment calls about a learner's ability. The educator merely records what he sees, which will indicate whether a specific criterion was achieved or not. When using the yes/no ratings, no credit is given for tasks or skills not performed at all. In addition, no credit is given for those tasks or skills performed not meeting minimum requirements, as could be the case with the 0–3 method of scoring. Let's look at an example of a performance checklist used for testing a practitioner's competency in the performance of proper handwashing. Additional subsets can be added for evaluating performance in more detailed or advanced skills within a given curriculum.

Multiple-Category Grading

Multiple-category grading incorporates scoring of more than one area of learner assessment. This provides a broader understanding for the learner of the various specific areas of performance that need to be assessed. In the example provided, the educator could use the performance checklist instructions for rating each category (Figure 12–7). The educator would determine if the learner *did perform* or *did not perform* the task properly and rate the task as "yes" or "no" or rate the category on a scale from 0 to 3.

multiple-category grading
an evaluation chart that incorporates scoring of more than one area of learner assessment.

HAND WASING PERFORMANCE CHECKLIST

INSTRUCTIONS: The performance criteria have been developed to reflect the skill being performed at the absolute minimum level of competency. While observing the learner, the educator will enter a "checkmark" for *yes, the learner correctly performed the individual criterion.* Conversely, the educator will leave it blank if *the learner did not correctly perform the individual criterion.* Upon completion of the evaluation, the educator will divide the number correct into the total number of criteria to obtain the score on a 100 percent scale and apply the correct grade according to the institution's grading policy.

HANDWASHING ASSESSMENT

_____ Wet hands with warm running water.
_____ Applied and distributed soap.
_____ Vigorously rubbed hands together for 20 seconds.
_____ Brushed nails with clean, disinfected nail brush for about 60 seconds.
_____ Thoroughly rinsed hands under warm running water.
_____ Blotted hands with disposable towels.
_____ In the absence of foot controls or automatic shutoff, used paper towel to turn off faucets.
_____ Used paper towels to handle door knobs.
_____ Properly disposed of paper towels.
_____ Optional step: Applied hand lotion.

Point Grading

point grading
grading that assigns specific weights or points to each criterion or task, which allows the educator to place emphasis on the more important tasks during evaluation.

Point grading assigns specific weights or points to each of the criteria, which allows the educator to place emphasis on the more important tasks to be completed during the evaluation. This also ensures that the learner receives credit for performing the more difficult or more important tasks correctly. For example, some educators maintain that infection-control practices are more important than the performance of specific tasks. Refer to the example of a point-grading procedure for client/communications (Figure 12–8).

CLIENT/COMMUNICATION	POINTS
Greeted client warmly with a smile.	5
Introduced self.	5
Called client by name.	5
Extended arm for handshake.	10
Escorted client to chair.	10
Ensured client was seated comfortably.	10
Performed pre-service consultation.	10
Listened attentively to client.	10
Asked intelligent, relevant questions.	10
Was open to client suggestions.	10
Put client at ease during consultation.	10
Accurately recorded comments on card.	5

Figure 12–8 Point Grading – Client/Communications

Rubrics

Rubrics are similar to Likert scales and are used in education for organizing and interpreting data gathered from observations of student performance. It is a clearly developed scoring document used to differentiate between levels of development in a specific skill performance or behavior. Rubrics list clear performance criteria that allow the instructor to perform an objective evaluation of a student's performance. This type of grading tool helps to ensure that two different instructors evaluating the same practical skills performance will assign the same grade. A rubric may also be used as a self-assessment tool to aid students in their skill performance development.

An example of how students might rate themselves or how they might be rated by an instructor is as follows:

(1) **Development Opportunity**: There is little or no evidence of competency; assistance is needed; performance includes multiple errors.
(2) **Fundamental**: There is beginning evidence of competency; task is completed alone; performance includes few errors.
(3) **Competent**: There is detailed and consistent evidence of competency; task is completed alone; performance includes rare errors.
(4) **Strength**: There is detailed evidence of highly creative, inventive, mature presence of competency.

Space is provided for comments to assist students and/or instructors in developing a plan for improving performance and achieving a higher rating. See Figure 12–9 on page 264 for an example of a rubric for Handwashing.

Academic Advisement and Counseling

Accrediting bodies require that students have access to **academic advisement** from members of the faculty, including referral to professional assistance, if necessary. In addition, students whose academic or attendance progress is unsatisfactory must be advised and provided with any needed assistance. Educators will be called upon to provide information and advice to learners on subjects such as employment and continuing education opportunities. Learners will also need to be advised about any number of other topics, such as planning for and completing the occupational education programs they pursue.

Educators should schedule regular sessions with every student to discuss their academic progress through the course or program of study. Those sessions may be scheduled monthly, quarterly, or on a semester basis depending upon the policies and structure of the institution. Such sessions should provide for a meaningful exchange between the educator and the learner. They should be designed to summarize how the student is doing in practical skills performance, written or theoretical progress, and progress toward course completion in attendance. Other areas that an educator may wish to address include the learner's professionalism, attitude, communication skills, ability to interact with others, and compliance with the institution's standards of conduct. In every case, a conference or face-to-face meeting with the student will be required.

Rubric
a clearly developed scoring document used to differentiate between levels of development in a specific skill performance or behavior; it may also be used as a self-assessment tool.

Development Opportunity
in some rubrics, "development opportunity" indicates that the student displays little or no evidence of competency; assistance is needed; performance includes multiple errors.

fundamental
in some rubrics, "fundamental" indicates that the student displays beginning evidence of competency; task is completed alone; performance includes a few errors.

competent
in some rubrics, "competent" indicates that the student displays detailed and consistent evidence of competency; task is completed alone; performance includes rare errors.

strength
in some rubrics, "strength" indicates that the student displays detailed evidence of highly creative, inventive, mature presence of competency.

academic advisement
the process of advising a student regarding his academic performance, including written grades, practical skills and attendance, and developing a plan for improvement, if needed.

private conference
a private meeting between the educator and learner that gives both the opportunity to discuss concerns (whether performance or behavioral) and potential solutions.

PERFORMANCE ASSESSED	1	2	3	4	IMPROVEMENT PLAN
Preparation					
1. Gathered equipment, supplies, disposables, and products.					
Procedure					
1. Wet hands with warm running water.					
2. Applied and distributed soap.					
3. Vigorously rubbed hands together for 20 seconds.					
4. Brushed nails with clean, disinfected nail brush for about 60 seconds.					
5. Thoroughly rinsed hands under warm running water.					
6. Blotted hands with disposable towels.					
7a. In the absence of foot controls or automatic shutoff, used paper towel to turn off faucets.					
7b. Used paper towels to handle door knobs.					
8. Properly disposed of paper towels.					
9. Optional: Applied hand lotion if desired.					
Post-procedure					
1. Inspected hands for visible microabrasions.					
2. If microabrasions were present, wore gloves for cleanup.					
Cleanup and Disinfection					
1. Cleaned and disinfected sink area as routinely scheduled.					
2. Properly disposed of paper towels.					

Figure 12–9   Handwashing Rubric.

IT'S WORTH REMEMBERING ✳

Using rubrics for self-evaluation often motivates the learner to work harder and achieve more sooner.

CONSIDER AND CONNECT

The environment for the conference should be as nonthreatening as possible. The educator and learner should sit face to face with no barriers between them.

Conferences. A **private conference** between the educator and the learner gives both parties the opportunity to discuss the problem and potential solutions (Figure 12–10). The educator must carefully prepare for such a conference if it is to be successful. Some factors the educator should consider for conference planning were discussed in Chapter 8, "Effective Classroom Management and Supervision," and are repeated here for ease of access.

1. Identify specific areas needing improvement, whether in performance or behavior.
2. Provide documented evidence of performance or chronic misbehavior.
3. Develop questions for the student to perform self-evaluation.
4. Establish concrete goals for improvement.
5. Identify specific consequences for failure to improve performance or remedy misconduct.
6. Plan for concluding the conference.

As we confirmed in Chapter 8, "Effective Classroom Management and Supervision," the purpose of the conference is to bring about change, not to intimidate or control. When progress or improvement has occurred, the educator has a wonderful opportunity to give recognition, approval, and positive reinforcement to the learner.

Often, if students are having difficulty at home or in their personal lives, their progress at school will be affected. The master educator will learn to identify problems that are of a personal nature and not suitable for discussion at school. In fact, he will be prepared to provide ready reference to those professionals or agencies that are qualified to counsel students with

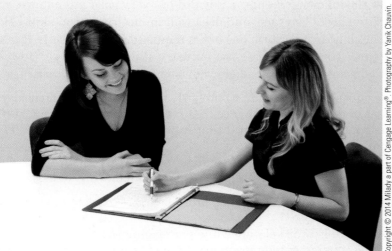

Figure 12–10   Conferences provide the educator and learner the opportunity to discuss problems and potential solutions.

specific personal problems. Educators will, however, be prepared to assist students in areas appropriate for their career training and development.

Agreements or Contracts. Verbal agreements are commonly used to follow up on violations of classroom rules. When you believe students will live up to their word, it is appropriate to remind them of your contract. A written contract adds meaning to the agreement made between the educator and learner. A simple written agreement or contract is prepared and signed by the educator and the learner. A signed agreement carries a greater commitment to the agreed-upon behavior. This agreement can be as simple as stating the conditions and length of the agreement in the comments section of a regular counseling form used by the institution.

Performance Meetings. A private meeting with a student is the perfect opportunity to outline all the areas in which the learner is meeting or exceeding standards set forth for performance as well as to define any areas that need improvement. Some questions that the educator may ask the student include:

1. Tell me how things are going for you in the program.
2. How do you think you are doing in attendance and why?
3. Are you happy with your academic written grades and why or why not?
4. Are you happy with your skills performance and why or why not?
5. What areas do you find the easiest?
6. What areas do you find the most difficult?
7. What specific areas do you feel need improvement?
8. How can I help you achieve that improvement?
9. Tell me three things you have achieved since we last met.
10. Is there anything else you would like to discuss while we are together?

The answer the student provides on the very first question may eliminate the need to ask some of the other questions listed. The master educator will use his own professional judgment in conducting the meeting and determining which direction the conversation needs to take.

Ultimately, however, the educator and learner should agree on a plan of action to improve the areas that are not satisfactory. Follow-up with regard to unsatisfactory performance is critical to the advising process. Let's consider the following scenario. Edward has very good attendance, an excellent written grade average, and does well in most practical skills. However, even though he can perform one of his requisite skills perfectly, it takes him nearly three times as long as the industry standard to do so. How would a master educator provide academic advisement in this situation?

1. The educator would want to properly recognize and acknowledge all areas of positive performance that meet or exceed minimum standards.
2. The educator would suggest that Edward's speed needs to increase significantly.
3. The educator must give the student a plan of action for improvement. A plan for improvement might include the following steps:

   a. Identify the rate at which a professional is expected to perform the task.
   b. Observe Edward closely while performing the task and determine if he is using any unnecessary, time-consuming steps or movements and advise him accordingly.
   c. Perform a specific number of timed exercises in a mock situation.
   d. Perform a specific number of timed exercises in a real-life situation.
   e. Schedule activities for the specific experience or task.
   f. Acknowledge his progress on each of the exercises and assignments so that appropriate feedback and guidance can be provided.
   g. If he has achieved the goals you have set for him, give him the deserved praise and recognition.
   h. If he has not, acknowledge his progress with positive reinforcement and agree upon a new plan that will result in continued improvement.

Academic advising is crucial to any student's progress through a course or program of study.

☑ Wrapping It Up

Educators in career education generally must be concerned with both the learners' knowledge of the theory behind their chosen discipline and also how well they can perform the practical skills required for competency and competitiveness in entry-level positions. Testing, both written and practical, is an effective form of measuring and evaluating student achievement. Therefore, master educators incorporate a variety of testing and evaluation methods into the training to ensure that all learners reach the desired degree of competency. Master educators will develop and implement a test plan to ensure that class objectives are appropriately evaluated and that appropriate weights are applied to subject matter according to their relevance and importance. In addition, committed educators will develop measurement criteria that reduce or eliminate subjectivity on the part of the educator or evaluator and focus on specific knowledge or skills abilities desired in student behavior. It is important for the educator to give regular and thorough feedback to students regarding their achievements. Plans for improvement are critical to the overall success of each student in the course. However, any plan will be useless if appropriate evaluation and follow-up are not applied.

In Retrospect

1. Explain the purpose of grading.

2. Explain what categories should be graded and when grading should occur.

3. List the characteristics of eight different types of grading styles.

4. Establish a test plan.

5. List advantages and disadvantages of various types of questioning used in evaluation.

6. Explain the purpose and use of Likert scales, rating scales, checklists, performance checklists, multiple-category grading, rubrics, and point grading.

7. Explain the basic principles and steps involved with academic advising of students.

EDUCATOR SPOTLIGHT

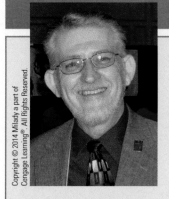

DANNY AUSTIN'S philosophy of what it means to be an educator is demonstrated by what he tells every student on their first day of class, "My goal is to make your goals come true." That task is accomplished by attention to detail in students' classroom time and their practical time and by talking to them individually. Mr. Austin believes that encouragement and praise are crucial to maintain student motivation, and he carefully chooses words of constructive criticism to help students achieve their goals and to not become discouraged.

Mr. Austin teaches from an intrinsic passion that he tries to also instill in his students if it is not already present. He believes that no student is unteachable. He believes that if he can start with student interest and cultivate passion, he is half-way there. He doesn't think of himself as an exceptionally smart man—it's just that he will stay with a problem longer than most. When a student doesn't get it, Mr. Austin analyzes his methods and tries something new until the student does get it.

The other strong philosophy that Mr. Austin believes in is that underlying theory determines what can be observed in real life. Students must understand the theory of a subject in order to draw conclusions from their observations. His methodology may not be the norm, but he sees the results each and every day when he hears students say, "I get it now." When Mr. Austin hears those words he becomes exhilarated and feels a deep sense of accomplishment that comes from knowing he makes a difference. It is so rewarding when students feel good about what they have learned and they truly understand it. In short, Mr. Austin feels that encouragement is key to starting and maintaining the learning process.

PART **2**

Basic Teaching Skills for Career Education in the Beauty and Wellness Disciplines

CHAPTER

13 Making the Student Salon an Adventure

Objectives (Desired Performance Goals):

After reading and studying this chapter, you should be able to:

- Explain a key benefit of having student salon revenue contribute to the institution's revenue.

- Describe the role of every institution team member.

- Explain why developing success habits while students are in school will contribute to their later success in the salon.

- Assist learners in developing a solid client base using referrals, rebooking, and ticket upgrading.

- List examples of how the institution team can work together to ensure the institution presents the best possible image.

- List basic standards that might be established for the effective operation of a reception desk and dispensary.

- Explain the most important record-keeping requirements of the student salon in the institution.

- Implement zone teaching.

KEY TERMS

Teamwork • 273

Rebook • 289

Repeat Services • 289

Referral • 290

Ticket Upgrading • 291

Downtime • 292

Portfolios • 294

Zone Teaching • 297

TASK • 298

! CRITICAL CONCEPT

Becoming competent in any area of performance is a process, not an event.

Practical Skills Training

THE ULTIMATE SUCCESS of any institution in the field of cosmetology may relate to how successfully the clinic is managed and supervised. Instructors should understand that throughout this chapter, the terms *clinic, student salon,* and *salon learning center* are used interchangeably. Institutions that provide training for professionals within the beauty and image industry have a distinct advantage over many other types of institutions. Our students receive a significant amount of their career training in a "hands-on" learning environment that is very similar to that of the actual salons and clinics in which they will become employed. With their "real-world" training experience, graduates make the transition from school to work far more easily than those students who have not had the same opportunity. Because the practical training received in the student salon is so vital to the graduate's success, it is both appropriate and advantageous for the master educator to ensure that the clinic is an exciting, well-managed, and well-supervised training environment.

Another advantage for institutions within the field of cosmetology is that in most states the student salons produce revenue that offsets the overall cost of tuition to students and contributes to the bottom-line profit of the institution. In other words, the more revenue generated in the student salon of an institution, the less revenue needed from other sources to meet the expenses of institution operations. In addition, many of today's institutions participate in federal financial aid programs that provide students with financial assistance for completing their career education. In such institutions, extensive regulatory oversight is provided by the U.S. Department of Education that requires "for-profit" institutions to, in fact, make a profit and maintain sound financial stability. The clinic revenue makes a strong contribution to meeting those financial stability requirements.

The salon learning center provides the venue for students to learn and practice skills in communication, business, retailing, problem solving, conflict resolution, and more. Surveys show that as much as 85 percent of our students' success comes from their people skills, their visual integrity, goal orientations, and their ability to communicate effectively with clients, co-workers, and employers. The opportunity to develop these attributes is presented in the student salon. After all, students can master technical skills on mannequins or other apparatus used for practical skills training. However, they can only practice their people skills and ability to communicate effectively by working with people. Therefore, the clinic or student salon is a critical part of each and every student's training.

The Student Salon Philosophy

Students should be taught from the very beginning of their course of study that their success as a student in the clinic will determine their entry-level success in the salon or their first place of employment. It must be made clear to them from the onset of training that the habits they develop while in school will be habits that follow them into the workplace. They can either

+ MASTER EDUCATOR

1. Imparts sound education and facilitates learning for all students through teaching, grading, coaching, and mentoring.
2. Assists students in developing a sound client base.
3. Promotes and generates student salon revenue that contributes to the overall success of the institution.

be *success habits* or *failure habits*. Your role as an educator is to teach your students success habits and behaviors that will serve them well as professionals. Students often take the position that they don't want to work hard in the student salon during their training because it makes the institution money and doesn't do anything for them. They indicate that they will do all the things necessary for success when they get into the salon and will earn all the profits for themselves. If our students take that position, we have failed to convey to them the value of their training and practice in the student salon learning center. We have failed to make our students realize that the benefits of changing their behavior now far outweigh their judgments about the institution making a profit.

The last decade has brought about dramatic changes in the financial structure of cosmetology institutions. Tuition costs have increased greatly since 2000. As a result, current research indicates that for optimum profit, institutions should attempt to generate student salon revenue that represents at least 25 percent of the overall operating income. That same research suggests that 15 percent of the student salon revenue should be generated from retail sales. The remaining 75 percent of overall revenue should be derived from student tuition collections, including registration fees and the cost of books and kits. Institutions should expect a minimum net profit of 10 percent. If a net profit of greater than 10 percent is achieved, institutions should consider sharing that profit with the employees who helped achieve it through bonuses or rewards, which can be based on performance incentives. If the institution's annual financial statement shows less than a 10 percent profit, everyone, including all staff members and faculty, needs to understand that change *must* occur. If the systems and procedures that the institution is following are not generating the financial stability required, then operations must be evaluated and a plan of action implemented to achieve the desired results.

All personnel play an important role in the evaluation and implementation process. Master educators certainly have a vested interest in achieving quality outcomes for the institution because their students are directly affected by those results. In other words, the goal of the institution and the personnel should be to maximize student salon profit while maintaining educational excellence.

Master educators make certain that the student salon is an adventure for the students. You must instill in your students the philosophy of *purpose, adventure,* and *learning.* Teach students to not settle for anything plain or routine. Instill in them the desire for learning and provide a dynamic student salon experience that will help them understand its importance to their career education. From the very beginning of the student's relationship with the institution, even in the admissions process, students should be taught that although their *assignment* is to graduate, one of their *primary goals* is to develop a solid client base. Achievement of that goal does not begin with graduation; it begins on day one of their training. Staff and faculty should begin referring to all students as graduates on the first day of classes. Some institutions go so far as to have students' pictures taken in cap and gown so the students can visualize themselves as successful graduates from the beginning of their training. Science shows that positive self-suggestion and visualization are highly effective in helping people achieve important life goals. Use of such valuable research will aid the master educator in helping the students achieve their own success.

The Essence of Teamwork

Merrium Webster's Dictionary defines **teamwork** as "work done by several associates with each doing a part but all subordinating personal prominence to the efficiency of the whole." Wow, what a powerful word! Let's put it in simple English as it might apply to a school in the beauty and image industry. For example: "Work done by students, educators, and staff members with each performing an essential part of the work without expecting to receive personal recognition or prominence as a result, but rather expecting the institution as a whole to be recognized as one of quality and excellence!" There is no part of a school in the beauty and wellness industry where teamwork is more needed or more valuable than in the student salon or client service center. It actively involves everybody in the institution at one time or another. Therefore, it is critical for each team member, students and staff members alike, to understand their individual roles and do everything in their power to help the other team members succeed as well. In order to accomplish the desired results, it must be made clear to all members exactly what is expected of them to achieve a highly successful student salon.

Students need to understand that their personal role includes:

- Gaining knowledge and building practical skills expertise;
- Developing a positive winning attitude and wearing a winning smile;
- Developing a sound client base of at least 300 clients during a year; and
- Generating student salon revenue that ultimately contributes to the overall success of the institution.

Educators need to understand that their personal role includes:

- Imparting sound education and facilitating learning for all students through teaching, grading, coaching, and mentoring;
- Developing a positive attitude and wearing a winning smile;
- Aiding students in developing a sound client base of at least 300 clients per year; and
- Promoting and generating student salon revenue that contributes to the overall success of the institution.

Other staff members need to understand that their personal role includes:

- Developing sound and efficient administrative practices that support the education provided in the institution;
- Developing a positive winning attitude and wearing a winning smile;
- Aiding students in developing a sound client base by constantly promoting the institution; and
- Promoting and generating student salon revenue that contributes to the overall success of the institution.

Do you see a pattern here? Often we attempt to put the responsibility on the shoulders of another team member, when, in fact, if we share a common vision and goals, we share common responsibilities.

CONSIDER AND CONNECT

Master educators must teach students to stretch and expand their minds by attaching themselves to a purpose and becoming adventurous. They will instill in them the desire for learning.

teamwork work done by several associates with each doing a part but all subordinating personal prominence to the efficiency of the whole.

IT'S WORTH REMEMBERING

Teamwork is the ability to work together toward a common vision; the ability to direct individual accomplishment toward institution objectives. It is the fuel that allows common people to attain uncommon results.

CONSIDER AND CONNECT

A team composed of members who are open to ideas, eager to communicate with each other, focused on team goals, and accept all members as valuable contributors is a *dynamic team*!

☑ The Profitable Student Salon

One of the first steps in building an exciting and profitable student salon is defining goals that are worthwhile, predetermined, and realistic. If one goal is for students to develop an annual client base of 300 clients, how many clients should they be expected to serve during a day or week? Accrediting agency information tells us that the average cosmetology school in the United States enrolls approximately 104 students annually, with an average of 75 percent enrolled in the cosmetology program while another 25 percent are enrolled in other programs such as nail technology or esthetics. In addition, historical data suggest that tuition for cosmetology begins at $10.50 per clock hour and $10.00 per clock hour for shorter programs, including the registration fee, books, and kit costs. Let's develop a hypothetical situation based on these statistical averages.

A 15-POINT PROFILE: MILADY SPA ACADEMY

1. Tuition (includes fees, books, kits):
   Cosmetology—1,500 hours: $15,750.00
   Nail Technology—350 hours: $3,500.00
   Esthetics—600 hours:$6,000.00

2. Historical retention rate: 78%

3. Enrollment (based on national averages by school and program)
   Cosmetology 78 students X 78% retention rate = 61 X $15,750 = $960,750
   Nail Technology 12 students X 78% retention rate = 9 X $3,500 = $31,500
   Esthetics 14 students X 78% retention rate = 11 X $6,000 = $66,000

4. Total tuition revenue (allowing for lost tuition due
   20 approximately 22% student withdrawals): $1,058,250

5. Desired student salon revenue* for year: $352,750

6. Amount of student salon revenue desired from retail:* $52,912

7. Amount of student salon revenue from services only: $299,838

8. School has approximately 81 students enrolled at any one time.

9. Level I students generally represent approximately 20% of student
   Body and schools can expect an 8%–9% absentee rate which leaves
   An average of 60 students assigned to student salon at any one time.

10. $299,838 divided by 50 weeks per year for average clinic revenue = $5,996.76

11. $52,912 retail divided by 50 weeks per year for average retail revenue = $1,058.24

12. $5,996.76 divided by 60 students for weekly clinic revenue per student = $99.94

13. $1,058.24 divided by 60 students for weekly retail revenue per student = $17.64

14. Clinic and retail revenue per student per week to achieve annual goal of = $117.58

15. $117.58 divided by 5 days per week for services and retail by student = $23.52

*Generally, 75% of a typical cosmetology school's revenue is derived from tuition and fees.
25% of a typical cosmetology school's revenue is derived from services and retail.
Typically, 15% of a typical cosmetology school's student salon revenue is derived from retail.

If the institution's student salon averages $13.50 per ticket, the student only needs to serve *two* clients per day in order to achieve the institution's student salon's goal. This puts the student's concept of "slave labor" into perspective, doesn't it? More important is the fact that students are not even obtaining the *minimum experience* they need to master the various practical skills required for success in their profession. One way to make this exercise meaningful to students is to survey the area's salons and determine the amount of their average ticket. For example, if the average salon ticket is $30 to $45 depending upon the market area, the graduate will only gross $300 to $450 based on the two-clients-per-day average. Assuming the salon retains 50 percent commission and payroll taxes average approximately 14 percent (which varies by employee), the graduate's take-home pay will average between $129.00 to $193.50 for a full week—certainly not enough to support oneself or family. If, on the other hand, the new graduate provides services to an average of six clients in the salon daily, the weekly take-home pay would range from $387.00 to $580.60 (or $19,350 to $29,025 annually).

Now, let's take this scenario one step further. Let's assume that all students serve *five* clients in the institution daily at a ticket average of $13.50. This generates student salon revenue of $337.50 by each student. That amount multiplied by the 60 students training in the student salon totals $20,250, which multiplied by 50 weeks in the year totals $1,012500. This author would suggest that if student salon revenue was increased by nearly 300 percent, all staff members and educators would experience significant pay increases and performance bonuses and student tuition would probably decrease! More important, the students would have actually *gained the valuable experience* necessary to make them highly competitive with seasoned professionals in the salon. Let's take this example to yet another level. What if we taught our students to retail and/or upgrade the client ticket by 22 percent to $16.50 per client. Our 60 students multiplied by 5 clients per day by 5 days per week by 50 weeks per year would equal gross student salon revenue of $1,237,500 per year.

If this scenario doesn't describe the ever-desired *win-win-win* situation, nothing does. The students win because they know how to make a good income their first day on the job. The salon who hires them wins, because they have new employees who are capable and ready to "hit the floor running" to generate revenue and increase salon profit. The institution owner wins, because the overall profit margin just soared for the institution and the institution has achieved its mission by graduating successful salon professionals. The institution's educators and employees win because the increased profit justifies and affords significant pay increases for staff. Why is it, then, that educators across the country feel "uncomfortable" with teaching students that they must develop a *sound clientele, retail products*, and *upgrade client tickets* while they are in institution? It has been said that if we change the way we *see*, we'll change the way we *be*. That saying was never more appropriate than it is when referring to how we teach students to view the student salon experience while they are in institution. Educators are doing their students a disservice if they do not explain scenarios such as this to their students.

What Does the Public See?

Master educators know that they play a key role in how the institution is viewed as a whole. They know that the image or perception of the institution held by the members of the public who enter its doors depends on the efforts of the entire school team. A dirty or disorderly reception area or student salon can seriously tarnish a community's image of the institution and the education it provides. The team should regularly evaluate the institution from the front door to the back door and look for safety, cleanliness, and comfort. If we are training graduates for careers in the beauty and image industry, it is only logical that we, as professionals, and our physical facilities present the best possible professional image at all times. The consuming public, including our students, is much more aware than ever before of the importance of infection and disease control as well as the need to make a positive first impression.

The team should periodically exit the front door and reenter as if entering the facility for the first time ever. They should see the reception area the way the clients who are walking in the door for the first time see it. A checklist is provided to assist you in this important evaluation.

RECEPTION AREA CHECKLIST

_____ Reception area neat, clean, and orderly.
_____ Reception area inviting and attractive.
_____ Reception desk neat, clean, and organized.
_____ Telephone clean, free of dirt and grime.
_____ Magazines current and stacked neatly.
_____ Plants watered, pruned, and leaves free from dust.
_____ Windows clean and shining.
_____ Retail display dusted and well-organized.
_____ Trash cans emptied and clean.
_____ Water fountain clean and sanitary.

☑ The Warm Reception

The challenge and opportunity of operating the reception desk is one of the most important jobs in the operation of an institution or professional salon. The attendant, whether an assigned student or a full-time receptionist, not only schedules appointments, but also acts as a link between the client and the institution. She also acts as a link between the public calling on the telephone and the institution. A positive, smiling attitude must be maintained at all times. That familiar expression that "you never get a second chance to make a positive first impression" certainly applies to the career institution environment. The reception area is the first thing clients and prospective students see when they arrive at the institution (Figure 13–1). Their perception should be a positive one. They should be greeted warmly, made to feel important, and generally experience a friendly, positive welcome.

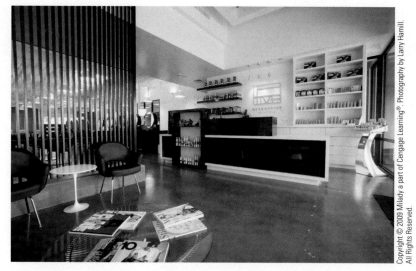

Figure 13–1   The reception area forms the first impression for clients and prospective students.

RECEPTION DESK OPERATION

Mission: To ensure the institution achieves its major goals, objectives, and continuing purpose by contributing maximum effort through competent completion of the duties and responsibilities assigned to the reception desk.

1. Smile, smile, and smile again.
2. Set up reception desk prior to opening the clinic.
3. Ensure that the following items are readily available at the desk:
   a. Appointment book (if institution schedules clients by appointment) or point-of-sale (POS) system
   b. Client register (if institution requires clients to sign in for services, which is highly recommended)
   c. Client tickets for services
   d. Client intake forms (client personal information and history)
   e. Client analysis and record forms
   f. Hold harmless forms or chemical release statements
   g. Daily revenue report (recommended for summarizing daily clinic activity)
   h. Student sign-in sheet (recommended in addition to routine "clocking" procedures)
   i. "Deposit Only" stamp for checks
   j. Returned check list for clients who have a "bad check" history
   k. Electronic debit, credit, or gift card machine
   l. Price list or menu of services with prices
   m. Price list for retail products
4. Never leave reception desk unattended (obtain a substitute when breaks are needed).
5. Greet all clients with a smile and offer immediate assistance.
6. Have clients sign in on the client register (if used by the institution).
7. Assign a ticket for the client and list all services scheduled for today.
8. Suggest an additional service (perhaps you notice that a haircut client needs an oil manicure; simply offer, "Would you like me to schedule you for a manicure to accompany your hair service today?" or "A conditioning treatment might really add some needed shine to your hair this week. Would you like me to advise your student stylist that you'd like to have one?"

(continued)

RECEPTION DESK OPERATION *(continued)*

9. Notify the student stylist that the client has arrived and hand her the client ticket.
10. NEVER leave a client waiting without personal attention for long periods of time.
11. Ask if the client would like something to drink, such as water, coffee, or a soft drink.
12. Whenever possible or when it is the client's first visit to the institution, formally introduce the student stylist to the client.
13. If the assigned student stylist is completing another service, assign another student to begin the service whenever possible.
14. NEVER assign a client to a student who is attending a scheduled theory class.
15. Schedule appointments based on client request, rotation of the students assigned to the student salon, availability of students for specific services, and training needs of the students as indicated by educators. (Institution policy may vary.)
16. Ring-up tickets and count change back to the client.
17. Request that clients rebook for a future service.
18. Offer retail or maintenance products to all clients.
19. Encourage clients to bring a friend for their next appointment.
20. During lulls, the attendant keeps the area clean, magazines arranged, styling books organized, retail displays dusted and neat, trash discarded, and so on.
21. Personal calls are not made or received by attendant while operating the reception desk, except according to policy.
22. Calls are directed to appropriate personnel; clear and accurate written messages are taken when necessary. For example, when a prospective student inquires about enrollment, the attendant *never* attempts to answer the questions. She simply states that she is a student in training and then asks the name and phone number of the caller and states that she will direct the call to the registrar.
23. Educators are never called out of class to take a personal or business call unless it is a bona fide emergency.
24. Walk-in applicants for enrollment are seated and institution policies are followed. At some institutions, there may be an introductory questionnaire that the applicant is requested to complete while the attendant notifies the registrar or admissions representative that a prospective student has arrived.
25. Attendant may be required to provide training in telephone procedures or reception desk procedures to students being oriented to the student salon.
26. Register is closed out at end of day and the daily revenue report (as applicable to the institution) is completed accurately.

Master educators will ensure that every student is taught the important steps of managing a successful reception desk, from the proper way to answer the telephone to the correct operation of the cash register. It is recommended that students be assigned to train at the reception desk on a rotation basis, even if the institution employs a full-time receptionist. Certain standards must be set for behavior when training in this capacity. As with other rules and standards, it might be beneficial to get the students involved in establishing the standards appropriate for professional reception area procedures. Following is a detailed example of reception desk standards that have been adopted in some institutions. They can be modified or adapted, as appropriate, for the institution in which you teach.

Depending on the layout and policies of the institution, the reception desk attendant may also be required to perform several of the dispensary and laundry duties. This will vary from institution to institution.

High-Tech, High-Touch Safety

As previously noted, never before in our history has the public been more aware and conscious of the importance of disease and infection control. In the high-tech, high-touch environment found in institutions of cosmetology and related career fields, the professional practice of sanitation and disinfection is essential. Educators should assume a large role in ensuring that the student salon is maintained in a clean and safe manner at all times (Figure 13–2). Educators will ensure that all students understand the importance of performing required cleanup duties before and after serving each client. Educators will insist that students practice the highest degree of cleanliness throughout the day and leave their stations shining at the end of the day. Some institutions have even taken the restaurant approach by installing large dispensers of disinfectant wipes in the student salon for students to use to clean their work area before and after each client. Master educators will assign and monitor other general cleanup duties that will ultimately leave the student salon in the best possible condition for the next day's services.

As part of the routine rounds through the student salon, educators should also take note of the soiled towel bins. Educators will empty them frequently and assist the student on laundry duty with keeping the towels laundered, dried, and folded throughout the day. By setting this example, other students who are not busy will begin helping. Educators often assume that such menial tasks as washing and folding towels is the students' responsibility and beneath them. With that attitude and opinion, the status of master educator will never be achieved.

The example set by you, the educator, with regard to cleanliness and presenting a professional image in the student salon is critical to the future success of your graduates. Even if some salons fall below standard procedures in this area, the consumer will be the final judge. Clients will refuse to be served in an environment that is cluttered, dirty, and may cause the spread of germs. Instilling in your students the desire and commitment to a sparkling clean student salon or professional service facility is a challenge that must be met by every master educator.

The concerned, committed institution team will ensure that the facility and equipment are monitored regularly and needed repairs are reported to appropriate management personnel in a timely manner. The team should automatically take steps to correct any minor image concerns that need improvement. For example, students should be taught that if they are escorting their client to the front door after a service and notice that magazines have been strewn all over the area, they should simply straighten them on the way back to their station (regardless of whether they have been assigned that particular responsibility on that day). When an educator or other staff member is passing through the clinic and notices that the soiled towel bin is overflowing, she should automatically remove the soiled towels, take them to the laundry area, and begin the wash (even if specific students are assigned that task for the day). When an admissions representative is walking through the clinic and notices that a sign or poster is hanging askew, she should simply straighten it before proceeding to her destination. By taking actions such as these, staff members become role models for students. The students will then mirror their behavior and begin to automatically perform

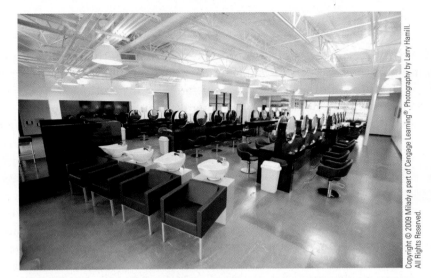

Figure 13–2   A clean, professional student salon is critical to the future success of graduates.

CONSIDER AND CONNECT

There's a saying that aptly applies to operating a successful student salon: "He who sees the need, does the deed." By completing the deeds one at a time throughout the day while also completing other job or training responsibilities, the deeds hardly feel burdensome or time consuming.

STUDENT SALON CHECKLIST

_____ Safe, clean, and comfortable.
_____ Equipment arranged in an orderly manner.
_____ Equipment in good repair.
_____ Signs and posters properly framed, neat, and hanging straight.
_____ Hair removed from the floor promptly and placed in a closed container.
_____ Floors and equipment free from tint stains.
_____ Mirrors clean.
_____ Stations free of paraphernalia and photos.
_____ Soiled towels disposed of properly.

such tasks, which will improve the image of the institution overall. When you think about it, if you perform any particular task needed (such as cleaning the telephone receiver and keypad) at the time you notice the need, there will not be any "big" jobs at the end of the day. Master educators will take every step possible to role-model exemplary behavior that students will ultimately mirror. Developing these kinds of habits will serve the graduates well when they reach a professional service facility.

Record-Keeping Requirements

For a successful student salon to run smoothly, certain client records must be maintained by students. Educators must ensure that each student understands the record-keeping responsibility and knows how to accurately complete all of the applicable forms. In institutions of cosmetology, a release form or hold harmless form is signed by clients for all chemical services. It is designed to release the institution and students from responsibility for accidents or damages. The form is even required by some malpractice insurance companies.

The release statement is not a legally binding document and therefore will not totally absolve the business of responsibility for what has occurred.

The release statement is used primarily to fully explain to clients whose hair, for example, is in questionable condition that their hair may not withstand the requested chemical service. It also encourages the client to be truthful about any prior chemical services that may affect the results of the current service being requested (Figure 13–3). Master educators will ensure that all students understand that it is critical to obtain the client's signature on the release statement *prior* to the service. This is an area where students can be somewhat negligent. If they fail to obtain the signature prior to the service and then there is a problem with the service, it is highly unlikely that the client will sign the release at that time. The release form should be a routine part of any chemical service at the institution, such as a chemical reformation or methacrylate nail extension service.

Another form of record keeping in the institution is the client intake form. Students should learn early in their student salon training to always record the client's personal information and history on the client intake form. Another important record is the client analysis and consultation form. It is important to keep an accurate record so that successful services can be repeated and any difficulties encountered in one service can be avoided in another. A complete record should be kept, containing all analysis notes, strand tests and whole-head results (if applicable, such as for hair coloring), timing, and suggestions for the next service. These records may be retained in hard copy or in an electronic file folder made available through the institution's point-of-sale computer system.

RELEASE FORM

I, the undersigned, _____.
                                                   (name)

residing at_____.
                                              (street, address)

_____.
                                         (city, state and zip)
                        about to receive services in the Student Salon of

_____.

and having been advised that the services shall be performed by students, who are supervised by instructors, in consideration of the nominal charge for such services, hereby release the school, its students, graduate students, instructors, agents, representatives, and/or employees from any and all claims arising out of and in any way connected with the performance of these services.

The Proprietor Is Not Responsible for Personal Property

Signed _____.

Date_____.

Witnessed_____.

THIS RELEASE FORM MUST BE SIGNED BY THE PARENT OR GUARDIAN IF THE CLIENT BEING SERVED IS UNDER 18 YEARS OF AGE.

Figure 13–3   Release statements are used to encourage truthfulness from clients as well as to protect the institution.

Accurate client records are also important to other student practitioners who may be providing different services to the client. A student may discover certain product sensitivities while providing a hair service and record that information on the client analysis and service record. That information may be vital to the esthetician student who will be providing skin care services. The same holds true for the esthetician student who serves the client first. All students must record accurate data for the benefit of anyone who may later serve the client. Students should write down what they learn and read the information each time they see a client. See Figures 13–4 and 13–5 for two examples of client record cards. Figure 13–4 reflects a combination client in-take form, analysis and consultation, client service history, and hold harmless agreement. Figure 13–5 is an example of a client record card used specifically

---

CLIENT RECORD
HAIR ANALYSIS, SERVICE HISTORY, AND HOLD-HARMLESS AGREEMENT

Client Profile

Client Name _____ Telephone_____

Address _____

1. Occupation: _____ 2. Hobbies: _____
3. How much time do you spend daily caring for hair, skin, and nails? _____
4. Describe your personal grooming regimen. _____

_____

5. How frequently do you have professional hair, skin, and/or nail-care services? _____

MEDICAL RECORD Please indicate if you currently have or have had in the past any of the following conditions.

Condition	No	Yes	Condition	No	Yes
Arthritis	____	____	Stroke	____	____
Cancer	____	____	HIV	____	____
Diabetes	____	____	AIDS	____	____
Heart problems	____	____	Pregnant now?	____	____
High blood pressure	____	____	Taking medications?	____	____

Please list and explain any other medical conditions that we should be aware of. _____

_____

If you answered yes to any of the above conditions or questions, please list what medication, if any, you are currently taking.

_____

HAIR, SCALP, SKIN, NAIL ANALYSIS

Hair texture: _____   Hair density: _____

Hair porosity: _____   Hair elasticity: _____

Scalp condition: _____   Hair condition: _____

Skin type: _____   Skin condition: _____

Nail shape: _____   Nail condition: _____

Prior relevant services: _____

SERVICE RECORD

Service performed: _____ Student/stylist: _____ Charge: _____

Procedure/formula used: _____

_____

Comments/results: _____ Instructor initials: _____

HOLD HARMLESS

My signature hereby acknowledges that I will not hold the salon/school, its proprietors, officers, agents, or students liable or accountable for any injury or damage that may occur as a result of the service(s) received.

_____   _____
          Client Signature   Date

Figure 13–4   Client record cards contain analysis notes, tests, processes, and results.

HAIR COLOR RECORD

Name _____ Tel. _____

Address _____ City _____

Patch test: ☐ Negative ☐ Positive   Date _____

Eye color _____ Skin tone _____

DESCRIPTION OF HAIR

Form	Length	Texture	Density	Porosity	
☐ straight	☐ short	☐ coarse	☐ sparse	☐ very porous	☐ resistant
☐ wavy	☐ medium	☐ medium	☐ moderate	☐ porous	☐ very resistant
☐ curly	☐ long	☐ fine	☐ thick	☐ normal	☐ perm. waved

Natural hair color _____

	Level	Tone	Intensity	Category
	(1–10)	(warm, cool, etc.)	(mild, medium, strong)	(B, W, S, R)

Scalp Condition

☐ normal   ☐ dry   ☐ oily   ☐ sensitive

Condition

☐ normal   ☐ dry   ☐ oily   ☐ faded   ☐ streaked (uneven)

% unpigmented _____ Distribution of unpigmented_____

Previously lightened with_____for _____(time)

Previously tinted with_____for _____(time)

☐ original hair sample enclosed   ☐ original hair sample not enclosed

Desired hair color _____

	Level	Tone	Intensity
	(1–10)	(warm, cool, etc.)	(mild, medium, strong)

CORRECTIVE TREATMENTS

Color filler used _____ Conditioning treatments with_____

HAIR-TINTING PROCESS

whole head _____retouch inches (cm) _____shade desired _____

formula: (color/lightener) _____ application technique_____

Results: ☐ good   ☐ poor   ☐ too light   ☐ too dark   ☐ streaked

Comments: _____

_____

_____

_____

_____

Date	Operator	Price	Date	Operator	Price

Figure 13–5 **Some institutions use a customized record card designed specifically for haircolor services.**

for hair color consultations. Whatever type of form your institution employs, you must make sure that students complete the forms accurately and in a timely manner. Effective record keeping will make a strong contribution to the efficiency and effectiveness of the institution's student salon training.

☑ The Efficient Dispensary

No student salon can function to its fullest ability without a well-stocked and efficiently managed dispensary (Figure 13–6). Positioning of the dispensary is essential to efficiency. In your institution, it should be centrally located so that it can be easily accessed by all students and supervisors at all times. The dispensary contains back-bar products and other products that are expected to be needed on a daily basis. It should also contain any tools and implements that may not be normal student kit items. For example, students may not receive perm rods or texture tools in their kit, but certainly must complete numerous texture services in the student salon. A typical procedure would be for the dispensary to house the perm service trays and a sufficient quantity and variety of perm tools to meet the needs of all texture services at one time. The student assigned to the dispensary for the day would be responsible for checking the appointment book and determining how many clients are scheduled for texture services that day. She would then pull the applicable client record forms for each client and set up the perm tray accordingly. She would place the appropriate product and tools according to the prior service on the tray. She would also add strips of cotton, end papers, and picks for wrapping and processing. Of course, the student performing the service will still complete a thorough client consultation, which may result in a product or design change, and the tray set-up may then have to be modified to accommodate the recommended changes of procedure.

Other responsibilities of students assigned to the dispensary might include:

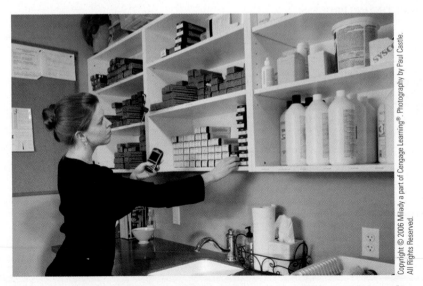

Figure 13–6   A well-stocked and efficient dispensary is essential to the successful operation of the student salon.

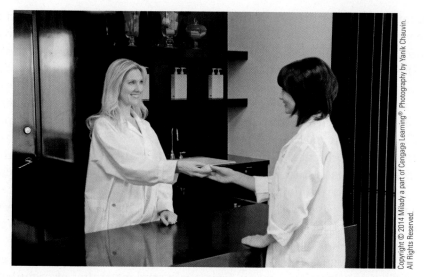

Figure 13–7 Dispensary attendants help prevent waste by dispensing appropriate product amounts.

* keeping the back-bar shampoo and conditioning rinse replenished
* changing the disinfectant soak solution as prescribed by the manufacturer
* performing regular inventory of both the dispensary and the stockroom
* recording and reporting inventory needs to appropriate personnel
* monitoring other student cleanup duty assignments
* obtaining needed products from the stockroom for all students
* checking-in product orders as they are received by the institution
* keeping all implements, such as perm rods, foils, cotton, brooms, and so on, in their designated location

At many institutions the dispensary responsibilities and laundry responsibilities are combined. In that case, the dispensary attendant would also ensure that:

* all towels are laundered throughout the day, properly folded, and stored in the appropriate place
* towels used for hair color service or sculptured nail services may be stored in a different place than those used for routine hair care services
* the dryer filter is cleaned before and after each load of towels are dried
* the lint around the dryer area is cleaned daily

Dispensary attendants must also be taught the importance of monitoring inventory control. They should help prevent other students from wasting product by dispensing appropriate amounts (Figure 13–7). They are responsible for maintaining the dispensary in a neat and sanitary condition at all times. Of course, dispensary procedures will vary from institution to institution. Educators should make certain that all students assigned to the student salon fully understand the responsibilities of dispensary duty so that when the schedule calls for them to be the attendant, the clinic will operate smoothly and efficiently.

Cultivating Satisfied Clients

We've discussed some of the more routine procedures for operating a successful student salon, such as record-keeping requirements and dispensary operations. The bottom line, however, is that how clients are handled from the moment they enter the institution until the time they depart is the most critical part of building a dynamic clinic.

Research studies reveal some important information about why clients leave. For example, 1 percent die; 3 percent move away; 5 percent develop other relationships, 9 percent leave for competitive reasons, 14 percent are dissatisfied with the product or service or the handling of a complaint, and a significant portion, 68 percent, leave due to an indifferent attitude by the service provider. Typically, a dissatisfied client will tell a minimum of seven people about their experience. The majority of complaining clients will return if the complaint is resolved to their satisfaction. Because it takes 12 positive service experiences to make up for 1 negative one, and a business spends six times more to attract new clients than it does to keep a current one, it makes sense to master excellent customer service skills.

We have discussed how clients are greeted by the reception desk attendant. The greeting they receive from their student stylist or technician is also key to developing a loyal customer. When student stylists come to the reception area to get their next client, they should be smiling. They should greet the client by name and introduce themselves if they have not met before or if the receptionist is unavailable to make the introduction. For example, they should be trained to greet their client by stating, "Good morning (afternoon), Mrs. Sanderson. My name is Sarah, how are you? I am looking forward to giving you your texture service today. Please come with me and we'll get started."

Recognizing First-Time Clients

Some institutions have developed special treatments or recognition for first-time clients. For example, the reception desk attendant determines that today is the first time a client has patronized your institution's clinic. She either informs the student stylist or uses a colored dot on the client ticket to indicate to the student that this is a new client. The student then uses a specially colored cape that is different from those used on all other clients (Figure 13–8). The colored cape signals to all students and staff that this is a "first-time" client. They can then make sure to acknowledge the client and make her feel welcome. The client feels extremely special because everyone in the facility is offering a personal welcome. Other procedures include offering a complementary service, such as a scalp massage, to all new clients or a free polish change for the nails. Whatever your institution's methods are, all clients should be made to feel special, appreciated, important, and welcome.

Tender, Loving Client Care

Many principles and concepts should be part of every student's career training. Such training will contribute greatly to building a dynamic, adventurous student salon environment for all students. Master educators might assign various activities and projects that allow students to reflect on their educational experience as well as take necessary steps to make it a more productive one.

The Student Image. The way students dress and groom themselves is a reflection of their own self-image, but also a reflection of the institution and clinic. It's the first thing clients will notice about a student. If the client is fa-

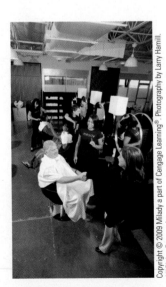

Figure 13–8   Consider using a different-colored cape for recognition of first-time clients.

DAILY QUESTIONS FOR STUDENT IMAGE

1. Is my clothing clean, pressed, and free of stains or damage?
2. Is my makeup tasteful and neatly applied?
3. Is my hair appropriately styled?
4. Are my hands and nails well-manicured?
5. If my fragrance appropriate for the institution's environment?

vorably impressed, it may result in repeat business and higher student salon revenue. Master educators will teach students to dress for the success they desire (Figure 13–9). Student appearance should be evaluated daily. Suggest to students that they perform a daily self-evaluation of their appearance and give themselves small rewards when they meet high professional standards.

The Student Attitude. Master educators know that a willingness to work hard is a key ingredient to success. Your challenge will be to convince students of the same. The commitment they make now in terms of time and effort will pay off later in the workplace. Students must develop an enthusiasm for getting the job done. That enthusiasm will become contagious, and when all students and educators work hard, everyone will benefit through

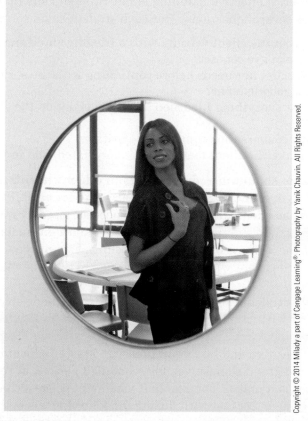

Figure 13–9   Students should evaluate their appearance daily and dress for the success they desire.

the success of the clinic. Suggest to students that they make a checklist for the following areas and keep a daily record for at least one week to see how they have performed:

- Professional appearance
- Positive attitude
- Punctuality
- Diligent practice of new techniques learned
- Regular class and student salon attendance
- Strong interpersonal and communication skills
- Contributing team member
- Helping others

After students have completed their self-evaluation, have them ask for feedback from a few other students whom they trust to be honest. Suggest they offer to do the same for the other students.

Interacting with Clients

We've stressed the importance of conducting a thorough client consultation prior to proceeding with student salon services. Master educators will remind students that the clients they serve are not just another head of hair, set of nails, or face. They will stress that the clients they serve are human beings who need pampering and need to be made to feel special. They will encourage students to make an effort to understand exactly what the client wants before they proceed. They will emphasize the need for the student to practice effective listening skills. Students should be taught to ask themselves several questions after each student salon service:

- Did I greet the client warmly with a friendly smile and handshake?
- Did I make eye contact?
- Did I discuss her needs before continuing with the service?
- Was I a good listener?
- Did I list everything I learned about my client on the client record card?
- Was my conversation upbeat and positive?
- Did I make the client feel needed, appreciated, and important?

Students should introduce clients to other students, especially those specializing in other disciplines such as esthetics or nail technology in the event that the client should ever seek those services. Students should keep the tour brief but informative. They should show enthusiasm when speaking about the various offerings of the clinic. The purpose of the tour is to familiarize the client with the surroundings so that she may be comfortable while there.

Finally, students should be taught to extend themselves when they are interacting with clients (Figure 13–10). Students extend themselves by doing or saying a little bit more than is absolutely required. It's a great way to make a positive and lasting impression. Master educators will challenge students to extend themselves for scheduled periods of time and evaluate the difference it makes. For example, you might suggest that with every person they come in contact with during the following week, they make a point of saying one pleasant comment that isn't expected of them. It could be a

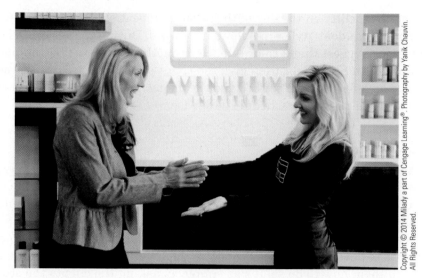

Figure 13–10 Students should learn to extend themselves by doing or saying something that is a little bit more than is required.

simple compliment, such as, "You have such lovely hands, Mrs. Albright." It might be nothing more than a kind word, such as, "I hope little Deanne's recital went well." These comments merely show the other person that the student has noticed her and has paid attention to her in some manner.

Building a Successful Clientele

We noted at the beginning of this chapter that the student's primary goal should be to develop a solid client base and learn key skills necessary for building a successful business in the salon. Now we will look at a number of different strategies for achieving that goal.

Rebooking Clients for Future Services

Upon completion of the service for any client, students should be taught to escort the client back to the reception area. If the client has prepaid for the service, the receptionist would be informed of any add-on services. The student stylist should then explain to the client that she enjoyed serving the client today and that she will look forward to doing so again. The student should ask if the client would like to **rebook** their next appointment at this time and should then suggest retail products that will help the client maintain the new look at home. The student might also suggest that the client bring in a family member or friend for the next service.

Encouraging Repeat Services

The institution's team can use a number of methods to build student salon revenue. One is rebooking, which is accomplished when the client is scheduled for another appointment before leaving the facility. Another method is **repeat services**. This refers to the client returning every four to six weeks for a haircut, but doesn't necessarily imply making the appointments before

---

IT'S WORTH REMEMBERING ✳

When a student extends herself, she makes everyone around want to come back for more. In addition, when students make someone else feel better, they feel better themselves. A happy clinic is a successful clinic.

rebook
refers to a client booking a future appointment before leaving the student salon or professional service facility.

repeat service
a service completed for a regular client such as a haircut scheduled every four to six weeks.

leaving the facility on the day of the service. Repeat services can be encouraged by the student stylist in a number of ways. During the service, the student might suggest that a color retouch or another cut would be appropriate in four weeks. She might then give the client a student card with a recommended date for the next service and the phone number of the institution so the client can call and reschedule with ease.

Client Referrals

referral

a client obtained from another client who has recommended that client to the student or professional for a service.

Another method for building student salon revenue is to obtain **referrals** from clients for their friends, neighbors, and relatives to patronize the clinic (Figure 13–11). Some have suggested that the single most important way for anyone to build a client base is to have the current clientele help, and it doesn't cost a dime in advertising. If we are establishing goals for our students to develop a client base of 300 clients during a year, then we need to teach them how to do so. It's as simple as asking the clients the student currently serves for their help.

When the student stylist completes the service and escorts the client to the reception desk, she simply hands the client three student business cards and says, *"I'm really glad you like the way your service turned out today (this can apply to hair, skin, or nail care services). I want to thank you for trusting me with your hair (skin or nails). I want to give you a few of my cards and ask you to share them with your friends or relatives. Would you do that for me? The more clients I can serve with a variety of beauty needs, the better my training will progress. I would really appreciate your help."* This is a very simple technique, and it has to be carried out in exactly this manner. Students can't simply hand the client a couple of business cards and say thank you and expect the client to do anything with them. Clients need direction. When they receive it, they will likely follow through for the student. It is human nature to want to help others. This simple request allows the client to feel important by helping the student.

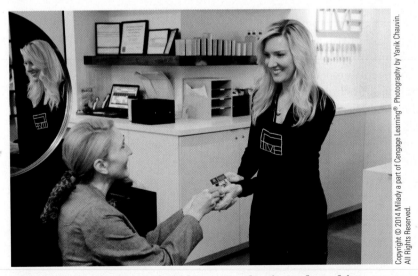

Figure 13–11   Students build a strong business by asking satisfied clients for referrals.

Student Persistence. Students should be taught to be persistent in the client-referral activity. Often they will start out doing what you've directed but then after a few weeks, they simply forget or fail to hand out the cards. While it is important for students to continue to hand out cards, it is also important that students do not hand out three cards to every single client every time they come in. That would get bothersome to the client. Handing out cards approximately every fourth or fifth visit is appropriate, however. Another good time for students to extend business cards is when they have made a significant change in the client's service. Perhaps the client has decided to have highlights put into her hair and it changes her appearance dramatically. Students should always be sure to offer business cards after such a service because the client's friends will be noticing and commenting on the change, which presents a perfect opportunity for the client to share your card with someone else and recommend your services. In fact, the student stylist might ask, "Julie (or Mrs. Harrison, as applicable), do you have a friend or relative that might enjoy having her hair highlighted in a similar manner?" Usually, the client will think of at least one immediately. The student should seize the opportunity to obtain another client. The student might continue by saying, *"Why not do both your friend and me a favor? Show her your hair and tell her you thought of her when you saw the results. Please give her this business card. I have designated a complimentary hair-color consultation on it."* Whenever possible, the student stylist should obtain the name and number of the potential client so that she can personally follow up in a couple of days with a phone call. Leslie Edgerton, author of *You and Your Clients, Milady's Human Relations for Cosmetology*, says that in one salon he owned, he had the following message printed on the back of all the stylists' business cards, *"The highest compliment you can pay us is for you to send us your very best friend."* He says the message came across, loud and clear, and many people commented on it and most of them sent their best friend to the salon.

The master educator might suggest students actually develop a *written plan* for client development. The students would write a list of the clients they are currently serving in the clinic. Then they would list the people they would like to contact about trying their services. They would identify how many new clients they would like to develop. They would create a plan with a goal of contacting a certain number of potentially new clients every week for at least one month. Certainly, they would schedule those who respond and follow up with a phone call after the service to see if they are still satisfied and if they would like to schedule another appointment (if appointments are allowed in the institution).

Upgrading Client Tickets

Another procedure crucial in increasing student salon revenue is known as "add-ons" or **ticket upgrading**. We discussed it briefly in the behavior expected of the reception desk attendant. However, everyone in the institution should be aware of the importance of ticket upgrading and assist

> **CONSIDER AND CONNECT**
>
> *They* cannot quit handing out the cards and expect their clientele to grow. *You* cannot allow them to quit handing out the cards and expect your student salon revenue to grow.

ticket upgrade refers to the technician "adding on" additional services to what was previously booked for the client.

students in making that happen whenever possible. Ticket upgrading is nothing more than suggesting an additional service to that which the client is already scheduled to receive or adding a retail product to the ticket. For example, the client might be coming in for her monthly haircut. The student stylist might say, "Larry, I'm especially pleased with the way your haircut turned out today. I would really like to blow-dry style it so you can see how you should wear it during the week." The student might continue by adding, "In fact, I am going to apply this light gel product, which is going to make it much more manageable and hold the style longer. If you use this product at home in the mornings, styling your hair will be much easier and it will look nice longer. Let me show you how to apply the product and work it into your hair." What started out as a simple haircut ticket resulted in a haircut, a hairstyle, and a retail product sale for home maintenance.

Another example might be a facial client who comes in for a plain facial. The facial or esthetics student might say, "Mrs. Richardson, I notice that after your long golfing vacation in the Southwest your skin seems to be exceptionally dry. I would highly recommend a special herb mask designed especially for dry skin. The benefits will far outweigh the extra time and cost involved." The student might then suggest, "In fact, I want to show you a special moisturizer we carry that is formulated for your type of skin. Using it daily will make a big difference in how soft and supple your skin will feel." It is likely that the student has upgraded the ticket from a plain facial to a mask facial as well as added a retail product sale to the total.

Professional training allows the students to identify when real needs exist and what services and products are best suited to meet those needs. Frankly, it is much easier to increase revenue through increasing the client ticket average than it is to obtain large numbers of new clients to accomplish the same end. Let's reconsider the scenario we discussed in the 15-Point Profile earlier in this chapter of the new salon professional serving 30 clients weekly with a ticket average of $45. By upgrading the ticket a mere $10 to $55, the stylist's net annual income will increase by $6,450 per year. Master educators see the value of developing client-referral and ticket-upgrading skills in every student. Those same skills that will develop a dynamic student salon in the institution will help the graduate develop a dynamic clientele in the salon!

✓ Effective Use of Downtime

For a student salon to be considered dynamic, there should be no "downtime" for student stylists. However, if this so-called **downtime** is used effectively, it won't be long before all students are busy throughout the day when they are assigned to the student salon. In today's high-tech world, using a computer and e-mail can be highly effective. However, when using electronic media, there are some critical professional email etiquette tips that should be considered.

IT'S WORTH REMEMBERING ✳

Professional ethics mandate that the student stylist does not suggest services or products that are not needed by the client.

---

downtime salon time during which the student or professional is not serving a client; when used effectively, downtime becomes productive.

TIPS FOR PROFESSIONAL EMAIL ETIQUETTE

1. Be clear, concise, and spell correctly.
2. Read carefully and answer all the client's questions.
3. Answer e-mails promptly.
4. Do not attach unnecessary files or overuse the high-priority option.
5. Do not write in capital letters.
6. Minimize abbreviations and emoticons.
7. Do not copy a message or attachment without permission.
8. Do not discuss confidential information.
9. Read your email before hitting the "send" button.
10. Add disclaimers when necessary.

Some activities that can be performed by students during student salon hours when they do not have a client to serve are discussed next.

TOP 10 USES OF DOWNTIME

1. **Client Awareness Notes.** These are notes sent out to the student's or institution's regular client list to let them know about special promotions or events that will be going on in the student salon during the next few weeks or for upcoming holidays.

2. **Birthday Notes.** These are sent on a regular basis to clients whose birthday (or anniversary) will fall in the next few weeks. It's a simple acknowledgment of the event and a notice that the student is looking forward to serving them again in the near future.

3. **Client Appreciation Notes.** These notes are sent to regular, loyal clients to simply explain how much their loyal patronage is appreciated. A complimentary or discounted service might even be offered for their next visit to the student salon upon presentation of the card.

4. **Preferred Client Cards.** These cards are also given to regular, loyal clients and offer a complimentary service once they have paid for a predetermined number of services. For example, with every six paid haircuts, the client receives a complimentary haircut or manicure.

5. **Chemical Service Reminder Notes.** These notes are sent when the student stylist knows that it is time for a color retouch or that the previous texture service is likely no longer effective. They simply remind the client that it's time for the follow-up service and suggest a date or time that the client might come in.

6. **Client Referral Cards.** These are written requests containing business cards asking the client to refer friends, neighbors, and relatives for student salon services. A complimentary or discounted service might be offered for every three referrals received.

(continued)

TOP 10 USES OF DOWNTIME *(continued)*

7. **Making Reminder Calls.** These are brief phone calls to clients who are scheduled for important services in the next day or two. A simple reminder phone call reinforces the appointment, emphasizes the student stylist's professionalism and credibility, and ensures that the appointment will not be forgotten by the client.

8. **Acknowledgment Notes.** These are brief notes sent to client who is experiencing a special circumstance such as becoming pregnant, getting a promotion, receiving an award, becoming ill, graduating, retiring, and so forth. A quick email of acknowledgment sends a powerful message of caring.

9. **General Client Campaign.** This activity involves doing an email "blast" to every client in the institution's record file system. It might describe an unadvertised special that is only offered to regular clients. This can be especially beneficial during those times of the year when business routinely falls off. Clients should print the notice and bring it in to take advantage of the "special."

10. **Contact Inactive Clients.** Regular review of the student salon file system will reveal the names of clients who formerly came in regularly, but haven't been in for three or four months. Rather than wondering what happened to them (it's pretty simple—usually, someone else got them), steps should be taken to get them back. Have students send them a nice card or letter noting that they have been missed at the institution. Perhaps an incentive such as discount or a complimentary second service with a paid service could be offered to get the client back. The contact cannot hurt; the client has already gone elsewhere. The simple contact may say to the client that she really was appreciated and may cause her to give the institution another chance.

Master educators will place a great deal of emphasis on the importance of using student salon downtime effectively. Research shows that stylists only spend approximately 50% of their time on the job actually serving clients. They can increase that percentage significantly by actively building business during those hours and minutes that they are not occupied with clients.

The Professional Portfolio

portfolio
a folder or binder used to sell services or obtain employment that includes key items such as a resumé, certificates, awards, before-and-after pictures of services, pictures from photo shoots, and so forth.

Another important tool in building business is the development of professional portfolios by students. The **portfolios** can serve numerous purposes. They can be used when "selling" services to clients in the clinic. They are also effective in obtaining employment after graduation. The master educator will encourage students to begin enhancing their professional portfolio when they are first assigned to the student salon. Students should keep before-and-after photos of their best work professionally displayed in some type of attractive binder. Photos can be mounted on colored paper. Scrapbooking techniques can be used to create at appealing presentation of the student's work. Students should also keep photos of any design competitions or photo shoots that they might have participated in during their training. The portfolio is an attractive and convenient way for the student to display what she has learned during her training. Viewing a student's portfolio can give the client confidence in the student's ability to perform that special color or texture service that is being suggested.

PORTFOLIO CHECKLIST

√   Academic achievement certificates
√   Awards and recognitions
√   Current resumé focusing on accomplishment
√   Letters of reference from former employers
√   Advanced training certificates
√   List of trade shows or events attended
√   Membership certificates in industry and professional organizations
√   Statement of relevant civic affiliations and/or community activities
√   Brief essay explaining why this professional field was chosen
√   Before-and-after photos of services performed on models and clients
√   Photos of work created for photo shoots

Making the Student Salon an Adventure

We suggested at the beginning of this chapter that master educators should make the student salon experience an adventure for the students. Let's look at some systems and procedures that might help you do that.

Service Promotions

Get students involved in developing promotions for the institution that can be used throughout the year for special occasions (Figure 13–12). Assignments for students to create promotions correlate with their business skills training unit, and grades can be awarded accordingly. One such suggestion might be for the students to provide a written plan for promotions that could be used for a variety of holidays, such as Valentine's Day, Mother's Day, Father's Day, or Christmas. The plan should include factors such as the decor of the student salon and reception area, client-sales goals, product displays, services displays, and any other promotional materials that will make the event a success. Another way to make this type of promotion successful is to offer gift certificates and have a selection of cards available so the client does not have to make yet another stop on the way home to complete the gift selection process.

Contests

Contests are a great way for educators to boost student salon revenue. Any contest you suggest should involve both the students and the clients. For example, if the contest awards a prize for the student who obtains the most new clients through the referral process, clients will become involved and refer new clients because they will want their student stylist to win. If the contest awards a prize to the student who sells the highest dollar volume of retail products, the client might decide to help out by buying home-care products for herself, *and* she might also decide to purchase products for gifts in order to help the student win.

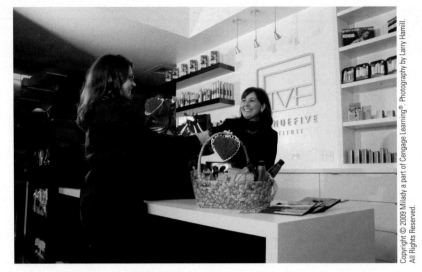

Figure 13–12   Have students create promotions for a variety of holidays throughout the year.

Have students design their own in-institution contests that include a theme, an energizer or pep rally to promote the contest, contest rules or guidelines, and suggested incentives/prizes or awards that would make the contest a success. One institution reports that it conducts a monthly Success Rally that includes identifying six areas of competition for each month. Records are kept to report which students complete the most haircuts, texture services, hair colors, sculptured nail applications, or facials, for example. Other categories for competition might include the highest ticket average, best attendance, most retail dollars, highest ticket sales, best attitude, or completion of the most sanitation duties. The students meet at the end of theory class on the first Wednesday of each month, where categories for the current month are established and the winners for the previous month are announced. Winners have the opportunity to compete for admission into the institution's honor student salon, where they receive added benefits over the regular clinic. The institution provides juice and donuts and a true success rally environment is established. Students and staff have lots of fun. Their enthusiasm extends to the student salon while they are serving clients.

Another such competition is to divide the students into two or three teams (depending on the number of students assigned to the student salon). The students then determine a name, a theme, and color scheme for their team. Students may receive special color-coded name tags to indicate which team they are on. Then a winning name is established that ties to the institution name. For example, for Milady's Spa Academy, the designated name might be *Milady's Spa Team*. Guidelines are established for awarding points to each team. Teams might receive five points if every member of the team completed all their daily cleanup duties. Five points might be awarded if every member of the team is present for the day, and so on. For every 15 or 20 points awarded to a team, they buy one letter of the winning name. The laminated letters are large and cut out of colored card stock. As each team earns letters, they post them in a designated place in the student salon. The first team to spell out the winning name wins prizes. Prizes might include school T-shirts, extra implements for student kits, and so forth. The assigned staff member to the team might win a half-day off with pay.

Another contest that can be extremely beneficial to students' training is one in which students are challenged to compete with each other for getting the most new clients for services they need to meet the training requirements. For example, it is reported that oftentimes cosmetology students begin doing hair in the student salon and fail to serve as many clients for facials or manicures because those services are assigned to the students specializing in those disciplines. Increase the client base for those services by having a student contest to bring the clients in. Provide quality rewards for the winning students.

Distributors are often willing to subsidize retail product competitions by providing prizes to students with the most retail sales of their product line. Prizes might include gift baskets of products or tickets to distributor-sponsored hair shows and classes. Whatever the competition, master educators will take steps to have some type of contest, promotion, or competition going on at all times.

Simple Surprises

Perhaps you have heard it said that when delivering dynamic customer service, you should under-promise and over-deliver. Teach your students that one of the ways they can accomplish this is by offering many small complimentary extras, especially when they are trying to create client loyalty through a long-term relationship. One simple surprise might be a complimentary scalp massage with every hair service. Another might be a five-minute hand and arm massage while the client receives a scheduled haircut. The nail technology area might have ultrasonic jewelry cleaners available to clean client jewelry while they receive their nail care services. Offering a hair color client a complimentary fringe trim and perimeter cleanup between haircut appointments is usually appreciated by both male and female clients. Why not have bottled water and even snack crackers or energy bars available for clients? The cost is minimal and will make a difference in developing customer loyalty.

Student Salon Teaching

The student salons in many of our nation's institutions are quite large in size. Larger campuses have as many as 60 to 80 students or more assigned to them at any one time. Therefore, it is important that the team of educators understand what area they are responsible for and which students they will be supervising.

The Three Elements of Zone Teaching

Some institutions have assumed what has been referred to as the **zone teaching** approach. Each student salon educator or supervisor is assigned to a specific number of stations and students for which she will be responsible. Three key elements are involved in zone teaching. The first element requires

> **IT'S WORTH REMEMBERING** ✴
>
> Competitions and promotions create enthusiasm, excitement, and a sense of adventure for students, especially those that are designed and implemented by the students themselves.

zone teaching
a method of student salon supervision that considers three elements—student and client safety; client comfort; and practical teaching.

the supervising educator to walk through her assigned zone and check the area for safety. She will be checking for any obstacles such as extension cords or frayed electrical cords that might present challenges during the operation of the clinic. This step occurs in no more than a few minutes for the seasoned educator who is well familiar with the environment. The next element of the process is to walk through and check for comfort (Figure 13–13). This might simply be offering clients water or a cup of coffee or making sure that drapes are properly applied and the client is ready to receive the service. The third element is then to teach. Certainly, supervising the student salon involves teachings students. It is recommended that each educator develop a routine of teaching that follows a student-to-student-to-student pattern. By routinely checking all students assigned to your specific zone on a patterned and regular basis, you avoid the frequently heard complaint made by students that they can never find an instructor when they need one. Of course, based on the services that are being performed in the student salon, the educator may not always be able to assist students in the exact order of their station placement. Assisting a student with a chemical service may take precedence over helping a student who is performing a routine blow-dry style, for example.

It is relevant to remember that all students who have been advanced to the student salon and client services should have taken and passed a **TASK** (Technical Assessment of Skills and Knowledge). Therefore, they have had basic skills training in essentially all the practical services they will be expected to provide. However, the educator will need to ensure that additional training and supervision is provided to help students fine-tune skills and increase their speed as well as learn new and more advanced techniques that might not have been taught in prior phases of study.

TASK Technical Assessment of Skills and Knowledge; a practical and written test performed at various levels of training to determine the student's level of competence.

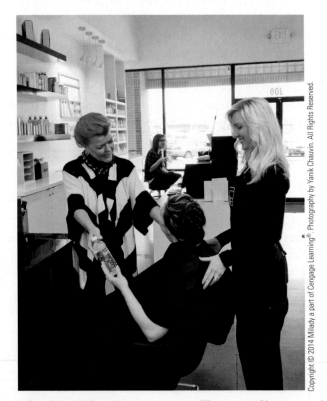

Figure 13–13   Student salon instructors will see to client comfort.

Supervising Multiple Students

Master educators will learn to observe a significant number of students at one time. They will learn techniques such as using student salon mirrors to observe several students at any one time (Figure 13–14). They will become proficient at observing details of a student's procedure as they merely pass by on their way to assist another student who needs the processing of a texture service checked. They will teach students how to check their own haircuts by using partings opposite to those used when performing the actual cut. They will ask the student to check the haircut while they observe rather than taking the shears and comb from the student's hands and checking the cut. Such a procedure often results in the educator taking over the haircut and completing it. This is not an appropriate teaching and learning method. The only way students can learn to perform completed, precision cuts is if they perform them from start to finish.

Master educators will also develop the art of knowing when to start a student on a procedure such as a haircut and when to allow the student to do it. For example, a new student assigned to the student salon may need the educator to establish the guidelines for the student to follow. On the other hand, more advanced, experienced students should be able to establish their own guidelines. Educators need to develop the skills necessary to monitor the performance of a number of students at the same time. This will allow the educator to intercede in a given service before too much damage is done that cannot be rectified. For example, if an educator observes a student wrapping a texture service with frequent "fish-hooked" ends, it is essential that she intercede and have the student correct the problem *before* the wrap is processed. If the educator is not making frequent rounds through the student salon and teaching in a student-to-student pattern, such behavior might be overlooked, resulting in a disastrous texture service and a dissatisfied client.

Master educators will ensure that all students are thoroughly trained in how to formulate, mix, and apply hair color properly. They will ensure that

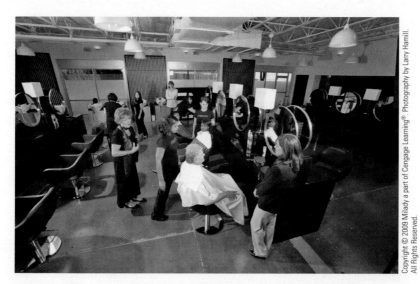

Figure 13–14   The student salon instructor supervises several students effectively.

students know how to apply color to the hair, rather than to the floor or the client's clothing or the hydraulic chair back and arms. If, however, a student does manage to apply color to some location other than the client's hair, the master educator will make certain that the student knows to *immediately* remove the product before unsightly and sometimes irreparable stains occur. Institution owners who constantly complain about how messy their students are and how difficult it is to keep floors cleaned and waxed should understand that the responsibility lies more with the educators than the students. A master educator will make sure that students know how to apply color properly and maintain their work area in a professional and sanitary manner.

Master educators will develop a method for assessing skills performance in the student salon that ensures each service is completed satisfactorily. For example, many institutions use a "satisfactory/unsatisfactory" or "meets minimum competency/does not meet minimum competency" method for assigning grades to clinic services. This ensures that each client service is reviewed by an educator. Some institutions, in fact, do not count any services that were not performed satisfactorily toward course completion or meeting graduation requirements. More formal, detailed methods such as rubrics or practical skills competency evaluation criteria are then used for grading at various levels or hours points during the program.

Tools of the Educator

Educators will be called upon to perform demonstrations of a wide variety of services when supervising students in the clinic. Master educators will plan ahead for these events by having available their own kit of implements and materials that may be needed for such demonstrations. A true professional will maintain a personal inventory of professional equipment for use in such situations (Figure 13–15). In doing so, she will be setting

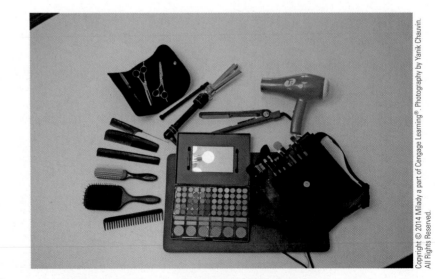

Figure 13–15   A professional educator will maintain personal equipment for student salon or classroom demonstrations.

a perfect example for students and will ultimately be able to present a much better demonstration by using her own tools. When a master educator performs a haircut demonstration, she will get the broom and sweep up the hair she has cut rather than ask a student to do it for her. This sets the example for students that they must sweep up the hair immediately after completion of the cut. Generally, when an instructor begins sweeping up the hair, an observing student will volunteer to do it. If that is the case, it is acceptable to allow the student's assistance, but the educator should never ask students to do it.

Wrapping It Up

Salon owners today are seeking graduates who look sharp, have the ability to perform high-level technical skills, know how to successfully communicate and interact with clients, know how to retail, know how to build a solid client base, and who contribute to the overall profit margin of the salon. By employing the techniques and procedures set forth in this chapter, the master educator will be providing quality training in each of those very important areas and ensuring that all graduates are highly competitive in entry-level professional abilities. Make the student salon experience an adventure for your learners—make it exciting and rewarding. Generate a spirit of enthusiasm that greets every client who enters your student salon. Involve the entire institution team in the challenge of creating a dynamic student salon. In doing so, all involved will benefit and win.

In Retrospect

1. What is a key benefit of having student salon revenue contribute to the institution's revenue?

2. Describe the personal role of every institution team member.

3. Explain referrals, rebooking, and ticket upgrading.

4. Explain why developing success habits while students are in school will contribute to their later success in the salon.

5. List examples of how the institution team can work together to ensure the institution presents the best possible image.

6. List basic standards that might be established for the effective operation of a reception desk.

7. List basic standards that might be established for the effective operation of a dispensary.

8. Explain the most important record-keeping requirements of the student salon in the institution.

9. Describe the three elements of zone teaching.

Objectives (Desired Performance Goals):

After reading and studying this chapter, you should be able to:

- Explain the importance of preparing for employment.

- Write an achievement-oriented résumé and prepare an employment portfolio.

- Complete a typical employment application and be prepared to complete an effective employment interview.

- Explain strategies to maintain employment once it is obtained.

- Explain the importance of keeping accurate school records.

- Explain the importance of the reception area to a school's success.

- Demonstrate good school telephone techniques.

! CRITICAL CONCEPT

Educators are not born; they are made through study, learning, and growth.

Preparing for Employment

IF YOU WANT to enjoy the success of other master educators, you need to be prepared for the opportunities that await you. One of your primary goals when you chose to become an educator was to be able to obtain gainful employment in a field that you enjoy. You're putting in your time in school; you're learning the basics of education. When you near graduation, it is the time for you to pursue employment in this exciting field. During your training, you have obtained a great deal of knowledge about how a career school is operated. That knowledge will aid you in your pursuit of the "right" school for you. It will also help you respect the need to deliver worthy service for value received in an employer–employee relationship.

As with other practical disciplines, more positions are available for educators within the field of cosmetology and related disciplines than there are educators who wish to fill them. This situation provides almost limitless opportunities for you, the aspiring educator. However, you still must research and discover the various available options before you take the giant first leap and commit to the first job offered.

You should answer a number of questions before you begin your employment search. What do you really want from your career in education? What particular disciplines within the beauty industry do you wish to teach? What are your strongest teaching skills, and in what ways do you wish to use them? What personal qualities do you bring to the table for a successful career in education? In this chapter we will attempt to help you answer these questions as you continue your journey to success. One of the first steps you can take is to complete the Personal Inventory of Characteristics and Skills found in Figure 14–1.

After you have completed the Inventory of Personal Characteristics and Teaching Skills and identified the areas that need further attention, you can determine how to focus the remainder of your training. In addition, you should have a better idea of what types of institutions you want to consider for employment and what types you are best suited for.

During your training, you may have the opportunity to network with various industry professionals who are invited to the school as guest speakers. Be prepared to ask them questions about what they like most—and least—in their current positions. Ask them for any tips they might have that will assist you in your search for the right position. Your willingness to work hard is a key ingredient to your success. The commitment you make now in terms of time and effort will pay off later in the workplace, where your energy will be appreciated and rewarded. Having enthusiasm for getting the job done can be contagious, and when everyone works hard, everyone benefits.

How To Get the Job You Want

There are several key personal characteristics that will not only help you get the position you want but also will help you keep it. These characteristics include the following points (continued on page 308):

+ MASTER EDUCATOR

1. Prepares an achievement-oriented résumé that sizzles with excitement.
2. Prepares a thorough and appealing performance portfolio.
3. Thoroughly prepares for each employment interview.

IT'S WORTH REMEMBERING ✳

If you choose the most suitable position for your first job, your career will be launched on the fast-track for success.

INVENTORY OF PERSONAL CHARACTERISTICS AND SKILLS

PERSONAL CHARACTERISTICS	EXC.	GOOD	AVG.	POOR	PLAN FOR IMPROVEMENT
Loyalty to institution					
Open to counsel from colleagues					
Pursuit of continuing education					
Effective time management					
Organized work methods					
Orderly and authoritative					
Self-confident					
Ethical and strong character					
Dependable					
Flexible and adaptable					
Cooperative					
Team player					
Able to work independently					
Patient and self-controlled					
Professional image					
Courteous					
Compassionate					
Consistent					
Desire and motivation					
Enthusiastic and energetic					
Imaginative					
Effective communication skills					
Winning personality					
Positive attitude					

Figure 14–1   continued

TEACHING SKILLS	EXC.	GOOD	AVG.	POOR	PLAN FOR IMPROVEMENT
Lesson-plan development					
Use of educational aids					
Presentation skills					
Classroom management					
Clinic supervision					
Effective grading performance					
Teaching and learning methods					
Achieving learner results					

After analyzing the above responses, would you hire yourself as an educator in your own institution? Why or why not?

State the short-term career goals that you hope to accomplish within the next 6 to 12 months.

State the long-term career goals that you hope to accomplish within the next 1 to 5 years.

Ask yourself: Do you want to teach in a small community or large city? Are you compatible with a sophisticated, exclusive, and advanced training institution or are you compatible with an institution that provides basic training in the various disciplines within the field of cosmetology? What types of learners are you able to communicate with most effectively? Do you want to start out slowly, working closely with a mentor, or do you want to jump in and throw everything into your career in education immediately? Will you be teaching in the future or is this just a stopover place in your career? Do you want to teach part time or full time? How ambitious are you and how many risks are you willing to take?

Figure 14–1   An inventory of characteristics and skills to identify strongest teaching skills.

- **Motivation.** This means having the drive to take the necessary action to achieve a goal. Although motivation can come from external sources—spousal or peer pressure, for instance—the best kind of motivation is internal.
- **Integrity.** When you have integrity, you are committed to a strong code of moral and artistic values. Integrity is the compass that keeps you on course over the long haul of your career.
- **Good Technical and Communication Skills.** While you may be better in either technical skills or communication skills, you must develop both to reach the level of success you desire.
- **Strong Work Ethic.** In the beauty business, having a strong **work ethic** means taking pride in your work and committing yourself to consistently doing a good job for your students, clients, employer, and school team.
- **Enthusiasm.** Try never to lose your eagerness to learn, grow, and expand your skills and teaching ability.

work ethic
taking pride in your work and committing yourself to consistently doing a good job for your students, clients, employer, and school team.

Résumé Development

A résumé is used to summarize your education and work experience and tell potential employers at a glance what your achievements and accomplishments are. Some basic considerations when preparing your professional résumé are as follows:

- Keep it simple and to one page if at all possible.
- Print a hard copy from your electronic version, using good quality paper.
- Include your name, address, phone number, and e-mail address.
- Present your recent, relevant work experience.
- Present your relevant education and the name of the institution from which you graduated.
- Present your abilities and accomplishments.
- Focus on information that is relevant to the position you are seeking.
- Include required personal information.

The average time a potential employer will spend scanning your résumé to determine if you should be granted an interview is about 20 seconds. Thus, you must market yourself in such a manner that the reader wants to meet you and ask how you have accomplished what your résumé states. Don't make the mistake of detailing your prior duties and responsibilities; instead focus on your achievements. Accomplishment statements should always expand upon your basic duties and responsibilities. The best way to do that is to quantify the information by adding numbers or percentages whenever possible. If you have never worked in a cosmetology school, consider the following issues with respect to your training as a student instructor. You might ask yourself:

- How many students were in my classes on average?
- How many students have I supervised on the clinic floor?
- How many clients did the student salon I supervised serve each day or week?
- What percentage of my students graduated from their course of study?
- What percentage of my students passed the state licensing examination?

- What percentage of my students obtained employment in career-related positions?
- What kinds of successes have my graduates enjoyed, such as winning competitions, going on to become a platform artist, and so forth?

This type of questioning can help you develop accomplishment statements that will generate employer interest. There is no better time than while you are in school to achieve significant accomplishments that will impress a potential employer. Even though your experience may be minimal, you still must present concrete evidence of your skills and accomplishments. This may seem a difficult task at this early stage in your working career. However, by closely examining your training performance, extracurricular activities, and/or part-time or past jobs, you should be able to create an attention-getting résumé. For example, did you receive any honors while enrolled in the teacher training course? Did you receive special recognition for your attendance or academic progress? What was your attendance average while in school? Did you work with the student body to organize any fundraisers? If so, what were the results? Answers to these types of questions may indicate your people skills, personal work habits, and your personal commitment to success.

Since you haven't completed your training yet, you still have the opportunity to make some of the listed examples become a reality before you graduate. You want to complete your education, obtain your certificate or license to teach, and become gainfully employed as an educator. You have the opportunity to make that success happen now. For further clarification, let's look at some strategies that are helpful in writing your résumé.

The Dos and Don'ts of Résumés

You will save yourself from many problems and a lot of disappointment right from the beginning of your job search if you keep a clear idea in your mind of what to do and what not to do when it comes to creating a résumé. Here are some of the things you should do when writing your résumé:

Insert Complete Contact Information. Use concise, clear sentences and avoid overwriting or flowery language. Consider changing your personal e-mail address if it is not professional. For example, jane.doe@yahoo.com is much more professional than foxyjane4u@yahoo.com.

Make It Easy to Read. Use concise, clear sentences and avoid overwriting or flowery prose.

Know Your Audience. Use the vocabulary and language used by your potential employer.

Keep It Short. Keep the overall length to one or two pages and no more.

Stress Accomplishments. Emphasize past accomplishments and skills used to achieve desired results.

Focus on Career Goals. Highlight information that is relevant to your career goals and the position you are seeking.

Emphasize Transferable Skills. The skills mastered at other jobs that can be put to use in a new position are **transferable skills**.

Use Action Verbs. Begin accomplishment statements with action verbs such as *achieved, coordinated, developed, increased, maintained,* and *strengthened* rather than with a personal pronoun.

IT'S WORTH REMEMBERING ✳

Just think how your positive performance while you are still *in school* can improve your résumé! Make success happen during your training.

---

transferable skills
the skills mastered at other jobs that can be put to use in a new position.

Make It Neat. A poorly structured, badly typed résumé does not reflect well on you.

Include Professional References. Use only professional references on your résumé and make sure you give potential employers the person's title, place of employment, and contact information.

Be Realistic. Remember that you are just starting out in a field that you hope will be a wonderful and fulfilling experience to work in. Be realistic about what employers may offer to beginners.

Always Include a Cover Letter. This assumes you have targeted and visited schools in advance, as advised in this chapter.

Note Any Skills with New Technologies. Include software programs, web-development tools, and computerized salon management systems.

Now, let's look at some of the things that you should not do when developing your résumé.

Avoid Salary References. Don't state your salary history or reason for leaving your former employment.

No Photos. Don't enclose a photograph (you may look like someone the reader dislikes).

Don't Stretch the Truth. Misinformation or untruthful statements will inevitably catch up with you.

Avoid the Personal. Don't list hobbies or memberships that are not business related.

Don't Expect Too Much. Don't hold any unreasonable expectations of what a résumé can accomplish. The potential employer is looking to hire a person, not a résumé!

If you are still uncomfortable with writing your own résumé, there are numerous resources that can be of assistance. For example, Milady U's Online Professional Development Courses are a perfect tool for students nearing the end of their program. Job Preparation (CED 410) includes education in résumé preparation, interviewing skills, personal communication, and more. In addition, Milady offers another online product called Beauty and Wellness Career Transitions, which also offers assistance in résumé development. Other Web sites such as Monster.com and CareerBuilder.com offer assistance in this area. When responding to electronic job boards, keep the same guidance in mind that we have discussed with regard to résumés. Keep your input clear and concise and use action verbs that depict significant accomplishments.

Carefully review Figure 14–2, which presents an achievement-oriented résumé for a recent graduate of the instructor training course.

Employment Portfolio

When preparing for work as an educator within the field of cosmetology, an employment portfolio can be extremely beneficial. In fact, an employment portfolio is your opportunity to brag about yourself and let your career accomplishments shine. The actual contents of the portfolio will vary from graduate to graduate. However, you should include the following items if they are available:

* Diplomas, both secondary and postsecondary
* Awards and achievements while in both the practitioner course and the educator training course

Harvey H. Educator
125 Apache Silver Court
Lost City, Illinois 76006

A barber/cosmetology instructor with honors in attendance and teaching skills who is creative, reliable, and works well with other educators and learners of all ages and backgrounds.

ACCOMPLISHMENTS AS A STUDENT INSTRUCTOR

Academics
*Achieved an "A" average in theoretical requirements and excellent ratings in practical teaching requirements; maintained 98% attendance for course.

Achievements
*Student of the Month for best attendance, attitude, academic grade average, and appearance.

*Supervised student salon team that won the in-school competition for highest clinic and retail revenue.

Administration
*Supervised a student salon team that developed a business plan for opening a twelve-chair, full-service salon; project earned an "A" and was recognized for thoroughness, accuracy, and creativity.

*Served as President of the Student Council and organized fund-raising activities to support "Jerry's Kids" and contribute to the institution's continuing education fund. Under my leadership, raised more than $4,000.

Teaching
*Supervised record-breaking, dynamic clinic of 43 students; increased clinic revenue by 18% weekly; increased retail sales by 23%.

*Taught theory classes for: barbering, cosmetology, manicuring, and esthetics; students achieved an overall grade average of 85% while in my classes; same students achieved a 90% completion rate.

Special Projects
*Reorganized school's dispensary, which increased inventory control and streamlined operations within the clinic.

*Catalogued the school's reference center of texts, books, videos, and periodicals by category and updated the center's inventory list; revised the "check out" procedures for easier access by learners.

*Developed and implemented a field-trip program in which learners were able to visit at least six different kinds of industry establishments throughout their course of study.

EXPERIENCE

2002–2005   Lord and Taylor's Department Store: retail sales, fashions, and cosmetics.
2006–2007   Putting on the Ritz Salon: full-service salon stylist.
2007–2008   Milady Academy of Cosmetology, Student Instructor

EDUCATION

2000–2001   Lost City Community College, General Studies and Business Classes
2005–2006   Milady Academy of Cosmetology, Barber/Cosmetology Course
2007–2008   Milady Academy of Cosmetology, Student Instructor Training Course

References available on request.

Figure 14–2   Your action-oriented résumé should convey your achievements and accomplishments.

- Current résumé focusing on accomplishments
- Letters of reference from former employers
- Synopsis of continuing education and/or copies of actual training certificates
- Statement of professional affiliations (memberships in industry organizations)
- Statement of relevant civic affiliations and/or activities
- Before-and-after photographs of technical skills services you have performed
- Evaluations you have received as a student instructor
- Your philosophy of teaching within the cosmetology industry
- Any other relevant information

Once you have assembled your portfolio, ask yourself whether it accurately portrays you and your career skills. If it does not, identify what needs to be changed. If you are not sure, run it by a neutral party for feedback about how to make it more interesting and accurate. This kind of feedback is also useful when creating a résumé. The portfolio, like the résumé, should be prepared in a way that projects professionalism.

- For ease of use, you may want to separate sections with tabs.
- If you are technologically savvy, you might want to create a digital portfolio or an online showcase of your work. However, don't expect potential employers to take the extra time to visit a Web site or view a DVD. Bring along a printed copy of everything you want the employer to see.

When you write the statement about why you chose a career in cosmetology, you might include the following elements:

- A statement that explains what you love about your new career in cosmetology education
- A description about the importance of teamwork and how you see yourself as a contributing team member
- A description of methods and ideas you would use to increase service and retail revenue

☑ Targeting the School

Chances are that you hope to pursue employment with the very institution in which you have trained. In fact, you may have a pre-enrollment agreement with the school that commits you to a certain period of employment after graduation. If that is not the case, you will need to pursue employment elsewhere. Before beginning your school search, consider the following:

- Accept that you probably won't begin where you ultimately want to be. It might not be possible for your first job or position to be where you want to end up.
- Do not wait until graduation to begin your search. If you do, it is probable that you will take the first offer you receive, and that may not be the most suitable school for you.
- Locate a school that serves the type of students and clients you wish to serve. You may not be afforded the opportunity of starting exactly

where you want to be; however, your experience there will be more beneficial to you if it relates to your ultimate career goals.

- Obtain a list of area schools. The Yellow Pages will be your best source for this list. You may desire to relocate to another area as well. The local library has available the phone books you would need to compile your list.
- Watch television advertisements for the various institutions. Most schools advertise for students and clinic clientele. Watch for consistency; evaluate the quality of the ad; consider what market they are targeting in the ad; and so forth.
- Check out Web sites and social networking sites for various types of schools. If you contact them, do not waste their time. Get right to the point that you are student instructor planning for future employment.
- Keep the institution's culture in mind. What is the dress code? What are the student and client demographics? Look for a school that will be best for you and your goals and talents.

Graduates of the student instructor training program may not find a position as an instructor immediately upon program completion. You should be aware that the content of this training program has also prepared you to be more effective in numerous positions other than teaching. The study of communication skills, conflict management, team building, presentation skills, success strategies, customer service, and more will serve the graduate well in almost any future position. So, as you begin your job search, you may wish to apply the strategies found in this chapter to establishments other than institutions.

Observe the Target

An indirect method of job hunting is a method called *networking*. It allows you to establish contacts and distinguish between schools. If at all possible, make contact with the institution while you are still a student instructor in training. Your first contact will be by telephone and you should follow these guidelines:

1. Call and use your best telephone manner.
2. Ask to speak to the owner, manager, or personnel director.
3. Convey confidence and self-assurance.
4. Give your name and explain that you are preparing to graduate from the instructor training program at the institution you are attending.
5. State that you are researching the local school market for potential educator positions and that you need just a few minutes to ask a few questions.
6. Ask if the school is in need of any new educators at this time and how many are currently employed.
7. Ask if you can make an appointment to visit the institution and observe its operations sometime during the next few weeks.

A school may be reluctant to have you come in and observe while you are attending another institution. However, you can explain that there is no opening available at this time where you are enrolled and that you are extremely interested in pursuing your career in education and that you would appreciate the opportunity to observe another professional institution in operation. Depending upon the school representative's reaction, you may want to schedule a less formal observation by scheduling a clinic appointment, such as for a manicure. What better way to observe how an institution operates than to be a client who is receiving its services? (Figure 14–3). If the institution is agreeable to your scheduled observation appointment, be sure to confirm the appointment with a typed or hand-written note on good-quality paper. The note might simply say:

> *Dear Ms. (or Mr.) _____,*
>
> *I appreciate the time you spent with me on the phone earlier today. I am looking forward to meeting with you and visiting your institution next Friday at 2:00 p.m. I am eager to observe your school, staff, and students at work. If you should need to reach me before that time for any reason, my home phone number is _____. See you on Friday.*
>
> *Sincerely,*
>
> *(your name)*

The School Visit

When you visit the institution, you may want to consider using a checklist to ensure that you observe all the key areas that might ultimately affect an employment decision (Figure 14–4). The checklist will be similar to the one suggested for field trips to area salons.

You may want to keep the checklist on file for future reference and comparison to those evaluating other institutions. Even if you did not like the school or wouldn't consider working there, write a brief note thanking the school representative for his time. Never burn your bridges; rather, build a network of contacts who have a typical thank-you note follows on page 316.

Arranging the Employment Interview

After you have graduated from your course of study and completed the first two steps in the process of securing employment, targeting and

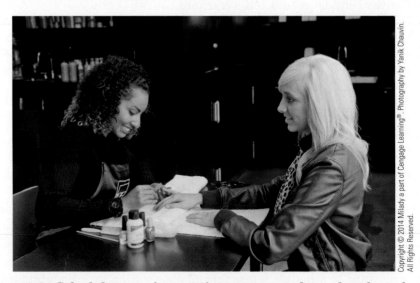

Figure 14–3   Schedule a service appointment to conduct a less formal observation of the school (photo of person getting a manicure).

SCHOOL-VISIT CHECKLIST

When you visit a school, observe the following areas and rate them from 1 to 5, with 5 considered the best.

_____ **School Image:** Is the school's image consistent with and appropriate for your interests? Is the image pleasing and inviting? What is the decor and arrangement? If you are not comfortable or if you find it unattractive, clients or potential students are likely do so as well.

_____ **Professionalism:** Do the employees present the appropriate professional appearance and behavior? Do they give their students and clients the appropriate levels of attention and personal service or do they act as if work is their time to socialize?

_____ **Management:** Does the school show signs of being well managed? Is the telephone answered promptly with professional telephone skills? Is the mood of the institution positive? Does everyone appear to work as a team? Do the students appear to be happy?

_____ **Client Service:** Are clients greeted promptly and warmly when they enter the reception area? Are they kept informed of the status of their appointments? Are they offered magazines or beverages while they wait? Is there a comfortable reception area for waiting?

_____ **Classrooms:** Are they clean, neat, bright, cheerful, and well organized? Do they contain appropriate educational aids for use by educators?

_____ **Clinic:** Is it clean, neat, bright, cheerful, and well organized? Is the equipment appropriate for the courses being taught? Are there sufficient work stations for all students assigned there?

_____ **Reference Center:** Does it contain reference materials sufficient in quantity and variety to support all the courses offered? Is it organized and easily accessible by all learners?

_____ **Educator Work Area:** Is there an appropriate office or area designated for educator preparation such as writing lesson plans, grading tests, preparing counseling records, and so forth?

School Name _____ School Manager _____

Date _____ Comments: _____

_____

_____

_____

Figure 14–4   A school-visit checklist will allow you to observe key areas affecting your employment decision.

observing schools, you are ready to more actively pursue employment. The next step is to contact the institutions where you are interested in teaching by sending them a résumé with a cover letter requesting an interview. Refer to the accompanying example of a résumé cover letter on page 315.

Make sure to mark your calendar for a suitable time to call and follow up on the résumé cover letter and schedule an interview appointment. The institution may not have an opening and the owner, manager, or personnel director may not wish to schedule an interview at this time. If that is the case, be polite and ask that they retain your résumé on file for later reference should an opening arise in the future. Be sure to thank them for their time and consideration. They may tell you that they are not hiring at this time, but that they would be happy to conduct the interview for future reference. If so, take advantage of the opportunity to do so. It will give you valuable interview experience. If the school does want to schedule the interview, several preparatory steps should be considered, as discussed next.

EXAMPLE OF A TYPICAL THANK-YOU NOTE

Dear Ms. (or Mr.) _____,

I appreciate the opportunity to observe your institution in operation last Friday. I know how valuable your time and that of the other employees is. I was impressed by the efficient and courteous manner in which each faculty member handled their classes. I was also impressed by how your students have been trained to treat their clients in such a courteous and professional manner. The atmosphere was pleasant and the mood was positive. Should you ever have an opening for an educator with my skills and training, I would welcome the opportunity to apply. You can contact me at the address and phone number listed below. I hope we will meet again soon.

Sincerely,

(Your name, address, telephone)

An example of a thank-you note to an institution at which you probably would not seek employment is as follows:

Dear Ms. (or Mr.) _____

I appreciate the opportunity to observe your institution in operation last Friday. I know how busy you and all your staff are and really appreciate the time that you gave to me during my visit. I realize that it can be somewhat disruptive to have visitors observing your activities. I hope my presence didn't interfere with the flow of your operations too much. I certainly appreciate the courtesies that were extended to me by your staff and students. I wish you and your school continued success.

Sincerely,

(Your name)

EXAMPLE OF A RÉSUMÉ COVER LETTER

Your Name

Your Address

Your Phone Number

Ms. (or Mr.) _____

School Name

School Address

Dear Ms. (or Mr.) _____,

   We met in August when you allowed me to observe your institution, staff, and students while I was still in instructor training. Since that time, I have graduated and have received my license, which allows me to teach barbering, cosmetology, manicuring, and esthetics. I have enclosed my résumé for your review and consideration.

   I would very much appreciate the opportunity to meet with you and discuss either current or future career opportunities at your institution. I was extremely impressed with your staff and school, and I would like to discuss with you how my skills and training might add to the achievement of your institution's mission and objectives.

   I will call you next week to discuss a time that is convenient for us to meet. I look forward to meeting with you again soon.

Sincerely,

(Your name)

Interview Preparation

1. Make a list of needed items that are typically requested on an employment application.

   a. Social Security number
   b. Driver's license number
   c. Names, addresses, and phone numbers of former employers
   d. Name and phone number of the nearest relative not living with you

2. Interview wardrobe. Your appearance is crucial, especially since you are applying for a position in the image and beauty industry. It is recommended that you obtain one or two "interview outfits." You may be requested to return for a second interview—hence the need for the second outfit. Make sure the outfit is comfortable, in perfect condition, and of a style and color that are flattering to your shape and personality (Figure 14–5). Consider the following:

   a. Appropriateness for the position
   b. Well-fitted and comfortable
   c. Clean and pressed
   d. Shoes clean and in good repair
   e. Jewelry basic and minimal

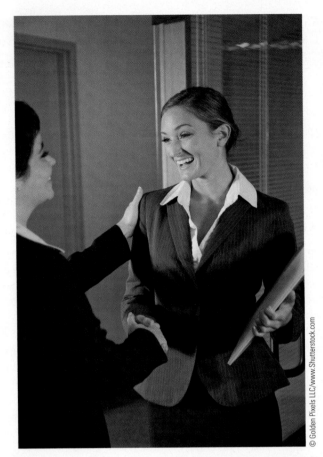

Figure 14–5 Ensure your interview attire is comfortable, stylish, and appropriate.

    f. Hairstyle current and appropriate for face shape and features
    g. Makeup current and appropriate for face shape and features (if female)
    h. Clean shaven or beard properly trimmed (if male)
    i. Carry handbag or briefcase, never both
    j. Appropriate fragrance—choice should be subtle and not overwhelming or bold

3. Supporting materials:

    a. Résumé. Even if you have already sent one, take another copy so that it will be readily available.
    b. Facts and figures. The list of names and dates of employers, education, references, and so on.
    c. Employment portfolio.

4. Answers to anticipated questions. Certain questions are typically asked during an interview. It would be beneficial to give thoughtful reflection to your answers ahead of time. Such questions might include:

    a. What did you like best about your practitioner training?
    b. What do you like best about your new career in education?
    c. Are you prompt and regular in attendance?
    d. Will your school director confirm that?

e. In which teaching skills areas do you feel you are strongest?

f. Which areas do you consider to be your weakest?

g. Are you a team player? Please explain.

h. Do you consider yourself flexible? Please explain.

i. What are your career goals?

j. What experience have you had as a practitioner before pursuing a career in education?

k. Since you have worked in the salon sector for more than one year, what was your average annual income?

l. What days and hours are you available for work?

m. Do you have your own transportation?

n. Are there any obstacles that would prevent you from keeping your commitment to full-time employment?

o. What assets do you believe you would bring to this institution and position?

p. Who is the most interesting person you've encountered in your work/education experience and why?

q. Describe any time in the past when your work/school load became too heavy and you had to revamp your schedule.

r. How would you handle a problem client? A problem student?

s. How do you feel this institution can help you attain your career goals?

The Interview

On the day of the interview, make sure that nothing will interrupt or disrupt your ability to complete a successful interview. Certain behaviors should be practiced and observed:

- Always be on time. If you are unsure of the location, be sure to find it the day before so there will be no reason for delays.
- Project a warm, friendly smile. Smiling is the universal language.
- Walk, sit, and stand with good posture.
- Be polite and courteous.
- Do not sit until asked or until it is obvious that you are expected to do so.
- Do not smoke or chew gum, even if either is offered to you.
- Do not lean on or touch the interviewer's desk. People are often territorial and do not like their personal space invaded without invitation.
- Do not fidget. You must concentrate on appearing confident and create a positive first impression.
- Speak clearly. The interviewer must be able to hear and understand you, especially if you are expected to be heard clearly by your students.
- Answer questions honestly. Think the question and the answer through carefully. Do not speak before you are ready and do not speak for more than two minutes at a time.
- Acknowledge the interview with thanks.
- Never criticize former employers.

Another critical part of the interview is when you are invited to ask the interviewer questions of your own. You should think about those questions ahead of time and bring a list if necessary. This will show that you are organized and prepared. Some of the typical questions that you might want to consider obtaining answers to are as follows:

- Is there a job description, and may I review it?
- Is there an operating procedures manual for the institution, and is it available to all employees?
- What systems are in place to ensure a successful institution?
- How frequently does the institution advertise for students and clinic clients?
- What are the student outcomes for the institution (i.e., completion, licensure, and placement rates)?
- How long do educators typically work here?
- Are employees encouraged to grow in skill and responsibility? How?
- Does the institution offer continuing education opportunities?
- Is there room for advancement?
- If so, what requirements must be met to achieve the next or higher level of compensation?
- What benefits does the institution offer, such as paid vacations, personal days, medical?
- When will the position be filled?
- Should I follow up on your decision or will you contact me?

By obtaining the answers to these suggested questions, you will be in a position to compare the information you have gathered with that from other schools and choose the one that offers the best package of current income and career development. As with your previous meetings, write a thank-you note. It should simply thank the interviewer for the time he spent with you. Close with a positive statement that you want the job (if you do). If the interviewer's decision comes down to two or three possibilities, the one expressing the most desire may likely get the job. Also, if the interviewer stated you should call to learn about the employment decision, then by all means do so.

The Employment Application

When you are applying for employment for any position, you will be required to complete an employment application even if your résumé contains much of the same information. Your résumé and the list you have prepared prior to the interview will assist you in completing the application efficiently and accurately. A sample form is provided in Figure 14–6 that you may want to complete in preparation for your upcoming employment interviews. The form the institution uses may differ, but it is very likely that it will request almost identical information.

✓ Success on the Job

You have done it! You are now employed as an educator within your chosen field of study. As you have learned as you have progressed through this text, you will be faced with a great number of challenges in your career as an educator. It is important to learn as much about the institution, its policies and procedures, the other personnel, the student body, the curriculum, and

TYPICAL EMPLOYMENT APPLICATION

Applicants are considered for all positions, and employees are treated during employment without regard to race, color, religion, sex, national origin, age, marital or veteran status, medical condition, or handicap.

PERSONAL INFORMATION   Date_____ SSN _____ Phone _____

Last name   First   Middle

Present street address   City   State   Zip

Permanent street address   City   State   Zip

If related to anyone employed here, state name: _____

Referred to salon by: _____

EMPLOYMENT DESIRED

Position _____ Date you can start _____ Salary desired _____

Current employer _____ May we contact? _____

Ever applied with this company before?   Where?   When?

EDUCATION

NAME AND LOCATION OF SCHOOL	YEARS COMPLETED	SUBJECTS STUDIED

Subject of special study or research work:

What foreign languages do you speak fluently?   Read   Write

U.S. military service   Rank   Present membership in Nat'l Guard/Reserves

Activities (other than religious): civic, athletic, fraternal, etc.

Exclude organizations for which the name or character might indicate race, creed, color, or national origin of its members.

Figure 14–6   Complete a sample employment application to prepare for the interview.   *(continued)*

FORMER EMPLOYMENT List below last four employers beginning with the most recent one first.

DATE: Month/Year	Name, Address of Employer	Salary	Position	Reason for Leaving
From:				
To:				
From:				
To:				
From:				
To:				
From:				
To:				

REFERENCES Give below the names of three persons not related to you whom you have known for at least one year.

Name	Address	Business	Years Known

PHYSICAL RECORD

Please list any defects in hearing, vision, or speech that might affect your job performance.

_____

In case of emergency, please notify:

_____

Name	Address	Telephone

I authorize investigation of all statements contained in this application. I understand that misrepresentation or omission of facts called for is cause for dismissal if hired.

Signature _____ Date _____

INTERVIEW RESULTS

INTERVIEWER NAME AND COMMENTS

INTERVIEWER NAME AND COMMENTS

INTERVIEWER NAME AND COMMENTS

Figure 14–6 **Complete a sample employment application to prepare for the interview.**

teaching in general as soon as possible. Following are a few reminders to help you make the most of your new position.

The Institution

Access a copy of the institution's operating procedures at the earliest opportunity. Review them carefully and completely. Make sure you have a good working knowledge of all general policies and procedures. Familiarize yourself with any applicable general guidelines for employment and make sure that you follow them explicitly. Determine which regulatory agencies have oversight over the institution and become familiar with their standards and rules as soon as possible. Determine what your compensation package will be, what company benefits are available, and how personal days or vacation days will be handled. Learn how you will be compensated and understand the payroll deductions that will be withheld from your paycheck. Educators are usually compensated either by hourly wage or salary and may be paid weekly, biweekly, or monthly. You may already be familiar with the various deductions, but a brief summary is provided here as a reminder. Withholdings and other deductions may include:

* Federal income tax—determined by your total earnings, your marital status, and the number of dependents you have.
* State income tax—if applicable in your state; the same factors determine the withholding amounts as for federal income tax.
* FICA—Social Security tax that is matched by your employer.
* Employer taxes—your employer must pay certain taxes to comply with state and federal laws, such as FUTA, Federal Unemployment Tax; SUTA, State Unemployment Tax; FICA, Federal Insurance Contribution Act.
* Worker's compensation—insurance paid by the employer to cover the employee if injured while at work and temporarily unable to work.
* Miscellaneous deductions—as an employee you may authorize your employer to withhold certain amounts from your paycheck for a variety of reasons, such as repayment of a student loan or contribution to a savings account. In addition, if the school offers a medical insurance plan as a benefit, the school may only pay a portion of the premium and the balance would be deducted from your paycheck.

The Curriculum

Study the school's curricula and familiarize yourself with the types of lesson plans currently in use. Make sure you are aware of the schedules, course outlines, course requirements, standards required for satisfactory academic progress, grading procedures, and practical skills grading criteria for every course taught. The more familiar you become with this information, the less likely it will be for you to make needless mistakes in your early employment stages.

Stay in Balance

Although going above and beyond the job requirements is an asset and a plus for you, recognize when you have given too much. Don't push your-

---

IT'S WORTH REMEMBERING ✳

Once you begin your new job, you must consider each work day as training in your journey to become a master educator.

IT'S WORTH REMEMBERING ✳

A master educator will go the "extra mile" and do more than what is asked or required.

CONSIDER AND CONNECT

Ask the person criticizing your performance what he would suggest or if he could help you do better in that particular area.

IT'S WORTH REMEMBERING

It has been said that ability is what you're capable of doing, motivation determines what you do, and attitude determines how well you do it.

self so hard trying to make a good impression that you begin to lose needed sleep or become so fatigued that you are unproductive while on the job. You must remain healthy and energetic if you are to serve your institution well. Make sure to incorporate an appropriate balance of rest and relaxation into your work week. Try to exercise daily, get enough rest, wear well-fitting and comfortable shoes, drink plenty of water, and eat a balanced diet. Avoid excess alcohol and tobacco and remain drug free. You will need every ounce of strength and stamina to get your new career in education off to a supercharged start. Remember, both your body and mind can accomplish amazing things if you take proper care of them.

Becoming a part of a new organization's "family" can be difficult. Practice the people skills and effective-listening skills that have been discussed throughout this text. If you receive criticism early in your employment, don't take it too personally. Consider it from a professional perspective, determine if it is valid, and decide what you should do to improve.

By responding with openness, honesty, and a sincere interest in doing better, you will earn respect and very likely an offer of assistance.

If you should find yourself a member of a school team that is rife with petty disagreements and infighting or jealousy, keep a positive attitude. In any business or position, attitudes can be contagious. You may begin your new job as an educator with a tremendous attitude and high hopes and then meet head on with a "veteran" educator who has gripes about everything from the inconvenient staff parking to the types of soft drinks sold in the vending machine. Some people just live in a "black box" and want everyone else to join them there. They tend to gravitate toward newcomers because of their vulnerability. Don't let it happen to you! Remind yourself that your career is what you make it. You can choose to be miserable or you can choose to approach the rest of your life and career with a positive attitude. And since attitudes, even positive ones, are contagious, you may even bring the veteran grumbler around to your way of approaching life.

Fundamentals of Business Management

As you become more and more proficient in your skills as a teacher, curriculum manager, supervisor, and advisor, you may decide to reach for one of the many exciting opportunities that exist for school owners or directors. Like climbing Mount Everest, and all the physical and mental challenges that entails, opening your own school is a huge undertaking. Regardless of the type of school you hope to open, you should carefully consider some basic factors, such as:

1. Consider hiring a qualified consultant with expertise and sound experience in school ownership, administration, and regulatory oversight compliance.
2. Location—Having good visibility and accessibility are two of the most important factors in predicting the success of a business. The location you select should reflect your target market, have access to plenty of

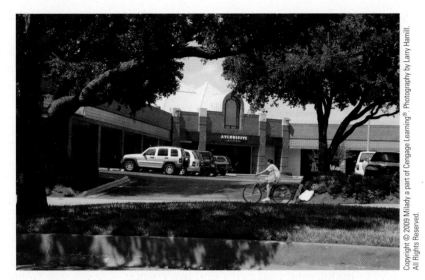

Figure 14–7 **Good visibility and accessibility are important factors for business success.**

parking, and be far enough away from competing schools to avoid too much competition (Figure 14–7).

3. Written agreements—Before you open a school, you must develop a **business plan**, a written description of your business as you see it today, and as you foresee it in the next five years (detailed by year). If you are considering obtaining financing, it is essential that you have a business plan in place first. The plan should include a general description of the business and the services it will provide; area demographics (e.g., average income in your proposed area, average cost of services, number of schools within a 10-mile radius); expected salaries and cost of related benefits; an operations plan that includes pricing structure and expenses such as equipment, supplies, repairs, advertising, taxes, and insurance; and projected income and overhead expenses for up to five years. A certified public accountant (CPA) can be invaluable in helping you gather accurate financial information. The Chamber of Commerce in your proposed area oftentimes has information on area demographics.

4. Business regulations and laws—When you decide to open your school, or rent a booth, you are responsible for complying with any/all local, state, and federal regulations and laws. Since the laws vary from state to state, it is important that you contact your local authorities regarding business licenses and other regulations.

5. Insurance—When you open your business, you will need to purchase insurance that covers malpractice, property liability, fire, burglary and theft, and business interruption. You will need to have disability policies as well. Make sure your policies cover you for all the monetary demands you will have to meet on your lease.

6. School operation—You must know and comply with all federal Occupational Safety and Health Administration (OSHA) guidelines, including those requiring that the ingredients of cosmetic preparations be available for employees. OSHA creates material safety data sheets (MSDS) for this purpose.

business plan
a written description of your business as you see it today, and as you foresee it in the next five years (detailed by year).

7. Record keeping—You will need to keep accurate and complete records of all financial activities that go on in your business.
8. School policies—All schools should have written policies they adhere to. These ensure that all students, clients, and associates are being treated fairly and consistently.

Types of School Ownership

A school can be owned and operated by an individual, partnership, or corporation. Before deciding which type of ownership is most desirable for your situation, research each thoroughly. Excellent reference tools are available, and you can also consult a small business attorney for advice.

Individual Ownership

If you like to make your own rules and are responsible enough to meet all the duties and obligations of running a business, individual ownership may be the best arrangement for you.

The **sole proprietor**:

sole proprietor
one who owns all the assets of an unincorporated business.

- is the owner and, most often, the manager of the business.
- determines policies, and has the last say in decision making.
- assumes expenses, receives profits, and bears all losses.

Partnership

partnerships
a business enterprise owned by two or more persons who share the profits and losses proportionately.

Partnerships may mean more opportunity for increased investment and growth (Figure 14–8). They can be magical if the right chemistry is struck, or they can be disastrous if you find yourself linked with someone you wish you had known better in the first place. In a partnership, two or more people:

- share ownership, although not necessarily equally. One reason for going into a partnership arrangement is to have more capital for investment; another is to have help running your operation.

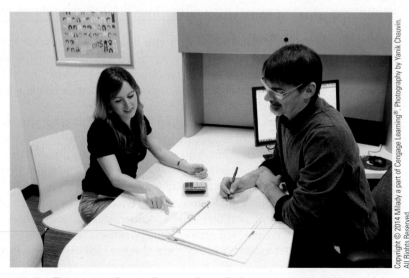

Figure 14–8   Partners share the work and the responsibilities.

- pool their skills and talents, making it easier to share work, responsibilities, and decision making.
- assume the other's unlimited liability for debts.

Corporation

Incorporating is one of the best ways a business owner can protect his personal assets. Most people choose to incorporate solely for this reason, but there are other advantages of a corporation as well. For example, the corporate business structure saves you money in taxes, provides greater business flexibility, and lets you more easily raise capital. It also limits your personal financial liability if your business accrues unmanageable debts, or otherwise runs into financial trouble.

Special Skills Needed

Should you decide to pursue the role of school director or owner, you must develop certain skills to do so successfully (Figure 14–9). To run a people-oriented business, you need:

- an excellent business sense: aptitude, good judgment, and diplomacy; and
- knowledge of sound business principles.

Smooth business management depends on the following factors:

- Sufficient investment capital
- Efficiency of management
- Good business procedures
- Cooperation between management and employees
- Trained and experienced school personnel
- Excellent customer service delivery
- Proper pricing of services (Figure 14–10)

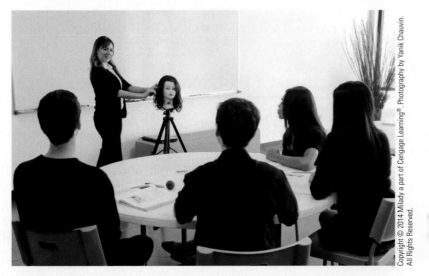

Figure 14–9   Smooth operations require qualified instructors.

HAIR

STYLE
Shampoo/Haircut/Blowout	$17
Men's Haircut	$15
Shampoo-Blowout	$17
Hot Tool Style (with service)	$15
Hot Tool Style (without service)	$25
Updo	$35+

COLOR
Permanent Color	$35+
Demi-Permanent Color	$35+
Highlights / Lowlights	$60+
Partial Highlights	$45+
Baliage Highlights	$55+
Streaks (per foil)	$10
Additional Color	$15+
Additional Toner	$15+

TEXTURE
Permanent Wave	$35+
Specialty Wraps (Root/Spiral/Piggyback)	$60+
Thermal Straightening	$155+
Relaxer- virgin	$45+
Relaxer- retouch	$35+
Sebastian Penetraitt Masque	$10
Kevin Murphy Born.Again Masque	$15
Global Keratin Treatment	$155+
Global Keratin Deep Condition	$25+

FACIALS

Ultimate Facial $30
Using Dermalogica products, this relaxing facial is customized to your specific skin type. Deep cleansing, exfoliation, extractions, massage, and a luxurious mask leave your skin clean, hydrated and glowing.

SkinCeuticals Deep Pore Facial $50
A deep cleansing facial with extractions using medical grade acne treatment products that help reduce oil production and heal skin impurities while preserving hydration levels.

SkinCeuticals Firming Facial $55
Vitamin C Facial – SkinCeuticals medical-grade firming line combats free radicals to provide a more visibly radiant complexion. Designed to give a firmer, more youthful appearance.
or
Intensive Hydrating Facial - Hydrating and firming serums are used under a cooling contour mask that increases circulation to aid in the penetration of products.

"Back-cial" $45
A back treatment with all the benefits of a facial to treat "bacne" and soothe and relax tired muscles.

SKIN TREATMENTS

Advanced Treatments

Chemical Peel $55 each
or $205 series of 5 treatments
Alpha Hydroxy Acids (AHA) are used to excelerate cell proliferation to treat acne scarring, sun damage, blemishing, fine lines and wrinkles. Skin is left smooth and brighter

Microdermabrasion $55 each
or $205 series of 5 treatments
A mechanical exfoliation that gently diminishes the appearance of fine lines and wrinkles creating a smoother, more youthful appearance.

Facial Additions
Add these enhancements to any of our facial services

Ultra-Sonic Exfoliation	$20
Brow or Lash Tint	$15
LED Light Therapy	$30
Jane Iredale Makeup Application	$40
Manual Extractions	$10
Gommage	$20
Exolift	$20

For the Eyes

Eyelash Extensions $80
Natural looking semi-permanent eyelash extensions that last up to four weeks.

Eyelash Extensions ReFill $40
Refill equates to no greater than half of original extension application.

Lash Tabbing $25

Waxing
Full Leg	$50
Half Leg	$30
Feet	$10
Full Arm	$40
Half Arm	$25
Under Arm	$25
Hands	$10
Brows	$15
Lip	$15
Bikini	$30
Face	$20
Nose	$15
Ears	$15
Chest	$30
Back	$40

Figure 14–10   Schools should take steps to ensure pricing of student salon services is appropriate.

The Importance of Record Keeping

As a business manager or owner, you must always know where your money is being spent. A good accountant and an accounting system are indispensable.

Good business operation requires a simple and efficient record system. Proper business records are necessary to meet the requirements of local, state, and federal laws regarding taxes and employees. Records are of value only if they are correct, concise, and complete. Proper bookkeeping methods include keeping an accurate record of all income and expenses. Income is usually classified as receipts from services and retail sales. Expenses include rent, utilities, insurance, salaries, advertising, equipment, and re-pairs. Retain check stubs, canceled checks, receipts, and invoices. A profes-sional accountant or a full-charge bookkeeper is recommended to help keep records accurate.

Purchase and Inventory Records

An area that should be closely monitored is the purchase of inventory and supplies. Purchase records help maintain a perpetual inventory, which pre-vents overstock or shortage of needed supplies in the classroom and clinic, and also alert you to any incidents of pilfering (petty theft by employees). These records also help establish the net worth of the business at the end of the year.

Keep a running inventory of all supplies, and classify them according to their use and retail value (Figure 14–11). Those to be used in the daily busi-ness operation are **consumption supplies**. Those to be sold to clients are **retail supplies**.

consumption supplies
those supplies used in the daily operation of the institution.

retail supplies
those supplies sold to clients.

Service Records

Always keep service records or client cards that describe treatments given and merchandise sold to each client. Either a card file system or software program will serve this purpose. All service records should include the

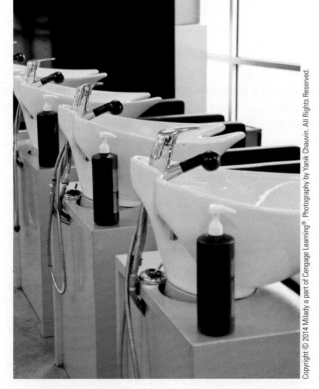

Figure 14–11   Supplies used in the daily operation of the school are known as *consumption supplies*.

name and address of the client, the date of each purchase or service, the amount charged, products used, and results obtained. Clients' preferences and tastes should also be noted.

☑ Operating a Successful School

The only way to guarantee that you will stay in business and have a prosperous school is to take excellent care of your students and clinic clients. Students as well as clients visiting your school should feel they are being well taken care of and should always look forward to their next visit. To accomplish this, your school must be physically attractive, well organized, smoothly run, and, above all, sparkling clean.

Planning the School's Layout

One of the most exciting opportunities ahead of you is planning and constructing the best physical layout for the type of school you envision. Maximum efficiency should be the primary concern. Items you will want to consider are what programs you want to offer, how many students you hope to maintain on an ongoing basis, and how many clinic clients you hope to serve on a daily basis. All of these factors will impact the design of the school and the overall efficiency of the facility. Once you have answered these questions, seek the advice of an architect with plenty of experience in designing schools. A reputable, professional equipment and furniture supplier will also be able to help you (Figure 14–12).

Personnel

The size of your school will determine the size of your staff and faculty. Large schools require receptionists, admissions personnel, administrative personnel, financial aid advisors, instructors, and educational directors. Smaller schools may have some combination of these personnel who perform more than one type of service. For example, the director of education may also serve as an instructor. The clerical support person may also serve as the receptionist. The success of a school depends on the quality of the work done by the staff.

When interviewing potential employees, consider the following:

- Level of skill (What is their educational background? When was the last time they attended an educational event?)
- Personal grooming (Do they look like you'd want their advice on your personal grooming?)
- Image as it relates to the school (Are they too progressive or too conservative for your environment?)
- Overall attitude (Do they seem more negative than positive in their responses to your questions?)
- Communication skills (Are they able to understand your questions? Can you understand their responses?)

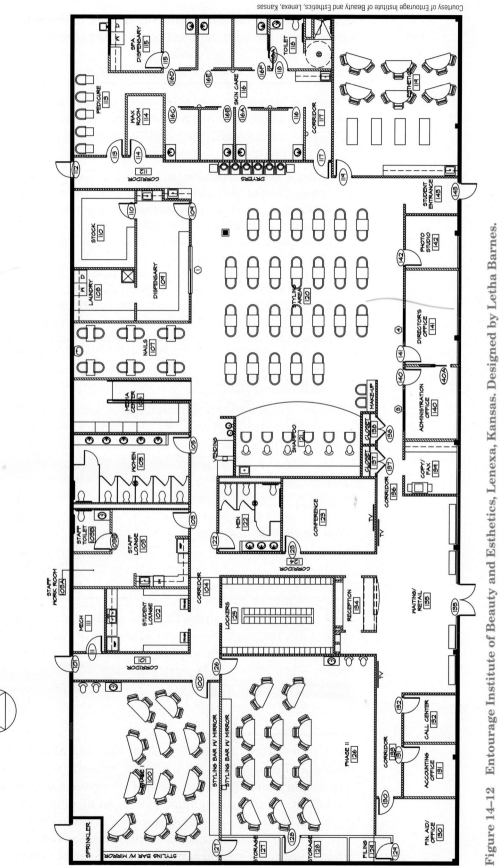

Figure 14–12 **Entourage Institute of Beauty and Esthetics, Lenexa, Kansas. Designed by Letha Barnes.**

Making good hiring decisions is crucial; undoing bad hiring decisions is painful to all involved, and can be more complicated than you might expect.

Payroll and Employee Benefits

In order to have a successful business, one in which everyone feels appreciated and is happy to work hard and service clients, you must be willing to share your success with your staff whenever it is financially feasible to do so. You can do this in a number of ways:

* Make it your top priority to meet your payroll obligations. In the allotment of funds, this comes first.
* Whenever possible, offer hardworking and loyal employees as many benefits as possible—either cover the cost of these benefits, or at least make them available to employees and allow them to decide if they can cover the cost themselves.
* Provide staff members with a schedule of employee evaluations. Make it clear what is expected of them if they are to receive pay increases.
* Put your entire compensation plan in writing.
* Create incentives by giving your staff opportunities to earn more money, prizes, or tickets to educational events and trade shows.

Managing Personnel

As a new school owner or director, one of your most difficult tasks will be to manage your staff. But this can also be very rewarding. If you are good at managing others, you can make a positive impact on their lives, and their ability to earn a living. If managing people does not come naturally, do not despair. People can learn how to manage other people, just as they learn how to drive a car or cut hair. Keep in mind that managing others is a serious job. Whether it comes naturally to you or not, it takes time to become comfortable with the role.

The Front Desk

Most school owners believe that the quality of the education and services offered are the most important elements of running a successful school. Certainly these are crucial, but too often the front desk—the "operations center"—is overlooked. The best schools employ professional receptionists to handle the job of scheduling appointments and greeting clients.

The Reception Area

First impressions count, and since the reception area is the first thing clients and prospective students see, it needs to be attractive, appealing, and comfortable. This is your school's "nerve center," where your receptionist will sit, retail merchandise will be on display, and the phone system is centered. Make sure the reception area is stocked with business cards, and have available a prominently displayed price list that shows at a glance what your clients should expect to pay for various services.

The Receptionist

Second only in importance to your faculty is your receptionist. A well-trained receptionist is the "quarterback" of the school's clinic, and will be the first person the client and prospective student will see on arrival. The receptionist should be pleasant, greeting each visitor with a smile. Efficient, friendly service fosters goodwill, confidence, and satisfaction (Figure 14–13).

In addition to filling the crucial role of greeter, the receptionist handles other important functions, including answering the phone, booking appointments, informing the student practitioners that a client has arrived, preparing the daily appointment information for the students, and recommending other services to the client. The receptionist should have a thorough knowledge of all of the retail products the school carries, so that she can also serve as a salesperson and information source for clients.

During slow periods, it is customary for the receptionist to perform certain other duties and activities, such as straightening up the reception area and maintaining inventory and daily reports.

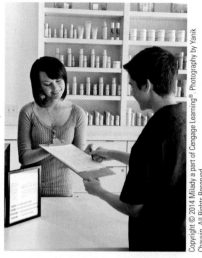

Figure 14–13 The receptionist handles many important functions within the school.

Booking Appointments

One of the most important duties the receptionist has is booking appointments, if you have set a policy for booking appointments for clinic students (Figure 14–14). This must be done with care, as services are sold in terms of time on the appointment page. Appointments must be scheduled to make the most efficient use of everyone's time. Under ideal circumstances, a client should not have to wait for a service and a student practitioner should not have to wait for the next client.

Booking appointments may be the main job of the receptionist, but when she is not available, the school director, clinic instructor, or assigned student practitioner can help with scheduling. Therefore, it is important for

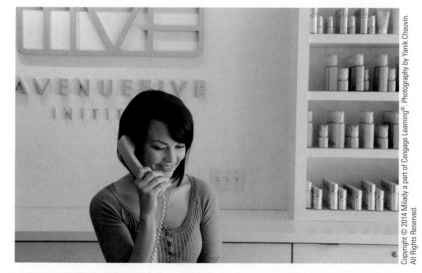

Figure 14–14 An important task of the receptionist is the booking of student salon appointments.

each person in the school to understand how to book an appointment and how much time is needed for each service.

Regardless of who actually makes the appointment, anyone who answers the phone or deals with clients must have a pleasing voice and personality. In addition, the receptionist must have the following qualities:

- An attractive appearance
- Knowledge of the various services offered
- Knowledge of the various programs offered and admissions personnel referral procedures
- Unlimited patience with both clients and school personnel

Use of the Telephone in the School

Much school business is handled over the telephone. Good telephone habits and techniques make it possible for the school owner and student practitioners to increase business and improve relationships with clients and suppliers. With each call, a gracious, appropriate response will help build the school's reputation.

Good Planning

Because they can be noisy, business calls to clients and suppliers should be made at a quiet time of the day, or from a telephone placed in a quieter area of the school.

When using the telephone, you should:

- Have a pleasant telephone voice, speak clearly, and use correct grammar. A "smile" in your voice is important.
- Show interest and concern when talking with a client or a supplier.
- Be polite, respectful, and courteous to all, even though some people may test the limits of your patience.
- Be tactful. Do not say anything to irritate the person on the other end of the line.

Incoming Phone Calls

Incoming phone calls are the lifeline of a school (Figure 14–15). Prospective students generally call in advance to obtain general information about the school and set up an appointment with the appropriate admissions representative. Clients usually call ahead for appointments with a preferred student practitioner, or they might call to cancel or reschedule an appointment. The person answering the phone should develop the necessary telephone skills to handle these calls. In addition, the following are some guidelines for answering the telephone:

- When you answer the phone, say, "Good morning (afternoon or evening), Milady Spa Academy. May I help you?" or "Thank you for calling Milady Spa Academy. This is Jane speaking. How may I help you?" Some schools require that you give your name to the caller. The first words you say tell the caller something about your personality. Let callers know that you are glad to hear from them.
- Answer the phone promptly. On a system with more than one line, if a call comes in while you are talking on another line, ask to put the per-

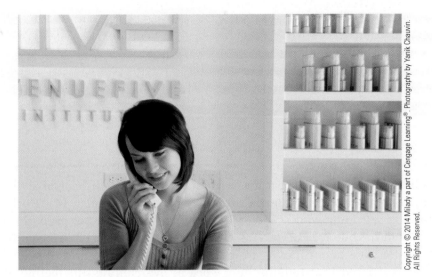

Figure 14–15   **Incoming phone calls are the lifeline of the school.**

son on hold, answer the second call, and ask that person to hold while you complete the first call. Take calls in the order in which they are received.

- If you do not have the information requested by a caller, either put the caller on hold and get the information, or offer to call the person back with the information as soon as you have it.
- Do not talk with a client standing nearby while you are speaking with someone on the phone. You are doing a disservice to both clients.

Booking Appointments by Phone

When booking appointments by phone, take down the client's first and last name, phone number, and service booked. You should be familiar with all the services and products available in the school and their costs, as well as which student practitioners are trained to perform specific services. Be fair when making assignments to ensure that all students receive maximum opportunity to gain expertise in every skill they will need for entry-level employment.

However, if someone calls to ask for an appointment with a particular student practitioner on a particular day and time, every effort should be made to accommodate the client's request if your school's policy allows for appointments. If the student practitioner is not available when the client requests, try one of the following to handle the situation:

- Suggest other times that the student practitioner is available.
- If the client cannot come in at any of those times, suggest another student practitioner.
- If the client is unwilling to try another student practitioner, offer to call the client if there is a cancellation at the desired time.

Handling Complaints by Telephone

Handling complaints, particularly over the phone, is a difficult task. The caller is probably upset and short-tempered. Respond with self-control, tact, and courtesy, no matter how trying the circumstances. Only then will the caller be made to feel that he has been treated fairly.

The tone of your voice must be sympathetic and reassuring. Your manner of speaking should convince the caller that you are truly concerned about the complaint. Do not interrupt the caller. After hearing the complaint in full, try to resolve the situation quickly and effectively.

☑ Selling in the School

An important aspect of the school's financial success is the sale of additional services and take-home or maintenance products (Figure 14–16). Therefore, you are doing your students a disservice if you are not properly training them in this area of service. Student practitioners often seem to feel uncomfortable about having to make sales of products or additional services. It is important to help them work at overcoming this feeling. When student practitioners are reluctant to sell, it is often because they carry a negative stereotype of salespeople—that they are pushy or aggressive—and they do not want to be seen this way themselves. Though some salespeople display such negative traits, remind students that many sales professionals are helpful and knowledgeable and make customer care their top priority. These people play a major role in the lives of their clients, and are valuable to them because they offer good advice.

Promoting the Student Salon in the Community

The latter part of this chapter has been dedicated to opening and developing a successful school. A significant part of that success will depend on the student salon, which contributes greatly to the bottom line of a school while also providing quality education to its students. A good way to create clinic business and goodwill is by speaking at community events or local

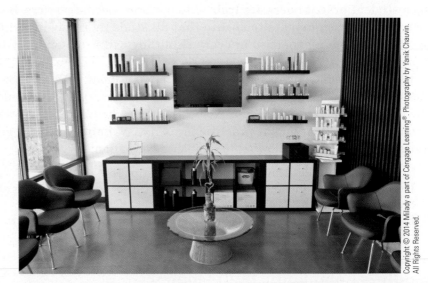

Figure 14–16   A large part of business success is achieved through retail sales.

colleges and universities. For example, women's organizations are often interested in learning more about image enhancement and may welcome guest speakers on related subjects. Master educators will volunteer to speak at such functions. They might even take a few of their advanced students along to assist and demonstrate. By offering complimentary image-consulting services or providing quick makeup touchups to participants at such events, the educator and students have gone a long way toward developing goodwill and encouraging attendees to patronize the student salon in the future. Often the organizations will create press releases that are published in area newspapers and depict the speaker and participants, which will result in additional free advertising and promotion for the school. It is essential, however, that if an educator takes on this role of public speaking, he thoroughly prepare for the engagement. He must remember the six Ps of teaching or presenting: Proper preparation and practice promote positive performance! The educator must prepare his presentation and practice it sufficiently before serving as the ambassador of goodwill for the school. *Without* the proper preparation, the presentation could do more harm than good to the school.

Master educators will look for other community service opportunities that will provide quality training and experience for their students as well as promote the clinic for the school. For example, the educator might arrange to take students to local nursing homes and provide complimentary services to residents. He might encourage promotions that honor certain working members of the community, such as law enforcement officials or firefighters, by offering them all services at half price. These types of activities are far more effective than spending hard dollars on planned advertising. Individuals that benefit from such promotions will send their friends, neighbors, and relatives to your clinic in appreciation of your treatment. In addition, if they are satisfied with your service, they will return even when the special promotion is not offered.

IT'S WORTH REMEMBERING ✳

In life, we must decide who and what we want to be—and then we have to do what we have to do to achieve that.

Wrapping It Up

You are about to embark on your exciting new career as an educator. Remember, educators are not born, they are made. By completing this course of study, you have taken your first serious step in becoming a master educator. Think ahead about your employment opportunities and use your time in school to accomplish exciting achievement-oriented activities that will make your résumé sizzle with excitement. By accomplishing exciting, quantitative goals while in school, not only will your résumé sizzle, so will you! Take the careful preliminary steps to prepare for employment: Develop a dynamic portfolio. Organize your materials, information, and questions in order to complete a high-impact interview. Once employed, take the necessary steps to learn all you can about your new position and the institution you will serve. Read all you can about the industry and the field of education. Attend trade shows and take advantage of every continuing education opportunity available. Become an active participant in making this great industry even better. Once you have obtained your license or certificate to teach, the doors of opportunity will continue to open.

In Retrospect

1. Explain the importance of preparing for employment.

2. List the key elements of an achievement-oriented résumé and an employment portfolio.

3. Explain strategies to maintain employment once it is obtained.

4. List key records that must be kept for the institution.

5. Explain the importance of the reception area to a school's success.

6. Explain why good school telephone techniques are important.

Objectives (Desired Performance Goals):

After reading and studying this chapter, you should be able to:

- Explain the importance of implementing a sound student-retention program.
- Write a mission and vision statement.
- Explain the role of administrative policies in institutional operations.
- Develop a unique institutional culture.
- Explain the effects of admissions and new-student orientation policies on student retention.
- Instill a sense of student ownership in the institution.
- Deliver effective curriculum content.
- Explain the importance of holding the highest level of enthusiasm when teaching.
- Deliver excellent student service.
- Explain the importance of professional development as an educator.
- Practice recognition and praise in the educational process.

! CRITICAL CONCEPT

So many students who have dropped out of high school or college say it is because the overall experience at the institution was negative. Master educators can make the learning experience a positive one.

The Importance of a Sound Retention Plan

retention plan
begins when a student walks in the door for the first time and continues until he or she graduates; it involves all institution personnel, regardless of position, and includes key elements such as establishing a vision and mission, sound ethical administrative policies, defining the school's culture, sound admissions procedures, a detailed new-student orientation program, instilling student ownership of the institution, developing and following a creative curriculum, employing energized educators, developing outstanding customer service, investing in the institution's educators, employing a praise policy.

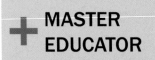

✚ MASTER EDUCATOR

1. Supports the sound administrative policies of the institution at all times.
2. Lives and breathes the established culture of the institution.
3. Provides energized education and instills the desire to learn daily.
4. Wraps every required student criticism in a praise sandwich.

A SOUND STUDENT-retention plan begins when the prospective student walks through the front door for the first time and continues until the student successfully graduates (Figure 15–1). The institution must be led by a set of agreed-upon and shared beliefs. To achieve this, every staff member must engage in defining and articulating the philosophy by which the institution will operate—they must control their own destiny, or someone else will.

Institutions have an ethical responsibility to be the best they can be and to live up to the claims they make to those students who are spending considerable money to attend them. Further, institutions are held to numerous standards by the various regulatory oversight agencies that govern them. Most of the agencies mandate a level of accountability with respect to the institution's performance outcomes. Institutions are expected to graduate a reasonable percentage of the students who enroll. They are also expected to provide the required assistance to ensure graduates successfully obtain licensure or certification in their chosen field of study and obtain gainful employment in that same field. Therefore, institutions today are challenged more than ever to put into place policies and systems that will facilitate the best possible education for their students. Only then will an institution enjoy a quality reputation and a successful student completion rate. *Total quality* spans the institution's entire system, giving priority to detection of concerns and correcting those concerns, establishing goals, monitoring results, and implementing more change as needed. Key elements of a sound student retention program follow.

Institutions, like students, have the potential to achieve great success, and that potential depends on many factors and variables. This chapter will take into consideration those variables and describe a set of specific

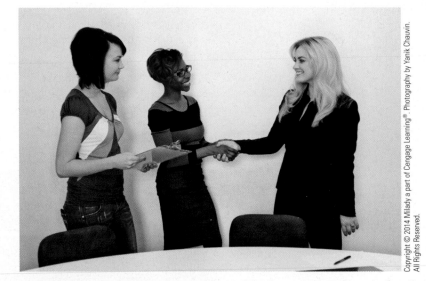

Figure 15–1 The retention plan begins with the prospective student's first experience at the institution.

KEY ELEMENTS OF A SOUND RETENTION PROGRAM

* Establishing a vision and mission
* Sound ethical administrative policies
* Defining the institution's culture
* Sound admissions procedures
* Detailed new-student orientation program
* Instilling a sense of student ownership of the institution
* Developing and following a creative curriculum
* Employing energized educators
* Developing outstanding customer service
* Investing in the institution's educators
* Employing a praise policy

IT'S WORTH REMEMBERING ✳

Students believe the institution can help turn their dreams into reality, and a dedicated institution will live up to those expectations.

strategies to help institutions retain students in school until program completion. Before you get started, faculty, staff, and management must ask themselves a set of collective questions, and everyone must agree on the answers:

1. Do we honestly want our institution to be the very best it can be?
2. Have we clearly defined our goals and implemented a plan to achieve them?
3. Have we broken out of the box in our way of thinking and performing?
4. Is everyone on the team communicating and contributing to the goals in a positive manner?
5. Does the institution have well-planned, organized systems and policies in place?
6. Is the institution financially sound, and is each staff member making a positive contribution to the fiscal and administrative practices?
7. Is there a plan B in place in the event that a serious flaw in plan A occurs?
8. Does the institution have a system of self-evaluation and continuous improvement in place?

It is recommended to schedule and facilitate an in-service day with staff to brainstorm about these questions and begin the process of developing the necessary policies to implement a strong and successful student-retention program. An institution's retention strategies must be planned. The art of planning for student retention is much like the principles of hair design. It includes creativity, concept design, form and shape, detail, and execution.

mission statement describes the identity of the institution; it says what the school is, what it does, what it hopes to accomplish or what it is trying to change, who it services, and where it provides its services.

Establishing the Vision and Mission ☑

Put simply, a **mission statement** describes the identity of the institution as it exists now. It says what the institution is, what it does, what it hopes to accomplish or what it is trying to change, who it serves, and where it provides its services.

The mission statement must align with the institution's culture. It should be published in the institution's catalog, printed, framed, and displayed in the institution. Once it is out there for all the world to see, the team will be compelled to live up to it.

THE MISSION OF MILADY'S CAREER INSTITUTE

The mission of Milady's Career Institute is to enrich lives by revealing the wonder, relevance, excitement, and value of creativity, laughter, and learning. This is accomplished by facilitating inspiring, innovative, and energetic education and business consultation services whenever and wherever they are needed with a sense of pride, respect, and integrity.

---

vision statement
outlines where the institution wants to be and concentrates on the future; it should be a source of inspiration and will provide clear decision-making criteria.

A **vision statement** outlines where the institution wants to be and concentrates on the future. It should be a source of inspiration. It will provide clear decision-making criteria.

EFFECTIVE VISION STATEMENT

* Is clear
* Paints a vivid picture
* Describes a bright and hopeful future
* Is memorable and engaging
* Includes realistic, achievable aspirations
* Rationally aligns with the institution's values and culture
* Is time-bound if it includes goals or objectives

Everyone on the institution's team needs to understand the vision and help it become assimilated into the institution's culture. Leadership members have the responsibility of ensuring everyone understands the vision and acting as role models by living and breathing the vision. This may require establishing short-term objectives and goals and encouraging the team members to create their own vision that is compatible with and supports the institution's vision.

Institutions that are already in operation have probably established a vision, but that doesn't mean it can't be changed or improved upon. Often, the vision changes when the institution adds a new program or relocates, for example. In any case, when change is going to occur, a plan should include the vision followed by the deliberate development of the institution's culture. The institution will need to establish an identity for itself and allocate resources in the budget to facilitate the changes. Finally, the institution will need to examine alternative courses of action. Everyone needs a backup plan. Thus, the institution's team will need to answer three key questions: Where are we today? Where do we want to be? How do we get there?

SAMPLE VISION STATEMENTS

- My vision is to take over my parent's business and work capably and conscientiously until the time comes when I can sell my institution and retire to Florida.
- My vision is to start an institution and achieve success. Once success has been achieved, I will open institution 2 and then institution 3 until I have opened successful institutions in every region of the country. The success of the institutions will facilitate my retirement to a chateau in the South of France.
- My vision is to start an institution that can serve as an example to other entrepreneurs willing to go into inner-city neighborhoods, where such small businesses have not proved successful in the past. I will enter into business alliances with other entrepreneurs and revitalize a neighborhood that had virtually been given up as a loss.

Source: Adapted from *9 Routes to Success for Institutions* by Robert K. Throop and Alan Gelb.

The institution must continually assess its performance against the stated mission and vision statements. It is recommended that the institution obtain feedback from key individuals as to how the institution is actually living up to its goals. The institution team, students, graduates, area salons that employ the institution's graduates, and members of the institution's advisory board are excellent resources for this type of feedback.

Sound and Ethical Administrative Policies

If an institution is to ensure that it effectively retains students until they graduate, it will have to effectively employ administrative policies and services as well as educational programs. The institution should publish and implement written policies and procedures that describe the various areas of responsibility within the institution (Figure 15–2). The institution must employ administrative personnel with the background and credentials sufficient to implement the institution's operating procedures. These personnel must be familiar with all the regulatory oversight requirements applicable to the institution and understand how those requirements apply to students. They must be available to advise students on important issues, such as sources for tuition payment assistance. The institution must operate in an ethical manner in all its policies, such as advertising and accounting. The institution must be committed to maintaining accurate student records to which students have reasonable access. While seemingly mundane, the administrative practices of the institution are every bit as important as the delivery of curriculum if the institution's mission, vision, and goals are to be reached.

CONSIDER AND CONNECT

A vision determined by the whole team will act as a net to support and protect the entire institution. A vision imposed from above may hinder the willingness of members to express themselves.

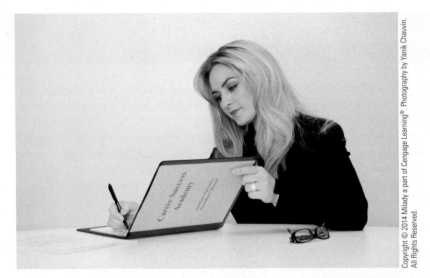

Figure 15–2   The institution's written policies and procedures serve as a guide to effective operations.

Defining the Institution's Culture

culture
the school's culture defines how students are trained, developed, and nurtured into professionals; the traits or distinguishing characteristics or qualities that make up the institution; the institution's personality.

Defining the institution's **culture** may be the most important step in the institution's retention plan. The institution's culture is what sets it apart from all others and represents the set of shared attitudes, values, goals, and practices that characterize the institution. The institution's culture defines how its students are trained, developed, and nurtured into professionals. It is ultimately the institution's culture that will cause its students to take psychological ownership of the institution. It is all the traits or distinguishing characteristics or qualities that make up the institution. In a word, it is the institution's personality. An institution needs to take a close look at its personality to determine if it is one that makes all those who walk through its doors feel welcome, needed, appreciated, and important, or if it portrays low morale or negativity. The individual personalities that make up the institution team contribute greatly to the overall institution personality. In its hiring practices, an institution must make sure it is choosing those people who share the vision and have the personality to support the institution's culture.

Surveys can be used to determine the working climate of your institution. The following survey is adapted from Milady's *9 Routes to Success*. For each of the statements, indicate how the statement applies at your institution by indicating "yes," "no," or "sometimes." The responses can help you determine whether the institution is organized or disorganized, formal or informal, innovative or traditional, and so forth.

Members of the institution's team need to determine what they want the atmosphere of the institution to be. Characteristics can vary. For example, team members should discuss the following traits of the institution's culture:

> **CONSIDER AND CONNECT**
>
> All institution cultures should be built around responsibility, respect, dignity, and compassion.

- Sober undertone versus lighthearted and freewheeling undertone
- Formality and structure versus casual informality

STATEMENT	YES	NO	SOMETIMES
The school tends to play it safe regarding innovation.			
Administrative staff relate warmly to staff and students.			
Conflicts are resolved; friendly relationships are reestablished.			
There are too many rules.			
Conformity to the rules is required.			
Risk taking is encouraged by the administration.			
Personnel are empowered to resolve complaints.			
Staff is encouraged to take initiative and work with little supervision.			
There are limited restraints on personnel.			
Staff members are treated equally and fairly.			
Staff meetings and effective communications occur regularly.			
The administration resists change and differing views.			
The administration praises effective performance by employees.			
The school is highly structured with little room for variation from the norm.			
The school facility is maintained in the best possible condition.			
The administration sets standards and criteria for performance evaluation.			
The administration is cool, distant, and formal.			
The atmosphere is one of excitement and enthusiasm.			
The atmosphere is one of structure and formality.			
Friendship among staff is encouraged.			
An atmosphere of helpfulness prevails.			
Risk taking is discouraged because all actions require prior approval.			
Working at this school can be challenging.			
Rewards and praise are more frequent than criticism.			
Policies are designed to promote high-performance goals.			
Excellent customer service is modeled and expected.			
Customer complaints are not a priority of the administration.			
Student satisfaction is an absolute priority.			
The administration invests in the school's teachers to ensure professional development.			
The administration expects instructors to arrange for their continuing education.			

- Calm, quiet atmosphere versus hip, buzzing, trendy atmosphere
- Traditional institution environment versus student-centered, discovery-oriented learning environment
- Clean, shiny, sparkling, and state-of-the-art facilities versus clean and adequate facilities

Once these choices have been made, the institution can set about creating policies and a language that supports that culture. Institutions today are electing to name their curriculum levels and classrooms and use that terminology whenever discussing those items. For example, an institution in Bedford, Texas, chose the family name of DuVall's School of Cosmetology. They then selected a tag line that used the initials (DSC) of the name: ***D****iscover the* ***S****kills to be* ***C****reative.* Further, they named their three levels of education accordingly, as discussed in the accompanying box.

DISCOVER THE SKILLS TO BE CREATIVE

Discovery: In this initial level of training, students will **discover** the underlying theory and the techniques for performing basic client services. Education is provided through interactive lecture, demonstration, technology, and hands-on practice.

Skills: In this vital level of training, students will develop and customize their **skills** to meet the needs of clients. They will become increasingly self-confident and proficient in their communication, consultation, and technical skills. Education is provided through interactive lecture, demonstration, technology, field trips, guest speakers, and hands-on practice.

Creative: In this exciting level of training, students will focus on state board preparation and developing the **creative** skills necessary for success in the workplace. They will focus on business-building knowledge, professional development, and career placement. Education is provided through interactive lecture, demonstration, technology, field trips, guest speakers, hands-on practice, and competency skills evaluation. They will *discover* the *skills* to be *creative* and successful in their new career.

IT'S WORTH REMEMBERING ✳

Ultimately, the institution's culture is portrayed through its physical image, its language, its attitude, its effectiveness, its education, and its people.

The institution's retention team includes everyone working for the institution, from the owners to the janitorial staff, and all must buy in to the desired institution culture. Studies show that it takes 11 positive people to overcome the negative force created by 1 negative person. That is strong testimony for the importance of ensuring that every person on the team is positive. People can be trained in skills, but it is much more difficult to train them to have a positive attitude or to be loyal, trustworthy, or compassionate.

☑ Admissions Policy

The institution must have a student admission policy that is consistent with its mission, vision, and educational objectives. We have already indicated that the retention plan begins before the student even enrolls. Institutions need to establish a thorough interview process that all prospective students are required to complete, regardless of how excited or ready to start they are (Figure 15–3). These potential students must be made thoroughly aware of what they are about to commit to. Depending on your state and students' schedules, they are about to make a 6- to 18-month commitment to education. Our adult learners have other responsibilities and priorities, and it would be a mistake for any institution to expect or demand to be the top priority. However, students must understand that school has to be one of their priorities once they enroll.

The admissions interview is an opportunity to give students all pertinent information about the institution and its programs.

Prospective students need to be made aware of information such as:

- Basic admissions requirements such as age and secondary education
- The complete costs involved in program completion

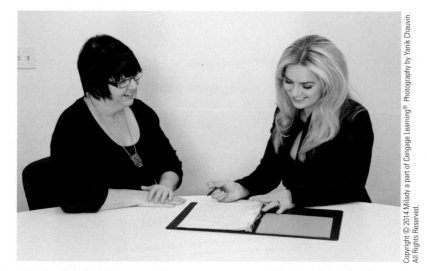

Figure 15–3 **A school's retention program continues with the first enrollment interview.**

- A thorough overview of the program including course syllabus, grading, and expectations
- What makes your institution a good choice
- A full explanation of institution policies and standards of conduct
- The institution's performance history with respect to completion, licensure, and employment rates
- The physical and safety demands for practicing their chosen profession
- Reasonable compensation they might earn in their chosen field
- Licensure or certification requirements and costs upon graduation

New-Student Orientation

Once all the requisite information has been delivered, a contract signed, and a start day scheduled, the student should be scheduled for a thorough new-student orientation program. A thorough orientation program is absolutely essential to student retention (Figure 15–4). If done completely and properly, it can be one of the best tools you have to prevent a later withdrawal. For a thorough discussion on developing a successful **new-student orientation program**, refer to Chapter 10, "Program Development and Lesson Planning," which includes the "My Promise" activity, which might result in the following student commitment.

new-student orientation program
a briefing designed to acquaint students with the institution's educational programs and objectives, administrative policies and procedures, and student support services.

MY PROMISE

I have taken the first step on my journey to success. I have given myself the courage to enroll in school. By taking this step, I have made the conscious decision that I want more for myself and for my family. This decision will allow me to accomplish my dreams. No one can take this dream away from me unless I allow it. I am my own greatest resource. I will complete my education. I can only fail if I give up.

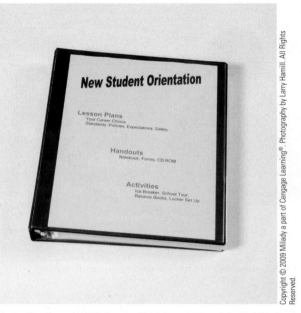

Figure 15–4   The institution should prepare and conduct a thorough new-student orient ation program for every new class.

☑ Instilling Student Ownership

The institution must establish and implement student-support services consistent with the institution's culture and encourage students to take psychological ownership of the institution, as mentioned earlier.

It is the institution's student-support services and culture that will have students referring other students to "my school." It is those services that will have students saying things like, "At my school, we do this. . . ." when they are in a social setting. It's that sense of ownership by students that will build the institution's reputation in the community, resulting in more students and more salon clients. Support services include the new-student orientation program already discussed; the provision of appropriate academic counseling; information and advice on licensing regulations, reciprocity with other states, and opportunities for further education; employment assistance when nearing graduation; and an internal grievance procedure for those times when things just aren't perfect.

transfer technique
a process that involves learners in decision making, establishing rules, and designing projects and contests, which ultimately results in the students taking ownership of the project or policy.

Many institutions employ the use of the **transfer technique** and have implemented a "You Speak, We Listen" policy. They recognize the need to involve their adult students in policymaking and culture-development decisions. We have established that adult students need some degree of control and mastery over their own lives. By involving them in the decision-making process, they will definitely take ownership of it, implement it, and monitor it with commitment. An institution should consider having monthly "rap" sessions with the students to get their feedback on how things are going and ask for their improvement suggestions. Institutions may also conduct periodic surveys of students to obtain their comments on the facilities, the educational process, administrative oversight, the inventory of supplies, the teachers, and more. In addition, institutions should consider an

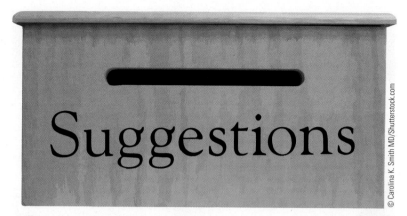

Figure 15–5 A suggestion box provides an avenue to receive valuable feedback from students.

old-fashioned suggestion box that can be accessed at any time by students (Figure 15–5). You might be surprised at the quality of the suggestions made there. Your policy can say that only those suggestions that are signed will get a formal response, and that frivolous requests, such as "watching soap operas in the student lounge," will not be considered.

Clearly, students need to feel they are active and important members of the institution. None of the other parts of your retention program will work unless the students are dedicated to the institution and support it fully. The students are the reason the institution exists, and that should never be forgotten. If you are unsure about the types of policies and standards that will create a culture the students will fall in love with, ask them. What better way to make them feel a part of the school family?

The Creative Curriculum

Generally, an institution's curriculum will be prescribed by the state regulatory agency and reviewed by the institution's accrediting agency. Programs must meet those required standards and elements and be of appropriate length to prepare graduates for gainful employment in their chosen field. They should be designed to incorporate appropriate academic learning with practical skills development. They must include a grading system that is fair and understood by all students.

It has been said that curriculum is primarily two parts: content and delivery. An institution can use the best textbooks and educational technology available, but if the teachers are unable to deliver that content in an engaging, enthusiastic, and interesting manner, the content will not likely hit the mark. On the other hand, the institution may have a group of dynamic educators on board, but if they are not provided with quality educational tools and resources, it is doubtful that students will get the full benefit of the information. Therefore, institutions must take great care in selecting the best possible textbooks, workbooks, and technology for student use and also hire and develop highly skilled educators. Milady is a comprehensive resource for quality materials.

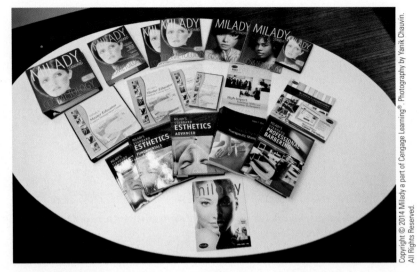

Figure 15–6   Design a creative curriculum containing all the elements to hold a learner's interest.

Educators should read and study Chapter 10, which deals with program design and development, and Chapter 11, "Educational Aids and Technology in the Classroom," which covers developing and using educational aids and technology in the classroom. In these chapters, institutions and educators will find helpful tools for designing a creative curriculum containing all the required elements for effective education (Figure 15–6).

Energized Educators

Institutions must employ a faculty of adequate size, with members who are fully trained, qualified, and experienced, to achieve the institution's mission and vision as well as all educational objectives. This book has been dedicated to providing the tools and knowledge needed to become what we refer to as a *master educator*. Certainly, it is unrealistic to summarize all of that information in a small section of this chapter. Suffice it to say that possibly the most important ingredient in a successful student-retention plan is the effectiveness of the education.

A critical part of the success of an institution relies on quality educators, who are the key to academic success for all learners. Institutions should give serious consideration to the educational model they want to adopt. In general, the educational model should focus on promoting the student's ownership of learning and demand the student's acquisition of knowledge and the development of skills and abilities appropriate to the career for which the student is preparing. Related actions of the teaching model should include:

* Encouraging independent learning for students
* Promoting teamwork among faculty and students
* Optimizing students' productivity
* Creating an atmosphere of excitement and love of learning
* Promoting and recognizing effective teaching activities

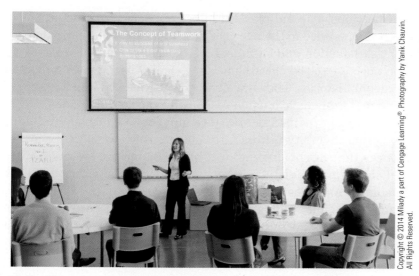

Figure 15–7 **Educators must have a high level of enthusiasm for their subject matter to retain learner attention.**

> ## CONSIDER AND CONNECT
>
> Teachers are the lifeblood of the institution. The faculty may represent the single most contributing factor in a student's decision to stay in school.

Educators must first develop the qualities and characteristics required of a career education instructor. Among those qualities are the ability to instill in learners a strong sense of self-esteem and a love of learning. We must then prepare and organize the elements for effective teaching and understand the importance of classroom management. The educator must have the ability to help students identify their learning styles so education can be delivered in the most effective manner. We then need to teach our students how to study and take tests with ease. Educators must develop and employ powerful teaching and learning methods that excite every learner. As will be discussed thoroughly in Chapter 17, "Learning Is a Laughing Matter," it is essential that humor be interjected into every single lesson presented.

As educators, we must hold the highest level of enthusiasm we can possess for the subject matter we are teaching (Figure 15–7). We cannot expect our students to be excited to learn material about which we are not enthused or committed to. Put simply, educators must have an undying passion for the field they teach and a sincere compassion and interest in their students.

Delivering Outstanding Customer Service

Customer service refers to the set of behaviors that a business or institution undertakes during its interaction with its clients. The first thing an institution needs to do is recognize that in an institution, both the students and the student salon clients are the customers, but the student customers always come first. We must ask ourselves three questions: Who are our students (age, culture, background, education, etc.)? What are their needs? How do we deliver what they expect? The characteristics of adult learners have already been discussed in Chapter 2, "The Teaching Plan and Learning Environment." A review of that information will be helpful when answering

customer service
the set of behaviors that a business or institution undertakes during its interactions with its clients and/or students.

these questions. The hallmark of effective service to students is the relevance of that service to the needs of the student population, as measured by student satisfaction and success. Adult learners bring diverse experiences and perspective to the classroom. They come with a range of personal and professional histories. They have elected to enter training for a specific reason, and definitely have outside responsibilities and priorities.

All services provided to students must take cultural, individual ability, and other diversity factors into consideration. We must be aware of the influences that might be related to these elements. If we are unsure, we should simply ask the student how those particular needs can best be accommodated. As educators, we need to recognize that good student service does not mean that students are "always right" and entitled to everything they want. It does mean providing them with the resources they need to make the most of the educational environment. Providing superior customer service for students can be accomplished by:

HELPFUL HINTS IN DEALING WITH ADULT LEARNERS

- See students as clients and respect them as such. Like any other customer, they have the right to expect a fair return on their investment.
- Respond to students as you would to colleagues. Discuss issues and offer resources and solutions. Adult students are actually our peers. We must avoid taking the traditional role enacted by teachers of much younger students.
- Incorporate the realities and ethics of the educational environment. Facilitate an understanding of ethical, accreditation, and other regulatory guidelines that define what we can realistically do as educators.

- **Responding with Immediacy.** This means that the educator responds to a student with verbal or nonverbal acknowledgement without delay. This will help sustain motivation in adult learners.
- **Providing Pertinent Information.** When students demonstrate an interest by asking for additional information, we need to make additional resources available.
- **Providing Relevant and Timely Feedback.** Meaningful feedback and comments are more useful to adult learners. Tailor comments to the individual student's goals and aspirations.
- **Being Available.** Being available for learners communicates concern and involvement. It shows a willingness to support them.

To provide quality service with adult learners, it is vital that we understand their point of view (Figure 15–8). Students don't really care about our problems and issues. They are interested in the teacher demonstrating with actions and words that they are cared for. Some strategies that may be helpful are as follows:

- **Listen.** Listening shows a total commitment to understanding the needs of the student.

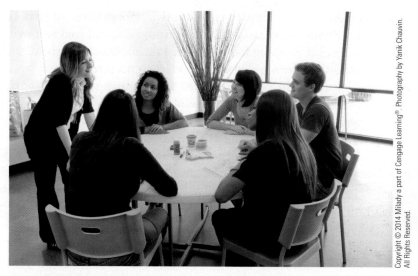

Figure 15–8 Educators must know their students and understand their point of view.

- **Have a Positive Attitude.** Attitude is an immediate reflection to the students of what their experience with you will be like.
- **Communicate.** Thorough communication is key; it builds trust and comfort.
- **Anticipate Needs.** Think about what students might want based on what they have already said and go above and beyond their expectations.
- **Follow up.** Excellent student service does not stop after information has been provided. Students should be asked if there is anything else they need or if they have more questions.
- **Show Appreciation.** Educators should let students know daily how much their business is appreciated. Without students, educators wouldn't have jobs. There is nothing that keeps students (and customers) more loyal than knowing they are appreciated and respected. Remember that students usually have a choice about where they go to institution.\

CONSIDER AND CONNECT

Customer service for students is the premise that educators provide students with reasonable choices and options based on a sound foundation of educational and institutional integrity.

Investing in Your Educators

Because faculty members come into daily contact with students and their effectiveness directly impacts student success, it stands to reason that every possible step should be taken to ensure that instructors are properly trained, motivated, further developed, and rewarded. The institution should have a written plan for continuing education of all educators requiring them to meet their state requirements for license renewal or their accrediting agency requirements for professional development. It is recommended that professional development training focus on teaching methodology and delivery skills as well as professional skills competencies. Even the best instructors can become complacent or fail to remain current with the newest methods or equipment. No educator should be exempt from regular observation.

Chapter 20 "Evaluating Professional Performance" of this textbook discusses improvement of performance through formal and self-evaluation. Please refer to that chapter for a self-evaluation checklist that instructors can use to take their own pulse with respect to performance.

Institutions should recognize that instructors need motivation, just like students. We know that genuine motivation is internal, but institutions can certainly create circumstances within which educators can remain motivated. Implementing the strategies already discussed in this chapter will certainly help to create a motivating environment. Having a clean, sparkling facility, allowing instructors to participate in designing the institution's vision and culture, and providing them with the best possible Milady tools and materials to use in the classroom will help keep educators motivated. The institution should be committed to providing employees a stable work environment with equal opportunity for learning and personal growth. Creativity and innovation should be encouraged to improve the effectiveness of the institution. Above all, employees should be provided the same concern, respect, and caring attitude within the organization that they are expected to share with students and salon customers.

Many resources are available through which an institution can invest in its educators. The American Association of Cosmetology Schools has an educational division, the Cosmetology Educators of America. Every year they hold a convention, usually in July, designed specifically for educators in the field of cosmetology and related disciplines (Figure 15–9). The education offered at this conference is phenomenal, and everyone leaves extremely motivated and excited to get back into their classrooms and share what they have learned. Interested parties can go to www.beautyschools.org for more information.

One effective method of recognition for teachers is the process of faculty training and development. Investment in teachers' skills and abilities is critical to achieving excellence in the educational environment. Many institutions across the country have incorporated the Master Educator program through the Career Institute as in-service training. Those institutions that have completed the program clearly and unequivocally state that they have seen an enormous improvement in the overall operation of their institutions. Their teachers are more motivated and have improved skills. Their enthusiasm and excitement is passed down to the students in their classrooms, who also become more motivated and interested in learning. As a result, these institutions have experienced a far lower turnover rate in teachers and an increased graduation rate for students. Such training creates a win, win, win situation.

For more information, institutions and educators may go to www.milady.com/careerinst to review educator profiles, course descriptions, and course schedules for public events. Whatever resource you choose to use for continuing education and professional development, it is important not to lose sight of its importance. This author recommends that educators invest at least 40 hours per year in professional development activities.

IT'S WORTH REMEMBERING

The institution should invest in teachers, and the educators should also be held accountable for improvement of their professional skills.

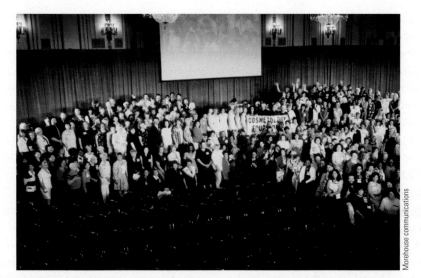

Figure 15–9 The Cosmetology Educators of America annual convention is a great source of motivation, inspiration, and professional development.

The P-R-A-I-S-E Policy

Institutions should use a systematic method of evaluating student performance and providing them feedback in theoretical knowledge, technical skills, and soft skills as well as overall progress through the course of study. Feedback for students should include a significant amount of praise.

Effective praise is more than simply saying, "good job." Strategies for praise that should be considered include the following:

1. **Do It Now.** Praise given immediately following positive performance has a stronger effect than delayed praise, especially for the younger generations in our classrooms.
2. **Be Specific.** General praise does not speak to the performance that deserved the praise. Avoid global praise and identify the specific reasons you are offering it.
3. **Connect It to Your Feelings.** It is important to share how the performance makes you feel as an educator. For example, "I feel so proud when I see how your hard work and practice pays off."

Past research shows that if educators want student performance to simply maintain the status quo, they should be praising four times for each criticism. In addition, if educators want to see improved performance and growth in the learner, they should deliver praise at least eight times for every criticism. Those researchers discovered that when they actually went into the classroom and observed, educators were only praising about one time for every eight criticisms—and we wonder why we have students dropping out of our institutions. Perhaps the single most important action an educator can take to prevent a student from dropping out of school is to find meaningful ways to praise a student's performance. More recent research now tells us that the right balance of praise to criticism is close to

10 acts of praise for every act of criticism. This is because praise is more powerful and it helps students know what to do, not just what not to do. The more a student acts in a praiseworthy way, the less criticism is necessary. It should be the goal of every educator to deliver praise at least 8 to 10 times more often than criticism. The praise needs to be sincere and true, which may not be an easy task. This is something that an educator will have to put conscious effort into.

Though praise is critical to the success of our students, it is also relevant to the institution's educators. Research in organizational behavior consistently shows that about 15 percent to 20 percent of an institution's faculty will be the top performers, and that another 15 percent to 20 percent will fall at the other end of the scale, with everyone else in between. About half of those in the middle will be passively positive, while the other half will be passively negative. A mistake many organizations make is to focus on the bottom 15 percent when, in fact, they should be focusing on the top 15 percent. By concentrating on and recognizing the top performers, those top educators will actually create an environment that pulls many of the others up to a higher level of performance. That is not to say that feedback and coaching should not be given to the bottom 15 percent; however, predominant attention should be paid to the motivators and energizers at the top. In other words, institutions should focus on their strengths and commit to managing their weaknesses.

THE IMPORTANCE OF PRAISE

P – Praise that
R – Recognizes
A – Accomplishment
I – Is
S– Spontaneous and
E – Effective

Trust is an essential component of the recognition process, and it may be necessary to use a collaborative effort to define trust for the institution. It needs to mean the same thing for the teachers as it does for the management. Once it has been defined and expected behaviors associated with trust have been clearly communicated, expectations can be set for performance. Everyone must agree on what behaviors work and what behaviors don't. Maintenance of trust will be achieved when teachers are recognized for performing as expected and beyond. In addition, teachers must be held accountable when not performing to expected standards.

You may have heard it said that the sweetest sound to anyone is hearing his or her own name. That likely takes second place to hearing one's own name followed by the words "thank you." In our culture, using a person's name while looking them in the eyes shows respect. It's a great first step in building a sound relationship. Giving positive feedback, encouragement, and praise when deserved will take the relationship a great deal further.

IT'S WORTH REMEMBERING ✳

It is not a quick or easy task to rebuild trust once it has been damaged. It is better not to lose it in the first place.

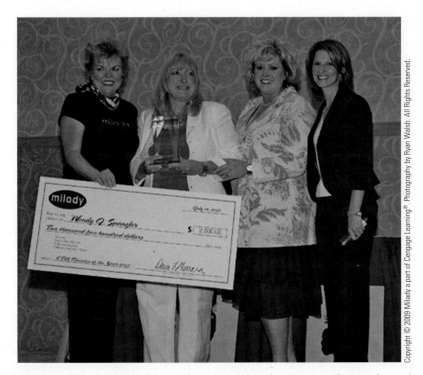

Figure 15–10 **The highest form of recognition in cosmetology education is the Educator of the Year award.**

Institutions can employ many types of rewards, from the simple to the complex, to recognize their top educators. Many institutions have a program in place to honor outstanding educators, such as Teacher of the Year or Teacher of the Quarter. (The American Association of Cosmetology Schools [AACS] cosponsors an annual award with Milady to recognize a national Educator of the Year (Figure 15–10). Readers can find more information about this award and how to be nominated at www.milady.com.) Many institutions offer bonuses and pay increases based on the achievement of advanced degrees or national certification, such as becoming certified by the Career Institute as a Master Educator. Additional bonuses may be paid based on the number of students an educator graduates with a specified grade and attendance average, or the number of their graduates who attain successful employment in their chosen career field.

Other rewards can be personalized for the individual teacher. Institutions should consider developing a questionnaire, much like the one in the accompanying box, that becomes a part of the new employee orientation process. This questionnaire provides key personal information about employees that will allow you to create a reward system that is meaningful to them personally.

If administration has the information gleaned from the questionnaire, it can select a gift or reward that is meaningful for the employee. Perhaps it will be a gift certificate to a favorite restaurant. It might be a book by a favorite author. It might be a bouquet of favorite flowers, and so forth. Such recognition is a way to say, "You're important to our institution. Thank you for being a valuable part of our team."

> As an employee of Milady Beauty Academy, having the following information will facilitate implementation of a more effective and appreciated mechanism for rewarding employees for a job well done.
>
> 1. What is your favorite hobby?
> 2. Who is your favorite author?
> 3. Do you like to go to movies? If so, what type do you enjoy most?
> 4. What is your favorite color?
> 5. What is your favorite flower?
> 6. What is your favorite restaurant?
> 7. What is your first choice of recreational activity when you have time off?
> 8. What is your favorite cologne or aftershave?
> 9. What is your favorite sport and/or sports team?
> 10. When is your birthday (month and day)?

☑ Wrapping It Up

Institutions and their management teams should never assume that achieving educational excellence is an easy task. First of all, it is clearly a sophisticated process, not a simple event. It is composed of many factors, including quality education and development of faculty and development and maintenance of a positive system of rewards, recognition, and trust, combined with the institution's goals, policies, procedures, and ongoing self-evaluation. Desire, commitment, and a dedicated team will make this an attainable goal.

In Retrospect

1. Explain the importance of implementing a sound student-retention program.

2. Explain the role of administrative policies in institution operations.

3. Explain the effects of admissions policies on student retention.

4. Explain the effects of new-student orientation practices on student retention.

5. Describe a few methods used to instill a sense of student ownership in the institution.

6. List some key techniques used in developing effective curriculum content.

7. Explain the importance of holding the highest level of enthusiasm when teaching.

8. List some key elements of delivering excellent student service.

9. Explain the importance of professional development as an educator.

10. Explain the importance of practicing recognition and praise in the educational process.

EDUCATOR SPOTLIGHT

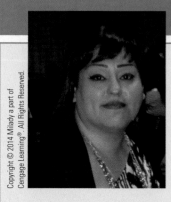

MS. MUNOZ is the recipient of the 2010 N. F. Cimaglia national Educator of the Year Award. She is the Director of Education at the Marinello School of Beauty in Bell, California. Ms. Munoz realized her passion for beauty when she competed in and won a local student style competition. From there, she decided to pursue a career in the beauty industry. As a student, she took such copious notes in her textbook that years later when she became an educator, she used that same textbook to help explain concepts to her students.

After graduating from school, Ms. Munoz worked in a salon for several years, but found her true calling—education—after attending a Cosmetology Educators of American conference in 1997. Inspired by her experience at the conference, she decided to become an educator. She has dedicated all the years since to cosmetology education. She prides herself on being a cheerleader in the classroom and strongly believes in the power of positive reinforcement. Her passion and unwavering devotion to cosmetology education is a reflection of the values put forth in *Master Educator*.

PART **3**

Professional Development for Career Education Instructors

Objectives (Desired Performance Goals):

After reading and studying this chapter, you should be able to:

- Explain the importance of effective communication.
- Identify the various types of relationships necessary to function successfully as a master educator.
- Practice effective listening skills and other steps necessary for building quality relationships.
- Identify the basic needs shared by learners of today.
- Explain the four critical principles to be used when correcting a learner's performance.
- Identify both destructive tactics and constructive tactics used when dealing with learners.
- Explain the purpose of the transfer technique.
- List the 10 steps an educator can take to cultivate a positive relationship with superiors.
- List the "golden rules" of human relations.

KEY TERMS

Relationship • 361

Mutuality • 361

Communication • 361

Praise • 365

Constructive
   Criticism • 365

Destructive Tactics • 366

Human Relations • 376

! CRITICAL CONCEPT

Master educators will become ambassadors of goodwill and cheerleaders for their colleagues, students, and the institution.

Relationships of a Master Educator

VARYING TYPES and degrees of relationships are necessary in order to function successfully as a master educator. A **relationship** refers to the state of affairs existing between those who have an aspect or quality that connects them as being or belonging or working together. Therefore, a master educator will have many professional relationships, including those with learners, other faculty members, administrative personnel, the industry, family members of learners, and the community or public. All are important.

Often, individuals believe that mere contact or acquaintance constitutes a relationship. If you only talk to a student while teaching a class or you only communicate with another educator during a monthly staff meeting, you do not have a relationship with those people; you have a mere acquaintance. In most cases, relationships are developed to the degree that you desire. You make a conscious (or unconscious) decision to allow your connection with someone else to grow only to the degree that you want it to.

Certain conditions must be met in creating and maintaining a true relationship. It is important to recognize that relationships do not result from doing nothing. Many educators expect certain relationships to occur just because they are teachers. They believe that since there are learners in their classrooms and they are the educators, good relationships naturally exist. That is a serious misconception. Relationships require personal investment; they are not automatic. In addition, the investment must be continuous and the relationship must be perpetuated. Finally, it is necessary to accept that confrontation is a natural part of a complete relationship. Reluctance or failure to discuss certain subjects prevents the development of a complete relationship. If one person always gives in to the requests of the other and never receives anything in return, a relationship does not exist. As a master educator, you will know that relationships require risk and effort but they will give you a great return on your investment. You will also accept the fact that you cannot have, nor should you want, a complete relationship with *everyone*. You will, however, need to develop varying degrees of relationships to work well with people. Remember, relationships are built on mutual communication and require mutual investment.

Communication Basics

Communication is the act of effectively sharing information between two people, or groups of people, so that it is satisfactorily understood. You can communicate through words, voice inflections, facial expressions, body language, and visual tools. When you and your students are communicating clearly about educational opportunities, your chances of pleasing and reaching the students grow tremendously. For more information on developing effective communication skills, refer to Chapter 6, "Communicating Confidently."

Meeting and Greeting New Students

One of the most important communications you will have with a student is the first time you meet him or her. Be polite, genuinely friendly, and inviting (which you will continue to be in all your encounters), and remember that your stu-

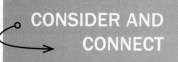

+ **MASTER EDUCATOR**

1. Takes the necessary risks to develop positive relationships.
2. Understands the needs of today's learners and works to nurture those needs.
3. Provides solutions rather than problems.
4. Respects and protects students, coworkers, and supervisors.

CONSIDER AND CONNECT

Relationships require **mutuality**.

relationship
refers to the state of affairs existing between those who have an aspect or quality that connects them as being or belonging or working together.

mutuality
the act of having the same relationship each to the other; being directed and receiving direction in the same amount; each party having the same commitment to the relationship.

communication
the act of transmitting information so that it is satisfactorily understood.

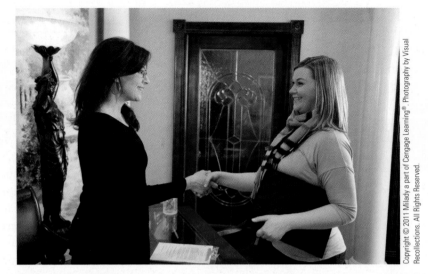

Figure 16–1   When first meeting students, be polite, friendly, and inviting.

dents are coming to you for an education (Figure 16–1). This means you need to court them every day; otherwise you may lose them to another institution.

To earn a student's trust and loyalty, you need to:

- Always approach a new student with a smile on your face. If you are having a difficult day or have a problem of some sort, keep it to yourself. The time you are with your students is for their needs, not yours.
- Always introduce yourself. Names are powerful, and they are meant to be used.
- Set aside a few minutes during orientation to take new students on a quick tour of the institution. Introduce them to staff and faculty members they have not yet met.
- Be yourself. Don't try to trick your students into thinking you are someone or something that you are not. Just be who you are. You will be surprised at how well this will work for you.

We have already established that an important ingredient for anyone attempting to build strong relationships is to talk less and listen more. That means establishing effective listening skills. Listening is an essential element of communicating. Often, people aren't good listeners because they simply do not recognize the value or worth of good listening.

☑ Educator-to-Learner Relationships

A master educator needs to know the learners' perceptions of the class, the assignments, the educator, and the other learners. An educator who wants good educator–learner relationships seeks feedback in order to make adjustments in teaching techniques and behaviors to meet the needs of individual learners. The master educator will take a proactive approach and follow specific steps to building relationships with students.

Be Genuinely Interested in All Learners. Schedule a five-minute meeting with four or five of your students each day. Before long, you would have had personal and private contact with each student in your class. The meeting does not have to cover anything vital but should

---

IT'S WORTH REMEMBERING ✳

Bear in mind that the degree of a relationship that is sought and achieved by you may or may not be desired by or acceptable to the other individual. So, you must never assume that simply because you are satisfied with a relationship, the other person is as well.

THE VALUE OF GOOD LISTENING

- **Listening increases learning.** What is learned is increased if you listen beyond words for deeper meaning; listen for facts found in the words; listen for specific answers to questions that have been asked; listen for the full context of the subject being discussed; listen to the *whole person*, considering temperament, attitude, emotions, intellect, speaking ability, and so on.
- **Listening reduces tension.** Listening allows the speaker to express a viewpoint or voice an opinion. It can clear the air of tension or adversarial attitudes.
- **Listening builds friendships.** The other individual will appreciate being allowed to talk and will like you for listening attentively. Everyone needs and wants to be able to express themselves.
- **Listening stimulates the speaker's ability.** An eager, alert, active listener helps the speaker present ideas more clearly and concisely.
- **Listening may solve problems for the speaker.** By allowing the speaker to "talk through" his problem with an attentive listener, you may allow him to clarify his own thinking about a topic and/or provide an emotional release for a difficult or controversial subject.
- **Listening results in better decisions and job performance.** By listening carefully, you draw upon the knowledge and experience of others, which can help you develop better judgment and gain additional important information about how to accomplish a task.
- **Listening leads to better cooperation from others.** When a speaker feels you are really interested in his problems, thoughts, opinions, and ideas, he will appreciate and respect you. He will also be inspired to cooperate and work with you in endeavors that are important to you.
- **Listening may resolve disagreements and solve conflicts.** You must understand the other person's point of view and opinions before you can agree or disagree with him intelligently. When both parties understand each other, they can work together to seek a solution to a problem or they can agree to disagree.

include asking the student if he needs anything or has any comments or concerns he would like to share with you. It should also include your making one specific observation about the student and a reminder for him to see you immediately if he needs help with anything. By requesting feedback from the student and by offering observations, mutuality will be established (Figure 16–2).

Be Cheerful. Before entering any classroom or meeting situation with a student, make a conscious effort to remove any glum expression and to enter with a smile. Learners are more interested in developing true relationships with educators who are of good cheer.

Know the Name of Every Learner and Pronounce It Correctly. It has been said that a person's name is the sweetest and most important sound in his language. Speak the learner's name clearly and warmly whenever you address him.

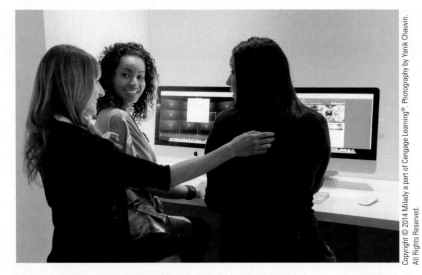

Figure 16–2   Informal meetings can be highly effective at strengthening educator–learner relationships.

Don't Do All the Talking. For mutuality to exist in any relationship, all participants must give and take, and that means they must communicate. As an educator, you might steer learners toward ideas and conclusions that build on your class or lesson, but it is beneficial if learners feel they are finding the answers needed.

Relate the Topic of Discussion to the Learners' Past Experiences. When you teach or converse in terms of their interests, relationships with students grow and learning occurs more easily.

Make Every Learner Feel Important. This can be accomplished by accentuating the positive. Praise learners at every opportunity: the correct answer, the quality practical work, the positive image, the enthusiastic attitude, the desire for success!

The relationship between educator and learner must be one of genuine interest and compassion. It isn't enough for the educator to simply be interested in all students; each student must feel confident that the educator is interested in him personally. An educator who seeks daily to recognize the needs of students and searches for ways to meet those needs is on his way to becoming a master educator. Some of the basic needs shared by learners of today are discussed next.

The Need for Acceptance as an Individual. Learners need to feel they are recognized and acknowledged for their own uniqueness. They must feel that the educator's empathy and compassion are genuine and sincere.

The Need for Knowledge and Understanding. Students must feel free to ask questions and give feedback. Every question asked must be given the attention and respect necessary to ensure clear understanding of the matter at hand.

The Need for Freedom from Guilt. All institutions must have standards and rules for ensuring order in the classroom. However, students should not be made to feel guilty about minor infractions or be constantly reminded of past infractions. The educator should assist the student in minimizing past unpleasant actions and give the student the opportunity for improvement in the future.

The Need for Freedom from Embarrassment. Errors or misunderstandings by the student should never result in that student being embarrassed, especially in front of his peers. A master educator will find a way to assume some of the responsibility to relieve the student of any unnecessary embarrassment.

The Need for Appreciation and for Belonging to the Group of Learners. All humans, including students, need to feel needed, appreciated, and important. They need to feel missed when they are absent. They need to feel they are important members of the class.

The Need for a Feeling of Accomplishment. All learners should be made to feel they are making progress, even it is slow. A master educator will help students build on small "wins" and feel confident that they are growing and progressing toward success.

The master educator will make every student feel that his contribution to the overall learning process is sincerely accepted and appreciated. Learners should be encouraged to give of themselves to improve and increase learning.

Praise. A master educator will devote his energies to the development of student self-esteem, self-confidence, and self-respect. That can be accomplished by giving **praise** or compliments to learners in ways that are well received and appreciated. Never send a mixed-message compliment to a student that also contains a negative or urges the student to "do more." A student will recognize that your comments aren't really praise but, in fact, criticism. The student will probably believe that you are dissatisfied with the work and want more effort.

praise
an expression of warm approval or admiration; strong commendation.

Also, the master educator will take the *initiative* to give praise and compliments to learners. If you compliment only when absolutely necessary, the praise won't be as well received or appreciated, and it won't generate positive feelings toward you as the educator. On the other hand, if you celebrate academic victories, including simple improvements, for every student on a regular basis, you and the students will be able to savor and enjoy the successes you helped create in the learning process. Positive educator–learner relationships will result.

Reprimand. Always remember that clarification and caring must precede confrontation if you expect to solve problems and generate good educator–learner relationships in the process. If a student's performance or behavior indicates the need for discipline or reprimand, use the clarification technique by saying, "Let me ask you. . . ." or "Do I understand what you are doing or saying . . . ?" By obtaining the answers to these or similar questions, you will demonstrate to the student your genuine interest and concern. Once you have obtained the answers, you can approach the issue or problem without the need for confrontation. This is another situation when good listening skills are essential. Take care to listen carefully to the student's responses rather than jumping to quick conclusions. Never formulate your questions or rebuttals before the student has finished speaking. To do so will result in a negative reaction on the part of the student. For more information regarding reprimands, refer to Chapter 8 is Effective Classroom Management and Supervision.

Constructive Criticism. It is easier to correct a learner's performance if you follow some basic principles. First, consider your instructions. Were they clear, concise, and easy to follow, or were they confusing and possibly

constructive criticism
a well-meant critique intended to help someone improve.

contributed to the student's inability to create the desired results? Second, when giving criticism always include a positive comment and consider using the word "and" instead of the word "but" when connecting the compliment with the criticism. Third, allow the student time to think about what you have said. Fourth, before giving any further advice, ask the student if it is wanted. You might say, "Can I offer some suggestions for developing a plan of action?" This allows the student to take ownership of her learning, but also reassures her that you are there to help her in any way possible.

Emotional Influence on Learning. Personal feelings and emotions play a critical role in the development of learning and in the development of strong relationships. Educators have a powerful influence upon the emotions of learners. Words, looks, gestures, and attitudes can make a learner feel inadequate and inferior. Conversely, the educator can use that same power to create feelings of confidence, importance, and worth among students.

destructive tactics tactics used to take away and/or harm an individual's creation, prestige, or self-esteem.

DESTRUCTIVE TACTICS

Without realizing what they are doing, some educators gratify their own egos by making students feel inferior by:

- **Generating student guilt.** This behavior makes the student feel he is letting the educator down. This emotion is created by the educator suggesting that he (the educator) has worked so hard to help the student and that the student has deliberately failed to respond or make an effort to appreciate the educator's great sacrifice. A master educator would never take this approach. No educator should ever indicate to any learner that it is just his job to help the student. Learners want educators to like them—to help students because they want to, not because they have to.

- **Talking "down" to students.** Educators sometimes use superior language or words that the learners do not understand. This tactic embarrasses the students when they don't understand the questions and are therefore unable to answer properly. A master educator will take care to ensure that he is clearly understood by all students in order to facilitate their learning as quickly as possible.

- **Focusing attention only on fast learners.** The most effective way to discourage or destroy a slow learner's confidence is for the educator to direct all teaching efforts toward the high achievers. This behavior may lead to students dropping out. The master educator, on the other hand, will develop his own teaching abilities and learn how to deliver the message to learners of all types and abilities.

- **Inappropriate or excessive praise.** Too much praise for a trivial or minor task can actually be detrimental. Learners will quickly recognize the extravagant praise as "phony" and insulting. The educator is actually suggesting indirectly that the student is incapable of any other task, and is therefore being praised for meaningless achievement. The master educator is sincere and genuine and will fashion all praise to be uplifting and truly applicable to the learner's achievement.

A CONSTRUCTIVE ENVIRONMENT

The following are characteristics of a constructive learning environment:

- **Students can express personal feelings.** The master educator will make sure every student has the opportunity to express his personal opinion and feelings on any subject. Respectful attention is given to an honest expression of the students' attitudes, ideas, concerns, and doubts. Under no circumstances is a student subjected to ridicule, regardless of how unrealistic or incorrect his statements may be.
- **Independent thinking is encouraged.** Students are encouraged to believe that it is educationally worthwhile to be individuals and to think independently. Students are encouraged to explore their own minds and express their own thoughts. They are made to feel that even if their ideas are outrageous, they may have merit, and students will never be humiliated as a result of expressing themselves.
- **Competitive atmosphere is avoided.** Competition has its place during the educational process. However, in a classroom filled with learners from different backgrounds and abilities, it can be disastrous. It will often serve to stimulate high achievers while discouraging lower achievers. Each student should be permitted to set his own learning pace. Competition should be encouraged in students with themselves rather than with others in the classroom.

Master educators realize that successful learning can only take place with the willingness and cooperation of students. No educational progress can be made in an antagonistic environment that perpetuates conflict or hostility between educators and learners. By fostering mutual respect and consideration in the educational environment, the educator has taken great strides in developing sound educator–learner relationships.

Educator-to-Educator Relationships

Teamwork is the ability for educators to work together toward a common vision. It is the ability to direct individual accomplishments toward organizational or institutional objectives. It is the fuel that allows common educators to attain uncommon results! One of the most important types of relationships an educator must develop is the relationship with other educators. **T**ogether **E**veryone **A**chieves **M**ore emphasizes the importance and effectiveness of developing a solid *team* of educators within the institution. Remember that you cannot be a loner and also be appreciated or accepted by everyone else. If you isolate yourself, others will not view you as part of the institution team. Other educators cannot relate to you if you purposely set yourself apart. In fact, they will generally feel more respect for educators who are inclusive rather than exclusive.

IT'S WORTH REMEMBERING

When educators come together, it is a beginning. When educators stay together, it is progress. When educators work together, it is success.

Behaviors for Building Strong Educator Relationships. A number of behaviors will help you build strong relationships with other educators, including the following:

- When another educator shines, share in the joy. The feeling of success is so pleasurable that it should be savored and indulged for awhile. Most of us have no problem enjoying praise and success for ourselves. However, it is often more difficult to enjoy the success of other educators. Their success might even spur feelings of resentment or jealousy of their accomplishments. Those emotions can be deadly not only for oneself but also for the other educators who are trying to enjoy an achievement. The following steps can help you enjoy the success of others:

  - Acknowledge and register approval of their success *now*. Remember, praise is like champagne, it should be served while it is still bubbling!
  - Become an advocate of the achievement. Train yourself to cherish and appreciate effort and accomplishment. This will help you grow, create, and nurture your own profession as an educator.
  - Inquire about details that led to the success. Become genuinely interested in how they attained their goals. They will appreciate your interest and you, in turn, will learn from their experience.
  - Don't chalk it up to "luck." It might appear that their success was no more than "being in the right place at the right time." Don't believe it. Even when opportunities arise, it takes a competent educator to create actual success.
  - Be aware of human nature. Don't abandon fellow educators when they win because you can't handle their success. They learn quickly who can share in their success and who cannot. If you're not there for them, they will pull away from you and your relationship will deteriorate.

- Talk about results versus work. When you are enjoying your own successes, discuss the results of the achievements rather than all the work you did to accomplish them. When you indicate "all the hard work" you did, you may be implying that you lack organizational skills or that you really wasted a lot of time getting to the end result. You'll be viewed more highly if you speak only about results and in a modest manner.

- Use the *transfer technique*. Master educators are quite persuasive. They have mastered a technique that gives ownership to others: the transfer technique. They know that there is a point in time when the ownership of a plan or idea must be transferred to another individual or to the group who will be working with it. Otherwise, group acceptance will decrease or diminish entirely. This is accomplished by involving the other parties in the development of a plan so that much of it is their idea.

- Appeal to another educator's ego. Everyone has special talents and a sense of importance. If they see you recognize those qualities, they will be pleased. Be sincere and compliment their real or hidden strengths from the heart.

- Never say, "Nobody tells me anything." Such comments cause bad feelings. Instead, ask sufficient questions to get the information you feel you are missing. Otherwise, you will be perceived as a grumbler or complainer and you will certainly send the message that you are *not* part of the institution team. Request more frequent staff meetings and suggest an agenda that includes all the information needed to function successfully within the institution.

- Never criticize the work of other educators. Comments like, "What do you expect . . . Ms. Holt has no real-world experience . . . how can she be effective?" can damage the institution's reputation and hurt yours in the process. Indicating poor performance on the part of others will ultimately reflect on you, and it will greatly damage your relationship with others.
- Don't hoard or protect information, materials, or equipment. A master educator will eagerly share his knowledge, thoughts, and ideas with all other educators. He will know that when he helps other educators become more successful, he will also become more successful. Another good rule of thumb is that if they share with you by loaning you something, always return it, whether it is big or small, important or insignificant.
- Don't "clam up" when angry. Silence will solve few problems and may foster bitterness. Instead, speak calmly and begin by clarifying your position. Be specific and reveal a sense of responsibility. If you should remain upset as you speak, stop yourself and explain that you need more time to think things through and you will continue later. The other party will be more receptive and you will be able to make your points more effectively when you're calm.
- Don't speak "off the record." Many a staff conflict has occurred as a result of the bad habit of saying different things to different people (Figure 16–3). Your fear then grows because you cannot remember what you've said to whom. It's good practice to avoid indicating to anyone that what you're saying is "off the record." Rather, you should make sure that everything you say can be repeated anywhere at any time.
- Never demand special privileges that are not available to all. This will cause disharmony and negatively impact good educator-to-educator relationships. Like students, educators want the policies that affect their environment to be applied fairly and consistently.
- Avoid faculty gossip. Students who hear you and another teacher talking negatively about a student or colleague will become distrustful and fear that you may feel the same way toward them. Try to always speak highly of others. If you cannot, don't say anything at all. As a master educator your behavior must be exemplary and set a high standard for students to look up to and follow.

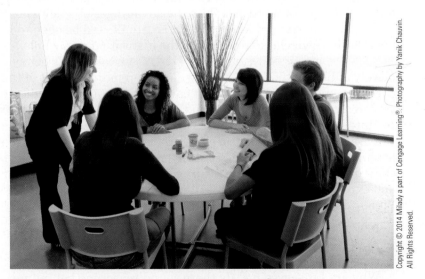

Figure 16–3   Never speak off the record with your students.

- Plan and implement educator "get-togethers." This can be an extremely effective way to build educator-to-educator relationships. Ask the other educators if they would like to plan a potluck luncheon or dinner once per month. This can offer a nice break from routine and encourage staff to socialize on regular basis.
- Learn to handle criticism well. All educators will receive some type of criticism from time to time. Whether or not you can handle it professionally will certainly impact how you are viewed by other educators. Here are some tips to help you handle any unpleasant criticism you might receive:

  - Be humble. This will keep the criticism from hurting so much.
  - Be open and honest. No one is perfect; therefore, admit your mistakes.
  - Put yourself in the other person's shoes. This will help you determine the cause of the criticism and may help you to deal with it more effectively.
  - Apologize if necessary. If, in fact, you have done something, perhaps inadvertently, that caused the criticism, make a sincere apology. If you haven't, an apology is not needed.
  - Don't whine, cry, or blame others. No one likes an educator who always puts the blame for any negative situation on others. Such behavior will cause you to lose the respect of all your colleagues.

- Stress the benefits of change. When introducing a new idea, concept, or policy to fellow educators, be aware of the roadblocks you may face. Others may view your idea with prejudice or be more concerned with self-serving interests. Such characteristics may interfere with their ability to evaluate the facts you present objectively. Be tactful and caring when presenting a new idea. Know that the benefits of change must outweigh the personal prejudices or prejudgments the other educators may hold or they will not change.
- See the "big picture" and be open-minded. Avoid tunnel vision. Some educators may see rules, for example, in relation to their own classrooms, but not see how they affect the entire institution. Most of us believe we encourage new ideas and are supportive of them. The truth is that often we tend to be overly critical of new ideas and change. We often look for the disadvantages rather than the advantages of a new concept or procedure. A master educator will listen, think, and be open to improvement for his own classroom and for the institution as a whole.
- Avoid the "but our institution is different" attitude. This behavior merely indicates that you are unwilling to remain abreast of the current trends within the field of education. It may also indicate that you are unwilling to face head-on the challenges you encounter with the intention of resolving them. This could suggest to your peers that you are out of touch with the ways professional educators solve problems. Adopting this attitude could eventually lead to your reluctance to experiment or to look to the future for ways to improve. Without vision and experimentation, growth will not occur.
- When you are about to disagree, ask yourself five questions:

  1. Does the end justify the means? (Is it worth disagreeing on this issue?)
  2. Am I really correct in this matter? (Should other factors be considered?)
  3. Why am I disagreeing? (Is there sound reasoning behind my disagreement?)

> ## IT'S WORTH REMEMBERING ✳
>
> A master educator will gather all the facts and present the benefits at the right time, in the correct manner, and for the right reasons.

4. Are there other solutions to the situation or disagreement? (What alternatives can you explore to resolve this without a confrontation?)

5. I wonder how I would feel if I were in the other person's shoes? (What have they been through that has caused their behavior in this situation?) Asking these very important questions in times of disagreement or confrontation can help prevent embarrassing behavior.

- Keep others informed and exercise your right to know. If you happen to be aware of information that other educators may not know, inform them of the relevant data. Not knowing important facts about the operation of your institution could turn an "ally" into a "foe" and cause staff friction. At the same time, make sure that you are kept informed by asking key questions while relating why it's important to you. Take care to never attack or criticize peers or supervisors for not keeping you "in the know." Remind the key people within your institution that they are very important to you and that you rely on them as a source of relevant and valuable information.

- Adopt the other person's position. It is not uncommon for educators to adopt the attitude that they aren't going to do anything for coworkers because no one ever does anything for them. That's a lower standard than what can be expected of a master educator. The master educator will adopt a higher standard and set the pace for other educators to follow. Otherwise, staff may regress to a low point. You can only get the best out of others by trying to be the best you can possibly be. That will not occur if you only act when others act first.

- Develop a high tolerance for frustration. A master educator will not "blow up" and lose control or pout and sulk when things don't go as hoped or planned. Master educators will hold their feelings in check and respond professionally so that their emotions don't interfere with their ability to work with and relate to other educators.

Learn to work effectively with other educators at your institution (Figure 16–4). A master educator will provide solutions rather than problems to fellow educators or administrators. He will not constantly identify, describe, or present problems to colleagues. If he does so, the chances are that he will not be liked, respected, or appreciated.

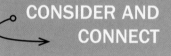

CONSIDER AND CONNECT

Master educators will assume the responsibility of offering at least three possible solutions to every problem brought to other educators. They will also ask for help in finding a solution rather than blaming others for the circumstances at hand.

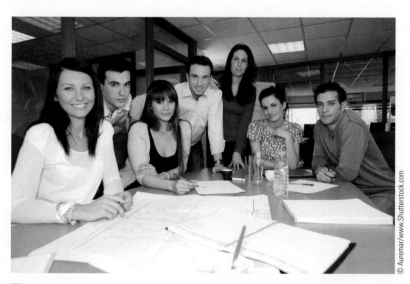

Figure 16–4 Regular staff meetings provide the perfect opportunity for building relationships with colleagues.

By working closely with other master educators, a powerful network is created—a network that should be able to effectively deal with any obstacle, hurdle, or challenge that may arise in the day of an educator.

 ## Educator-to-Supervisor/Employer Relationships

The master educator will strive to develop the best possible working relationship with his supervisor(s) to ensure that the mission and objectives of the institution are met and the needs of students are placed first. As a master educator, you will support the leadership of others and never disregard the authority of anyone in a leadership position within your institution. You must never degrade or countermand institution rules or objectives. As an educator, you have the freedom and opportunity to attempt to change rules, but you must follow them explicitly as written until they are changed.

In addition, the master educator will respect the curriculum offered and follow it diligently. As an educator, however, at times you may feel the curriculum needs to be changed or updated. If so, you have the same opportunity to recommend and help implement needed improvements. In doing so, you must follow the procedures set forth by the institution for such action. For example, you might prepare a detailed plan with specific recommendations for improvement and request an opportunity to present your plan to the appropriate supervisory personnel.

Steps for Professional Relationships with Superiors. There are other steps an educator can take to ensure a positive, professional relationship with one's superiors.

TOP 10 STEPS FOR POSITIVE RELATIONSHIP WITH SUPERIORS

1. Set high standards for professional performance and consistently achieve quality results on the job and in the classroom.

2. Verify questionable information or procedures to prevent unnecessary errors in performance.

3. Pay close attention to instructions and essential details.

4. Provide thorough and accurate reports when required.

5. Be observant—detect errors and correct them or make appropriate personnel aware of them.

6. Exercise initiative in starting and following through on assigned work; offer to help others when needed.

7. Initiate action to solve problems whenever possible without supervisory intervention while also keeping management informed about significant actions or problems.

8. Communicate ideas or the essence of problems clearly and concisely.

9. Develop and convey self-confidence at all times.

10. Follow faithfully all requirements of the educator position description and duties of the job.

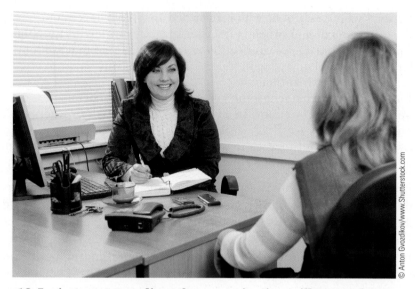

Figure 16–5 **A strong open line of communication will strengthen your relationship with your supervisor.**

By following these guidelines and developing all the qualities and characteristics required of a master educator as discussed in Chapter 2, "The Teaching Plan and Learning Environment," you will become an exemplary employee who is greatly appreciated by your supervisor or employer. Developing strong and open lines of communication will help in establishing sound relationships with your superiors (Figure 16–5).

Other Educator Relationships

As previously stated, a master educator will develop relationships with a wide variety of individuals and entities. He must consider the importance of his relationships with the family members of students, with the community he serves, and with the industry in general.

Educator-to-Family-Members Relationships. Educators in the United States must be aware of the Family Educational Right to Privacy Act of 1974 (FERPA), which is a federal law designed to protect the privacy of a student's educational records. The law applies to all institutions that receive funds under an applicable program from the U.S. Department of Education. FERPA gives certain rights to parents regarding their children's educational records. These rights transfer to the student or former student who has reached the age of 18 or is attending any institution beyond the high school level. Students and former students to whom the rights have transferred are called eligible students.

FERPA ensures that parents or eligible students have the right to inspect and review educational records and to request that an institution correct records believed to be inaccurate or misleading.

Generally, the institution and its employees, including faculty, must have written permission from the parent or eligible student before releasing information from a student's record. However, the law allows institutions to disclose records, without consent, to the following parties:

- Institution employees who have a need to know;
- Other institutions to which a student is transferring;

- Parents when a student who is over age 18 is still dependent;
- Certain government officials in order to carry out lawful functions;
- Appropriate parties in connection with financial aid to a student;
- Organizations doing certain studies for the institution;
- Accrediting organizations;
- Individuals who have obtained court orders or subpoenas;
- Persons who need to know in cases of health and safety emergencies; and
- State and local authorities to whom disclosure is required by state laws adopted before November 19, 1974.

Educators must know that they cannot discuss the performance of an eligible student with a family member without written consent from the eligible student, even if it seems totally harmless. For example, a mother may call the institution and wish to know what a student's grade average or attendance record is. The student may be an outstanding performer but has had some attendance problems recently. You feel that if you share that information with the parent, she might be able to encourage the student to get to institution on a regular basis. However, circumstances may exist in which the student does not want the parent to know that he was missing school. Under FERPA, you are not authorized to disclose educational records, such as grades or attendance, even to family members, without written authorization from the eligible student.

The Educator and Public Relations. A master educator will become an ambassador of goodwill for the institution he represents. He will become a cheerleader and not hesitate to brag about other educators, administrators, students, and the institution as often as possible to anyone who will listen. He will take every opportunity to relate good news about students' achievements or the positive educational environment found in the institution.

Four major factors will influence the public attitude toward any organization, including career education institutions:

- the various services and products offered by the institution;
- the ability of the staff, faculty, and, in the case of career education institutions, the students to deliver the services and products offered;
- the prices charged for the products or services rendered; and
- the believability of the publicity used to promote the other factors.

The ability of the staff and faculty to extend themselves to meet the needs of the public will play a large role in how the institution is perceived by its consumers. The public's perception about your institution begins with whether people believe the products and services are of good quality and are cost justified.

Educators may have the experience of being approached with concerns or complaints about their institution while attending a social function or other event (Figure 16–6). If the educator is not thoughtful, it can be easy to get caught up in the negativism. A master educator, however, will avoid that role at all costs. He will assume the role of facilitator and engage in active listening. He might respond with, "It sounds like you have been concerned about this issue for quite some time. Your comments suggest that you feel very strongly about it. Perhaps you have even given some thought

> ### CONSIDER AND CONNECT
>
> A master educator will take steps to develop a professional relationship with family members of learners while also taking proper measures to ensure that the rights to privacy for all eligible students are protected.

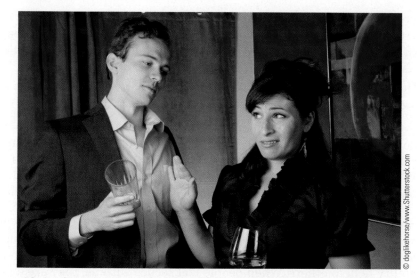

Figure 16–6   Assume the role of facilitator if approached at a social function with negativity about your institution.

to possible solutions to prevent it from happening in the future. Let me suggest that you contact Mr. Edwards, the campus administrator. I think he may be able to help you." By following this tactic, you neutralize the negativity. As a team player you would then alert Mr. Edwards of the conversation when you return to institution. Such notice will allow him to be prepared to turn a negative situation into a positive one.

Another element of public relations that an educator must consider is his role in community activities. Career education offers many opportunities for educators, students, and institutions to become involved with various charities, organizations, and needs within the community and society in general. Master educators will seek opportunities for their institution and students to provide complimentary services to the elderly, the ill, the unemployed, and more. Master educators will work with their institution to recognize key people in the community such as law enforcement officers, health care professionals, and firefighters. As a master educator you will remember that you are the institution's best public relations person. When you excel at public relations, you will establish better relationships in all areas.

Human Relations

No matter where you work, you will not always get along with everyone. It is not possible to always understand what people need even when you know them well. Even when you think you understand what people want, you cannot always be sure that you will satisfy them. This can lead to tension and misunderstanding.

The ability to understand people is the key to operating effectively in many professions. It is especially important in fields where customer service is central to success. Most of your interactions will depend on your ability to communicate successfully with a wide range of people: your boss, your coworkers, your students, your clients, and the different vendors who come to the institution. When you clearly understand the motives and needs of others, you are in a better position to do your job professionally and easily.

human relations
the study of how people relate to each other in group situations, especially at work, and how communication skills and sensitivity to other people's feelings can be improved.

Here is a brief look at the basics of **human relations** along with some practical tips for dealing with situations that you are likely to encounter:

- **Personal security.** A fundamental factor in human relations has to do with how secure we are feeling. When we feel secure, we are happy, calm, and confident, and we act in a cooperative and trusting manner. When we feel insecure, we become worried, anxious, overwhelmed, perhaps angry and suspicious, and usually we do not behave very well. We might be uncooperative, hostile, or withdrawn.
- **Social interactions.** Human beings are social animals. When we feel secure, we like to interact with other people. We enjoy giving our opinion; we take pleasure from having people help us; we take pride in our ability to help others. When people feel secure with us, they are a joy to be with. You can help people feel secure around you by being respectful, trustworthy, and honest.
- **Handling difficult situations.** No matter how secure you are, there will be times when you will be faced with people and situations that are difficult to handle. You may already have had such experiences. There are always some people who create conflict wherever they go. They can be rude, insensitive, or so full of themselves that being considerate just does not enter their minds. Even though you may wonder how anyone could be so unfeeling, just try to remember that this person at this particular time feels insecure, or he wouldn't be acting this way.

To become skilled in human relations, learn to make the best of situations that could otherwise drain both your time and your energy. Here are some good ways to handle the ups and downs of human relations:

- **Respond instead of reacting.** A fellow was asked why he didn't get angry when a driver cut him off. "Why should I let someone else dictate my emotions?" he replied. A wise man, don't you think? He might have even saved his own life by not reacting with "an eye for an eye" mentality.
- **Believe in yourself.** When you do, you trust your judgment, uphold your own values, and stick to what you believe is right. It is easy to believe in yourself when you have a strong sense of self-worth. It comes with the knowledge that you are a good person and you deserve to be successful. Believing in yourself makes you feel strong enough to handle almost any situation in a calm, helpful manner.
- **Talk less, listen more.** There is an old saying that we were given two ears and one mouth for a reason. You get a gold star in human relations when you listen more than you talk. When you are a good listener, you are fully attentive to what the other person is saying. If there is something you do not understand, ask a question to gain understanding.
- **Be attentive.** Each student or client is different. Some are clear about what they want, others are aggressively demanding, while others may be hesitant. Usually, you can calm upset students by agreeing with or affirming them and then asking what you can do to make them more satisfied. This approach is virtually guaranteed to work.

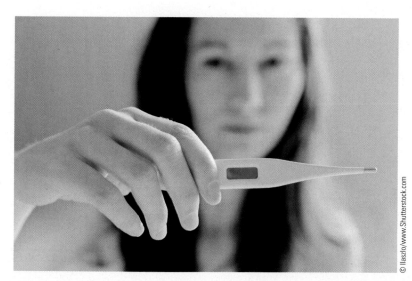

Figure 16–7 When in conflict or feeling down about yourself, stop and take your own temperature or evaluate your feelings to determine next steps.

- **Take your own temperature.** If you are tired or upset about a personal problem or have had an argument with a colleague or student, you may be feeling down about yourself and wish you were anywhere but at school (Figure 16–7). If this feeling lasts a short time, you will be able to get back on track easily enough and there is no cause for alarm. If, however, you begin to notice certain chronic behaviors about yourself once you are in a job, pay careful attention to what is happening. An important part of being in a service profession is taking care of yourself first and resolving whatever conflicts are going on so that you can take care of your students and clients. Trust can be lost in a second without your even knowing it—and, once lost, trust is almost impossible to regain.

THE GOLDEN RULES OF HUMAN RELATIONS

Keep the following guidelines in mind for a crash course in human relations that will keep you in line and where you should be:
- Communicate from your heart; problem-solve from your head (Figure 16–8).
- A smile is worth a million times more than a sneer.
- It is easy to make an enemy; it is harder to keep a friend.
- See what happens when you ask for help instead of just reacting.
- Show people you care by listening to them and trying to understand their point of view.
- Tell people how great they are (even when they are not acting so great).
- Being right is different from acting righteous.
- For every service you do for others, don't forget to do something for yourself.
- Laugh often.
- Show patience with other people's flaws.
- Build shared goals; be a team player and a partner to your clients.

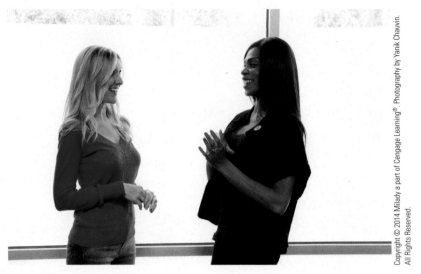

Figure 16–8   Effective communication is vital to building lasting relationships.

✓ Wrapping It Up

Master educators will be called upon to engage in and soundly develop relationships with learners and their family members, other educators, campus administrative personnel, and the community or public. They will know that a mere acquaintance does not constitute a relationship. They will recognize that risk and effort are required if a positive relationship is to be born and nurtured. They will know the values of good listening and work to develop effective listening skills. Master educators will take a proactive approach in developing positive relationships and follow established steps to do so. They will understand the basic needs of today's learners and work to meet and nurture those needs. They will avoid using destructive tactics that make students feel inferior and will employ constructive tactics that encourage learning and participation.

Master educators will, indeed, be contributing members of the institution team. They will adopt all the behaviors necessary to build strong relationships with the other educators at the institution. They will provide solutions rather than problems and will strive to create a powerful network among the educators with whom they work. They will believe in giving quality performance for value received on the job as an educator. They will support the leadership and respect the curriculum of the institution. They will respect and protect the privacy of students while taking appropriate steps to develop a professional relationship with the supportive family members of learners. And, finally, master educators will become ambassadors of goodwill and cheerleaders for their fellow educators and other personnel, students, and the institution. A master educator will recognize that he can be the best public relations person the institution has ever had.

> **⌐CONSIDER AND CONNECT**
>
> Master educators will use praise to help students develop self-esteem, self-confidence, and self-respect. They will use compassion to make reprimands and criticism more palatable.

In Retrospect

1. Explain the importance of effective communication.

2. Identify the various types of relationships necessary to function success-fully as a master educator.

3. Explain the values of good listening.

4. Identify six of the basic needs shared by learners of today.

5. Explain the four critical principles used when correcting a learner's performance.

6. Identify both destructive tactics and constructive tactics used when dealing with learners.

7. Explain the purpose of the transfer technique.

8. List the 10 steps an educator can take to cultivate a positive relationship with superiors.

9. List the "golden rules" of human relations.

Objectives (Desired Performance Goals):

After reading and studying this chapter, you will be able to:

- List the best conditions for learning.
- Define learning and laughter.
- Explain the theories of what makes us laugh.
- List the mental, physical, and work-related benefits of laughter.
- Explain the four stages of humor competence.
- Identify strategies for improving creativity.
- List ways to integrate humor in the workplace and classroom.

! CRITICAL CONCEPT

It has been long understood that when students are laughing and having fun, they learn more.

The Best Conditions for Learning

RESEARCH TELLS US that the best conditions for learning are those that allow the student to feel safe enough to take risks. All meaningful learning involves negotiating risk. These risks include the fear of finding out what we don't know, the risk of getting it wrong, and the risk of peer disapproval. For some students, simply raising one's hand in the classroom is a risk. The best conditions are created, of course, when the student elects to be there and wants to learn, as is most often the case with adult learners. As educators, we have the awesome responsibility of creating that needed sense of security. It has been determined that a shared positive experience can help accomplish this. For example, when students and teachers share humor and laughter, everyone feels safer and more comfortable. It is important to encourage joy and laughter in every classroom. There are many ways this can be accomplished to help make the classroom a positive and nurturing environment. Helping learners relish laughter and appreciate developing a sense of humor is a skill that is as important as reading, writing, and arithmetic!

Laughlab, a university project, determined some interesting facts about laughter and its effects, duration, and universality, as discussed in the accompanying boxed feature.

➕ MASTER EDUCATOR

1. Facilitates internal jogging to stimulate beneficial brain neurotransmitters.
2. Teaches learners to fake laughter that ultimately results in genuine laughter.
3. Uses laughter to engage both sides of the brain for more comprehensive learning.

FACTS ABOUT LAUGHTER AND ITS EFFECTS, DURATION, AND UNIVERSALITY

- Laughter produces endorphins that help us to handle pain and reduce stress. Our bodies produce a natural, morphine-like substance that operates on specific receptor sites in the brain and spinal cord. Endorphins reduce the experience of pain and screen out unpleasant stimuli. Thus, the presence of endorphins creates the feeling of well-being. Behavioral researchers have shown that as humans, we can actually stimulate the body's production of endorphins through just ***pretending*** to have a positive attitude and optimistic thoughts.
- People who laugh more tend to be liked more by their friends. It is a basic principle, but makes perfect sense. People want to be around happy people. None of us wants to be around someone who constantly gripes and complains.
- Teachers who use humor are liked more by their students. The preceding principles also apply in the educator–learner relationship. The more safe and comfortable students feel in our classrooms, the greater the likelihood that they will be more responsive to learning.
- Self-deprecation seems a safe way of using humor, but you must have a very positive relationship with your class before exposing yourself to a degree of "ribbing."
- The more positive and enduring a relationship you have with the class, the more risks you can take with humor. However, humor is highly individualized. What you find funny is not necessarily what your students will find funny. When in doubt, toss it out.
- Fake smiles differ from sincere smiles. When people find something genuinely funny, the zygomatic muscles around the mouth pull the lips upward and the eyes crinkle. When the smile is fake, it lasts longer, stops abruptly, and only involves the mouth. The cheeks aren't raised and the eyes don't crinkle.

IT'S WORTH ✳ REMEMBERING

Master educators will use humor to reach adult learners, who often need a lighthearted moment to ease the troubles they face throughout the day.

(continued)

A recent study concluded that humor helps teachers display a comfortable, secure attitude about themselves, the material they are teaching, and their relationship with their students.

FACTS ABOUT LAUGHTER AND ITS EFFECTS, DURATION, AND UNIVERSALITY

- There is great security in rituals—doing the same things, in the same way, at the same time—such as ending the day or week with a humor session.
- Students take their emotional cues from what they experience in the classroom, which makes the educator the principal orchestrator of students' emotions. Students will adopt the educator's mood as the prevailing mood for the day. This gives even more meaning to our responsibility to model the behavior we want our learners to mirror.

Candace B. Pert, a brain researcher, says that positive emotional experiences are much more likely to be recalled when we're in an upbeat mood, while negative emotional experiences are recalled more easily when we are already in a bad mood. Not only is memory affected by the mood we're in, but so is actual performance. Many studies have proven that laughter and humor can be helpful in delivering curriculum content by gaining and holding the attention of the learner and aiding in the retention of the information presented (Figure 17–1).

Learning and Laughter Defined

learning
to acquire knowledge, understanding, skills, or behavioral tendency by study, instruction, or experience.

laughter
1) the sound of laughing; 2) the cause of merriment, and to *laugh* is 1) to show mirth, joy . . . with a smile; 2) to find amusement or pleasure in something.

Webster's Collegiate Dictionary defines **learning** as "to acquire knowledge, understanding, skills, or behavioral tendency by study, instruction, or experience." It defines **laughter** as "1) the sound of laughing; 2) the cause of merriment," and *laugh* as "1) to show mirth, joy . . . with a smile; 2) to find amusement or pleasure in something." We must acknowledge that laughter and humor are not the same thing. Laughter is the physiological response to humor consisting of two parts. One part is a set of gestures and the other part is the production of sound. Our brains tell us to conduct both simultaneously

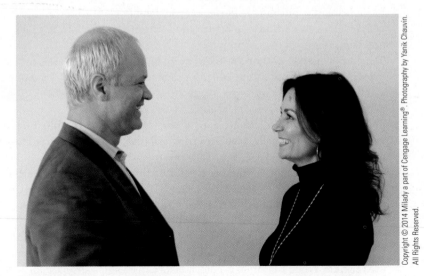

Figure 17–1   A genuine smile is reflected in the mouth, cheeks, facial lines, and eyes.

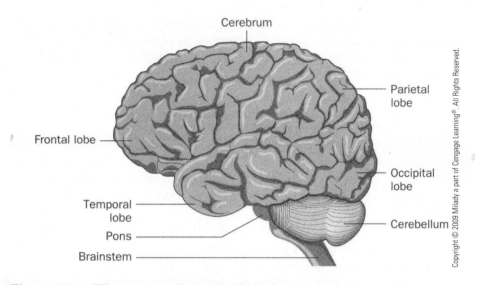

Figure 17–2　When exposed to something funny, the brain produces a regular electrical wave that moves through the cerebral cortex.

to produce a hearty laugh. According to the *Encyclopedia Britannica*, when we laugh heartily our bodies perform rhythmic, vocalized, expiratory, and involuntary actions. For example, 15 facial muscles contract and the zygomatic major muscle is stimulated. The respiratory system becomes upset, the larynx half-closes, tear ducts are activated, the mouth struggles for oxygen, and the face becomes moist and flush. The noises created from this process have a wide range, from a timid laugh to an outlandish guffaw.

Gelotology (from the Greek *gelow*, meaning laughter) is the formal name for the physiological study of humor and laughter and their effects on the human body. Though the relationship between the brain and laughter is not totally understood, researchers are gaining ground. For example, humor researcher Peter Derks traced the pattern of brainwave activity in subjects responding to funny material by connecting them to an electroencephalograph (EEG). He found that the brain produced a regular electrical wave moving through the cerebral cortex within four-tenths of a second of exposure to something funny (Figure 17–2). If the wave took a negative charge, the result was laughter. If a positive charge was maintained, there was no response. Gelotology forecasts that people who laugh a lot have improved health, better overall well-being, and a longer life.

The Purpose of Laughter

To many, the purpose of laughter is to make and strengthen human connections and relationships. More bonding occurs when people are laughing together. Philosopher John Morreall believes that a gesture of shared relief at the passing of danger may have resulted in the first human laughter. His perspective suggests that laughter may indicate a trust in our companions. A number of theories attempt to explain what actually makes us laugh:

- **Incongruity theory.** Laughter occurs when the outcome is different from what is expected.
- **Superiority theory.** Laughter, albeit inappropriate, occurs at the expense of someone else's mistake or misfortune causing us to feel superior.

IT'S WORTH REMEMBERING ✳

When we are enjoying humor and life, there is no time left for judgment and criticism.

gelotology
the formal name for the physiological study of humor and laughter and their effects on the human body.

incongruity theory
laughter occurs when the outcome is different from what is expected.

superiority theory
laughter that, albeit inappropriate, occurs at the expense of someone else's mistake or misfortune causing us to feel superior.

relief theory
laughter that occurs after a long period of tension, stress, suspension, or danger. This aspect of laughter is used in films quite effectively.

spontaneity theory
laughter that occurs as a result of an unplanned, momentary impulse.

- **Relief theory.** Laughter occurs after a long period of tension, stress, suspension, or danger. This theory is used in films quite effectively.
- **Spontaneity theory.** Laughter occurs as a result of an unplanned, momentary impulse.

☑ The Mental Health Benefits of Laughter

Laughter and humor make a significant contribution to both our mental and physical health. If we learn to take advantage of those benefits, we will gain the resilience needed to cope with daily challenges and open ourselves up for maximum learning opportunities. Let's take a look at some mental health benefits of laughter.

Less Stress. Reducing stress improves the body's physical health, and it also improves your mental well-being. The less you have to worry about or feel stressed about, the more balanced your mental attitude will be. Dr. Dale Anderson says that one solid minute of laughter is worth about 40 minutes of deep relaxation (Figure 17–3).

Reduced Anger and Anxiety. It has been said that you can't express two emotions at the same time. You cannot feel anger or anxiety while you also feel excitement and happiness. Think about it … and based on what we now know about endorphins, all we have to do is pretend to be happy and—voila—we become happy!

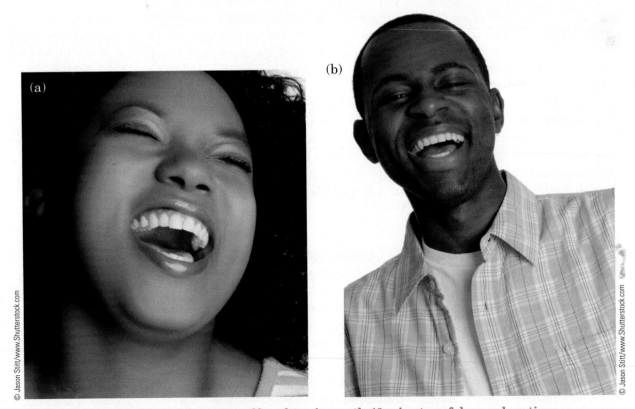

(a)

(b)

© Jason Stitt/www.Shutterstock.com

© Jason Stitt/www.Shutterstock.com

Figures 17–3a, b   One solid minute of laughter is worth 40 minutes of deep relaxation.

Increased Joy and Liveliness. Joy starts within. Joy confirms your self-worth and is reflected by a job well done and a positive attitude. If you've got a problem, why not write a silly song about it to increase your liveliness?

More Positive and Optimistic Mood. If we take an attitude of "playing" with serious events, life becomes so much more positive. There is a story about a gentleman who, in preparation for a serious surgical procedure, had his entire body shaved. When the operating room staff removed the sheet prior to the surgery, they discovered he had placed his toupee over his private parts. The result was uproarious laughter. This man was not stupid: He understood that laughter engages both sides of the brain and he wanted to ensure everyone in that operating room was thinking and performing at their maximum potential!

Greater Sense of Control. When we do some of the things we have been discussing here, we have a greater mastery over our own lives. Instead of letting the circumstances control us, we are controlling them. The next time you're experiencing high anxiety, give it a name like Nervous Nancy or Anxious Arthur. You might even take it one step further and develop a phrase or tag line to go with the name.

Emotional Release. Humans often store negative emotions such as sadness, fear, and anger rather than expressing them. Laughter can actually provide a harmless release of these emotions. Laughter is cathartic. Watching a funny movie or reading a hilarious book that produces loud rounds of laughter can wash away the negative emotions.

Work-Related Benefits of Laughter

In addition to the mental health benefits just discussed, laughter can also have a positive effect in the workplace, as discussed next.

Improved Team Building and Communication Skills. Laughter is the universal language. The message gets sent regardless of language, age, and cultural background. Consider the fact that "inside jokes" may lead to team-building. The first time a new employee laughs with a coworker is usually the first time he feels like part of the team in a new environment.

Better Conflict Management. It's much harder to disagree or argue with someone with whom you can also laugh. Humor helps us find a mutual ground.

Greater Morale and Job Satisfaction. Humor and laughter promote a much more "light hearted" environment within which to work. Plus, when you do a great job and everyone shares in your joy and success, morale soars for everyone.

Enhanced Creativity and Problem Solving. If you are negative and pessimistic, it is highly unlikely that you're going to be effective in coming up with creative new approaches to your daily challenges.

Resilience. Bouncing back and learning to adopt a lighter attitude to see the funny side of everyday situations gives you the resilience you need to cope on the tough days.

Stress Management and Productivity. We've already talked about how laughter can reduce stress. As another approach to our being in control, we can take proactive steps to reducing stress by doing things to manage issues and prevent crises.

CONSIDER AND CONNECT

A humorous suggestion to deal with anger is to write the name of the thing or the person who has made you angry on some masking tape and then tape it to the bottom of your shoe and walk all over it!

Physical Health Benefits of Laughter

Laughter also provides benefits for our physical health.

Strengthens the Immune System. We've established that our bodies produce endorphins that are also sometimes referred to as the "opiates of optimism." Endorphins encourage feelings of optimism and well-being, and those feelings reinforce positive attitudes. The process of choosing to stimulate our endorphin production is not unlike what Victor Frankl said when he wrote of his experiences in the Nazi concentration camps that everything can be taken from a man . . . but the last of the human freedoms is to choose one's own attitude in any given set of circumstances, to choose one's own way. What a powerful thought. So, to sum it up, laughter, good feelings, and endorphins strengthen the immune system and help reduce pain and unpleasant stimuli

Improved Physical Health. Laughter may lead to coughing and hiccups, which clear the respiratory tract. It also increases the concentration of salivary immunoglobulin A, which protects the body against infectious organisms entering the respiratory tract. It lowers the amount of residual air in the lungs, replacing it with oxygen-rich air. This reduces the level of water vapor and carbon dioxide in the lungs, thereby reducing the risk of pulmonary infection. Laughter provides an excellent source of cardiac exercise.

Reduces Stress Hormones. Laughter has been shown to lower the level of stress hormones (epinephrine, cortisol, dopac, and growth hormone) in the blood, temporarily lower blood pressure, and reduce pain. As Groucho Marx put it, "A clown is like an aspirin, only he works twice as fast."

Increased Weight Loss. Hearty laughter is like internal jogging because everything north of the diaphragm moves. The more you laugh, the more you move back and forth, getting a good body work out. The lungs take in more oxygen, breathing deepens, and the heart rate increases. Research indicates that 100 hearty laughs burn the same amount of calories as a 10-minute jog, 10 minutes on the rowing machine, or 15 minutes on an exercise bike (Figure 17–4). Laughing sounds like a whole lot more fun!

This Thing Called Stress

Stress has been defined as a physical, chemical, or emotional factor that causes bodily or mental tension and may be an aspect in the cause of disease. *Webster's Dictionary* goes on to say that stress is the inability to cope with a threat, real or imagined, to our well-being that results in a series of responses and adaptations by our minds and bodies. Stress is said to be the most common and rampant "physical disorder" in our country today. In fact, it has been classified as a worldwide epidemic by the World Health Organization. The medical costs alone have been estimated in the United States at well over $1 billion per year. Stress costs industry $150 billion per year in increased health insurance outlays, burnout, absenteeism, reduced productivity, costly mistakes at work, poor morale, and high employee turnover, as well as family problems and alcohol- and drug-related problems.

IT'S WORTH REMEMBERING ✳

Professor William Fry of Stanford University says that when laughter gets to the point where it is called "convulsive," almost every muscle in the body is involved. And that includes the important muscle called the heart!

CONSIDER AND CONNECT

It is hard to believe the impact stress has on the world when sometimes all it takes is some good gut-wrenching laughter to alleviate it!

stress
a physical, chemical, or emotional factor that causes bodily or mental tension and may be an aspect in the cause of disease; the inability to cope with a threat, real or imagined, to our well-being that results in a series of responses and adaptations by our minds and bodies.

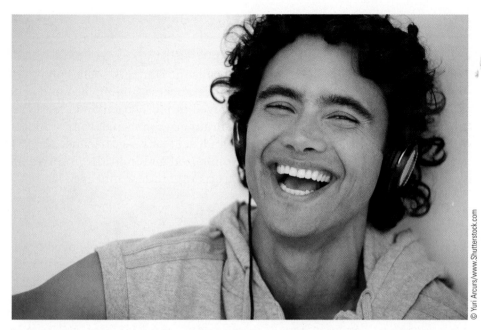

Figure 17–4   A hundred hearty laughs burn the same amount of calories as 10 minutes of jogging or rowing.

THE FOUR STAGES OF HUMOR COMPETENCE

In psychology, the four stages of competence relate to the psychological states involved in the process of progressing from incompetence to competence in a skill or ability.

1. **Unconscious incompetence.** The educator neither understands how to interject humor in the educational process nor recognizes the deficit, or doesn't have a desire to address it. At this stage, individuals don't appear to have a sense of humor, and the humor they do display is negative and demeaning.
2. **Conscious incompetence.** Though the educator does not understand or know how to effectively interject humor into the educational process, he does recognize the deficit and seeks ways to achieve higher levels in this area.
3. **Conscious competence.** The educator understands or knows how to interject humor into the educational process. He possesses both a sense of humor and sensitivity to humor. However, demonstrating the humor requires a great deal of effort and concentration.
4. **Unconscious competence.** The educator has had so much practice with using humor in the classroom that it becomes "second nature" and can be performed easily (often without concentrating too deeply). The educator's humor is spontaneous, warm, and appropriate.

The goal of every educator should be to grow to at least conscious competence. Eventually, your skills will become innate and your natural wit will abound.

unconscious (humor) incompetence
the educator neither understands how to interject humor in the educational process nor recognizes the deficit, or doesn't have a desire to address it. At this stage, individuals don't appear to have a sense of humor, and the humor they do display is negative and demeaning.

conscious (humor) incompetence
though the educator does not understand or know how to effectively interject humor into the educational process, he does recognize the deficit and seeks ways to achieve higher levels in this area.

conscious (humor) competence
the educator understands or knows how to interject humor into the educational process. He possesses both a sense of humor and sensitivity to humor. However, demonstrating the humor requires a great deal of effort and concentration.

unconscious (humor) competence
the educator has had so much practice with using humor in the classroom that it becomes "second nature" and can be performed easily (often without concentrating too deeply). The educator's humor is spontaneous, warm, and appropriate.

✓ Laughter Enhances Creativity

We have already established that laughter activates the limbic system of the brain. This system is important because it controls some behaviors that are essential to the life of all mammals, such as finding food and self-preservation. In humans, it is more involved in motivation and emotional behaviors. Thus, when both sides of the brain are connected, your students will do more brain work. On the other hand, acute stress can cause the two hemispheres of the brain to become disconnected and limit the brain's ability. Therefore, it is sound pedagogy to incorporate humor into each lesson.

What Is an Idea?

Before we can spend much time on improving our creativity, we need to explore how it actually starts. All great things and all great progress begin with an idea (Figure 17–5). By now it's probably clear to you that a common reference for this book is Merriam *Webster's Dictionary*, which defines an **idea** in a number of different ways, including: "a transcendent entity that is a real pattern of which existing things are imperfect representations" (now that tells us a lot!) and "a formulated thought or opinion" (that is a little more like it!). However, if you ask ordinary folks to define *idea*, you hear things like, "it's when you're thinking and the light bulb goes on" or "it's whatever the mind can conceive." In the world of brainstorming, we call it **hitchhiking**: taking the idea or information from another and hitchhiking or piggybacking off of it. A colleague once said, "There is really no new information, just old ideas with a new twist." When you think about it, that's the truth. Look at all the great recipes in the world. Most of them started with a basic recipe from grandma's kitchen and we took them and started adding ingredients and changing things until they became something uniquely new. If we look at all the great inventions in the world, we'll see that concept over and over. Henry Ford took the idea of a horse and buggy and the chain drive of a bicycle to design the first automobile. Reese combined peanut butter with chocolate to create the ever-popular candy. Eight-year-old Chelsea Lannon invented the pocket diaper in 1994, which holds a baby wipe and baby powder puff (combining items found in a diaper bag with the diaper). She got the idea while helping her mother with her baby brother while she was still in kindergarten.

As an educator, this author has been privileged to present to literally thousands of educators and professionals over the years. A routine part of those presentations have involved teams engaging in brainstorming and group activities. Without a doubt, the teams that came up with the most creative ideas were the teams that were having the most fun in the discovery process! The fun came first; the good ideas came second. Jerry Greenfield of Ben and Jerry's Ice Cream once said, "If it isn't fun, why do it?"

Inspiring an Idea

If we consider the traditional educational process, it is not designed to inspire creativity or critical thinking, is it? We have basically been taught to

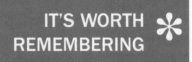

IT'S WORTH REMEMBERING

It has been suggested that life is simply too important to take it too seriously.

idea
a formulated thought or opinion.

hitchhiking
taking an idea or information from another and hitchhiking or piggybacking off of it.

IT'S WORTH REMEMBERING

Great ideas can come from anywhere.

look for only one key solution. Think of all the tests you have taken throughout school. The majority of them had only one correct answer per question. We may be doing our students a disservice by not asking them for multiple ideas on an issue rather than just one. Jack Foster, in his book *How to Get Ideas*, states that if we want to help our students become "idea prone," we must get them to accept two things. First, they must accept that what they think about themselves is the single most important factor in their success. Second, they must accept that human beings can alter their lives by altering their attitudes.

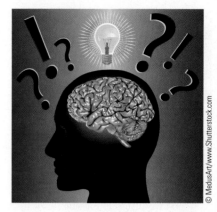

Figure 17–5 **All great progress begins with an idea.**

If learners begin to like themselves and alter their attitude to one of seeking knowledge and ideas in a positive light, there will be no end to their creativity. Positive self-talk can help a student get there. Perhaps we should have students write at least 10 positive self-talk statements to get them started. Five examples follow:

- I am energetic, always in a great mood, and well rested.
- I look great, and I feel even better; I am a happy person.
- I use my talent, my skills, and my sense of humor to make life grand.
- I wake up every day saying that it is a great day to be alive.
- I have an open mind that is creative and ready to rock and roll!
- I am talented, skilled, and powerful!!
- I can change the world!!!

The concept of self-talk is a powerful one. Our brains work something like a computer. If we tell the brain something over and over again, the brain begins to accept it as fact. So, our students have the option of telling themselves that they have no imagination and aren't creative, or they can tell themselves daily that they are creative, talented, and successful, either of which will become a self-fulfilling prophecy. We must also teach our students that positive self-talk must always be performed in the personal tense, the present tense, and with enthusiasm. None of the examples provided earlier indicates that the goal will be achieved in the future; instead all use the present tense. Then we must teach our students to visualize the praise and accolades they will receive when they actually accomplish the goal. They need to believe the ideas are already in their heads—not that they will eventually get them.

The Origins of Imagination

You may have heard your students say, "I just wasn't born with an imagination." Not true. Everyone is born with an imagination and the ability to be creative (Figure 17–6). If you have ever doubted that, give an ordinary stick to a four-year-old and stand back and watch. The stick will become everything from a horse to a sword, a magic wand to a gun, or a walking stick to something to write in the sand with. Perhaps we should take a lesson from this and never act our age, but play the role of a child and let the creative ideas flow. Psychologist Jean Piaget said, "If you would be more creative, stay the part of the child with the creativity and invention that characterizes children before they are deformed by adult society."

One of the ways we can aid our students in being more creative and having a more vivid imagination is by having them do things they don't normally do. Zig Ziglar said that a rut is nothing but a grave with the

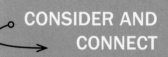

CONSIDER AND CONNECT

History repeatedly shows that having fun enhances creativity. As educators we must share that message so our students can get the powerful ideas they need to succeed.

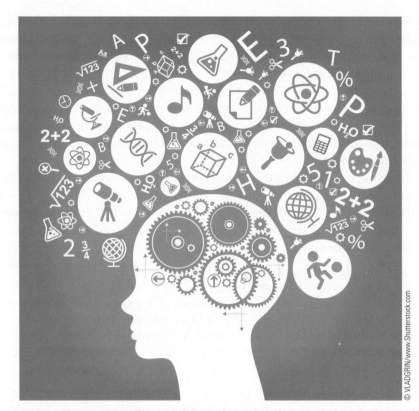

Figure 17–6   **Everyone is born with an imagination and the ability to be creative.**

ends kicked out. The fact is that most of us allow routine to take over our lives. One of the ways that we can break out of our rut is to try something different. Drive to work or school by a different route. Brush your teeth using your nondominant hand. Eat something totally unusual for breakfast. Read a magazine you've never heard of before. Learn something new like sign language or a foreign language. Study nature. Think of all you see and learn and experience. Play a vocabulary game with the dictionary instead of spending the evening in front of the television. Work on your observation skills: start to notice details about even simple things, such as which numbers on the phone have which letters of the alphabet.

What If?

We need to take care not to let the fear of rejection shut down our idea factory. We need to instill in our students that there are no bad ideas, and if one doesn't work, they can get another one, and it will probably be better than the last one. Our dynamic learners will ask this question naturally, "What if?" We need to help instill that curiosity in our other learners as well. When they learn a concept, we want them to think about what would happen if they combined that technique with another. It is when they start combining ideas that their creative juices will start to flow.

Another simple strategy must be conveyed to our students in the area of creativity development: ask and do. We need to instill in our students the passion for knowledge gained through asking questions. The more they learn about a subject, the more they can creatively apply the knowledge. Then they must take action. We need to get them thinking that there is always more than one answer to a problem. For example, one group of students was asked what half of 19 was and, after being challenged, the class came up with nearly 20 different answers ranging from 9.5 to 9 1/2 to "5," with the explanation for the latter response being that 1 and 9 equal 10, and half of 10 is 5. The point is that there is always another answer.

Many people find that they get their most creative ideas at a certain time or when they are performing a certain task. However, most of us experience blocks in the creative process from time to time. This can happen when students are studying or when they are trying to come up with a new creative approach to a problem. We need to teach them to stop working on that particular project, thought, subject, or idea and move on to something else. Rather than just relaxing, they should continue working on another important task so as not to stop the momentum of the mental process.

Finally, when helping our students to develop their creativity, we want to emphasize the importance of taking action. Too often, we have a great idea, we share it with someone who says, "That's a great idea," and we go on with our lives and never do anything about it. If that's the case, we might as well never have had the idea at all. We need to give ourselves a deadline, put together a list of required tasks, prioritize them into an action plan, and *take action*! When the "yeah buts" begin, we are the only ones that can do anything about them. For example, we have a great idea and we want to put it into action, but we never get it done. Isn't it human nature to come up with a "yeah but?" For instance, we might say, "Yeah but, I just didn't have enough time to make it happen" or "Yeah but, I just didn't have enough money to get it done." If that's the case, we need to get up an hour earlier every day, which basically adds a full work day to our week, or we need to borrow the needed funds to move forward. Whatever we do, though, we need to make sure we are having fun in the process.

Integrating Humor into the Workplace

We could all take a lesson from the world famous Pike Place Fish Market in Seattle, which, back in the 1980s, set forth a goal to be famous. The folks at Pike Place accomplished their goal not by spending a single dollar in advertising, but by interacting with their customers from the perspective of making a difference for them and improving their lives, not just selling them fish. They are dedicated to having fun and creating excitement while they work, and that has made them world famous. You can go to www.pikeplacefish.com and actually view webcams of these great people having fun while they work. They send a powerful message that could benefit us all.

CONSIDER AND CONNECT

When students experience a block in the creative process, they may need to stand up and walk away or give five minutes to daydreaming, but they should get right back into their work.

IT'S WORTH REMEMBERING

A spirited and fun work environment is branded with laughter. Happy team members are open to risk and challenge to make what they do even better.

EDUCATORS CAN CREATE A FUN WORK ENVIRONMENT

Try the following tips for creating a fun work environment:
- Keep goofy toys at your desk or workstation and play with them periodically.
- Use funny visualizations to help you keep things in perspective.
- Spend five minutes laughing on the way to work.
- Wear temporary, light hearted, or funny tattoos.
- Spend 10 minutes in a huddle with your coworkers before beginning the day, at least 3 of which are spent laughing as a group.
- Communicate with cartoons.
- Choose different funny hats to express your mood or attitude.

Integrating Humor into the Classroom

Since we have already established the importance of humor and laughter and how the brain works, it stands to reason that educators should carefully integrate humor into curriculum delivery. Following are some examples that might be implemented:

- **Build a "Mirth-Aid Kit."** Remember, mirth is gladness shown by laughter. Put together a nice big box with, perhaps, a red cross on it, and name it your Mirth-Aid Kit. Store all types of goofy items and toys in it, such as Groucho Marx glasses, finger puppets, silly hats, a red clown nose, a rubber chicken, stress balls, a Tickle Me Elmo toy, and/or other mechanical toys that dance or sing. Periodically throughout a class, pull something from the Mirth Aid Kit and use it.
- **Create a Joy Jar or Silly Sack.** Use humor to label the jar or sack, such as with a smiley face. Collect jokes and funny stories, making sure to keep them generic and rated G. Allow students to participate in collecting jokes and stories once you have explained the rules. Whenever the classroom mood requires a change of pace, have a student come up and pull out one of the entries and read it to the rest of the class.
- **Create an Inspirational Insights Container.** Like humor, inspirational stories can create feelings of safety, comfort, and warmth. This works just like the Joy Jar, but contains inspirational stories such as "children on love."
- **Show Video Clips.** Keep a watchful eye for great clips in movies and television that you can record and present during specific lessons. For example, the scene from *Beautician and the Beast* when the cosmetology clinic catches on fire might be fun to use when teaching safety.
- Wear a goofy hat for part of your presentation (Figure 17–7).
- Have students count how many times they laugh during a day.
- Have students list the positive things that happened the day before and share them with a partner.
- Schedule play time during the work day. It could be doing a five-minute line dance in the clinic or having a short relay race in the parking lot.
- Have your students give their curriculum projects funny names, like Elmer Fudd or Quasimoto.

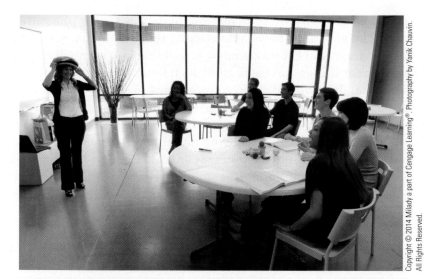

Figure 17–7   Create humor in the classroom by wearing a goofy hat.

- Suggest students wear a humorous T-shirt under their lab jackets to lighten them up (if the school's dress code permits).
- Incorporate elements of games into the classes, such as Jeopardy, Hangman, crossword puzzle competitions, Pictionary, or What's My Line?
- Award token prizes to volunteers and winners of competitions.
- Have students create different prize categories and create prizes for monthly awards for categories such as: Most Enthusiastic, Best Attitude, Funniest, Best Attendance, Best Grades, Best Partner, Most Prompt, Best Helper, and so forth. Let the students vote on the winners (except attendance and grades, of course).
- Create a selection of assignments and allow the students to choose the one they want to complete.
- Have students write silly songs about serious subjects, such as skin diseases.
- Encourage students to do at least one silly, nonconforming thing each day.
- Buy a CD of laughter, a laugh box, or a laughing toy and periodically play it throughout the day.
- Encourage student participation in creating fun and entertaining ways to learn.
- Wear fluorescent purple false eyelashes, or something equally unexpected, to class.
- Schedule hilarity breaks.

Wrapping It Up

In this chapter, we noted that science has found laughter to be a form of internal jogging that exercises the body and stimulates beneficial brain neurotransmitters and hormones. A positive outlook and laughter are good for our health. Children laugh about 400 times per day, while their adult counterparts only laugh about 15 times per day. Somehow, as we grow older, we manage to lose over 95 percent of our laughter. Now that is something to be sad about. The good side, however, is that it is simple to fix. All we have to do is fake a laugh, and before we know it, genuine laughter will abound and all sorts of great things will begin to happen to us.

Humor has been found to be so important in our lives that humorist and author Larry Wilde, Director of the Carmel Institute of Humor, founded National Humor Month in April of 1976. The aim of the program is to promote the value of humor in improving health and enriching the quality of life. How exciting that as educators we can contribute to the enriched lives of our students by using humor as an effective teaching tool! Wilde recommends that we should all take a humor break, laugh at ourselves, and create a funny file all our own.

In Retrospect

1. List the best conditions for learning.

2. Define learning, laughter, and laugh.

3. Explain the theories of what makes us laugh.

4. List the mental, physical, and workplace benefits of laughter.

5. Explain the four stages of humor competence.

6. Identify strategies for combining ideas and letting creative juices flow.

7. List ways to integrate humor into the workplace and classroom.

Teaching Success Strategies for a Winning Career

Objectives (Desired Performance Goals):

After reading and studying this chapter, you should be able to:

- List the six strategies and principles to achieve a winning career.

- List specific actions students can use to pay value to themselves.

- List specific actions students can use for self-motivation.

- List specific actions students can use for expecting to win.

- List specific strategies students can use to manage their goals.

- List specific methods students can follow to adopt a strong work ethic.

- List specific methods students can follow to value their clients.

! CRITICAL CONCEPT

Some succeed because they are destined to, but most succeed because they are determined to.

MASTER EDUCATOR

1. Teaches students the valuable soft skills necessary to achieve success in the workplace.
2. Teaches students to define what success means to them.
3. Inspires students to create a successful life and career by envisioning a future and building a plan of action to get there.

Success Is a Choice

IT HAS ALREADY BEEN established that only about 15 percent to 20 percent of our students' success will be achieved as a result of their highly polished technical skills while the other 80 percent to 85 percent will be derived from personal qualities such as strong goal orientations, visual integrity, people skills, and effective work habits (Figure 18–1). Thus, this chapter is dedicated to defining six success strategies that educators can instill in their learners to help them achieve the level of career success they all desire. In Chapter 1 of the *Master Educator*, the profile of a career education instructor was presented. Many of the qualities and characteristics discussed in that chapter are also relevant to the success of our students and graduates, so a quick review of that chapter might also be appropriate at this time.

Our first step is to congratulate our students for having made a life-altering decision to attend school and change their futures. How they manage that decision will determine what their futures hold. It is our responsibility to make them understand that the behavioral habits they develop *now* while they are in school will determine whether each student's career shines with success and prosperity or whether it is one of barely getting by and mediocrity. They must understand that the choice is theirs—just like it is our choice as teachers to achieve excellence or just be average.

The next step is to find out how our students view success. Merriam *Webster's Dictionary* suggests that success is reaching a desired outcome or result, such as the attainment of wealth, favor, or eminence. To effectively convey success strategies for students to achieve a winning career, you must first have students define what success means to them. Once that has been accomplished, you can effectively facilitate the strategies presented here. Let them know that you are speaking from experience by sharing with them a little about your own career and successes, thus establishing your credibility. Then the focus must be shifted back to the learners.

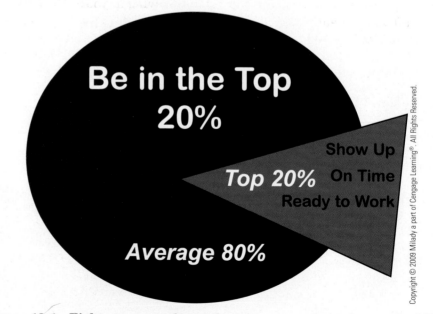

Figure 18–1   Eighty percent of a graduate's success depends on soft skills.

A great deal of research has been conducted throughout history to determine the qualities and characteristics that set highly accomplished, successful individuals apart from those who barely make it. This chapter will attempt to summarize much of that research into six principles or strategies your students can follow to achieve a winning career.

SIX STRATEGIES AND PRINCIPLES TO ACHIEVE A WINNING CAREER

1. Value Yourself.
2. Motivate Yourself.
3. Expect to Win.
4. Manage Your Goals.
5. Adopt a Strong Work Ethic.
6. Value the Client.

Value Yourself

We have noted numerous times in this text that if we could instill in our students a strong, healthy self-esteem and a love of learning, our jobs as educators would not be work anymore. It is exciting to think of the obstacles and challenges we would avoid if our students liked themselves and loved to learn. **Values** are the core thoughts and feelings we have about ourselves and about life (Figure 18–2). It is these values that lead us to make decisions and take actions. Highly successful people have a strong inner feeling of their own worth and value. They understand what they believe in and stand for. They like and hold themselves in high esteem. Behavior and performance are usually consistent with self-image. Our imagination creates and improves self-image. We have to be able to see ourselves doing something to actually do it. Knowing who you are and what you value gives you the ability to triumph over any adversity. Believing in yourself allows you to use all your potential to take the action needed to progress and achieve results. As with self-motivation, taking action strengthens feelings of self-value because of the sense of accomplishment. With confidence comes the willingness to take even bolder actions, which will likely result in greater achievement. The whole process is cyclical. It might be considered the winner's circle of self-esteem.

values
principles, standards, or qualities considered worthwhile or desirable.

IT'S WORTH REMEMBERING

Successful people like and accept themselves unconditionally and imagine the person they would most like to become. Then they become that person.

Self-Assessment for Valuing Yourself

Students must identify what they view as their core values and how they view themselves in order to build a strong self-belief and sense of self-esteem. They should ask themselves a series of questions, such as:

1. What are my five most important values?
2. Do I like myself as I am, or would I rather be someone else?
3. Does my ego overwhelm my humility?
4. Do I accept compliments and praise graciously?
5. Do I give compliments and praise sincerely?

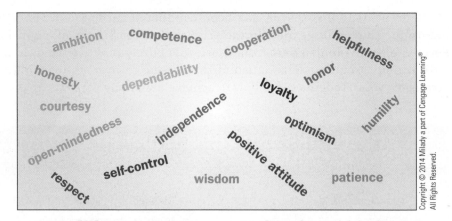

Figure 18–2   Values represent our core thoughts and feelings.

Actions for Valuing Yourself

After your students have performed the self-assessment, they need to identify actions for increasing their own self-worth. Examples include the following:

- **Sit up Front.** The next time you go to a class or a meeting, take a seat right in the front row (Figure 18–3). After all, your purpose in going is to listen, learn, and possibly interact with the speaker or teacher.
- **Practice Proper Posture and Look Your Best.** Stand tall, walk erectly, and practice professional deportment. This behavior portrays self-confidence, and when you act self-confident, your confidence grows. Regardless of peer pressure, look and dress your best at all times. Your appearance provides an instant outward projection of how you feel about yourself internally.
- **Set Personal Standards.** Put your five most important values in priority order and commit to living by them (Figure 18–4). Be mindful

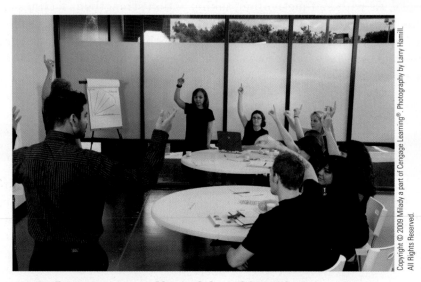

Figure 18–3   Improve your self-worth by taking a front-row seat.

My Values

As a professional educator, I am committed to the following five values:

Loyalty

Honor

Integrity

Dependability

Optimism

Figure 18–4   Identify and commit to living by your personal values.

of constantly improving your standards. For example, upgrade your personal grooming and image. Take stock of your lifestyle and identify areas for improvement. Work on improvement in your relationships.

- **Pay Value to Your Name.** State your name at the beginning of every phone call. Introduce yourself first whenever you meet someone new. Paying value to your own name when you are communicating helps you develop the habit of paying value to yourself as a human being.
- **Plan Your Growth.** Everyone should have a personal improvement plan in action at all times. Take the time to write down the actions needed for self-improvement and identify the knowledge you will need to accomplish them.
- **Say Thank You.** When someone pays value to you with a sincere compliment, accept it with a simple and courteous "thank you." People often minimize compliments because they are uncomfortable accepting them graciously. For example, someone might tell you they really like the dress you are wearing, and you respond with something like, "Oh, I think it makes me look 10 pounds heavier." Not only does this type of response disrespect you, but it also suggests to the person paying the compliment that it was meaningless.
- **Smile.** In every language and culture, a smile is understood. It is a universal symbol that, for the most part, indicates everything is okay. It makes the giver feel good and it makes the receiver want to give one back.

Motivate Yourself

Our students must cultivate an attitude of positive expectancy, develop an attitude of abundance, and create a definite purpose for their lives. As educators, we have the awesome responsibility of helping them understand that true motivation is internal. All the many external motivators such as pep rallies or inspirational speakers will only last as long as it takes to find out we have a flat tire waiting in the parking lot. The fuel for self-motivation lies in our dreams, ideals, and visions for the future. Self-motivation can be compared to the desire for change, excitement, and personal urges that are absolutely critical to success. It is unrealistic to rely solely on others to encourage us when we face difficult times. We need self-motivation to get us through and keep us from becoming depressed. We can't expect or count on others to encourage us to accept opportunity and challenge. We are, indeed, lucky if we have family and friends who do so, but if we depend on ourselves,

self-motivation motivation fueled by one's dreams, ideals, and visions for the future.

fear
a feeling of alarm or disquiet caused by the expectation of danger, pain, disaster, or the like; terror; dread; apprehension.

desire
a wish, longing, or craving; something longed for.

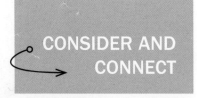

CONSIDER AND CONNECT

We must look to where we want to go or what we want to be and focus on the benefits of success. Then we must put together an action plan to get there.

we are less likely to be disappointed and we can better control the outcome. Self-motivation helps us plan and find direction in our lives, take up new activities, maintain enthusiasm about life, and have the courage to see things through in spite of negativity or setbacks.

Fear and **desire** are among life's greatest motivators. Our students need to recognize that fear can be destructive, but desire, if properly managed, will lead to achievement, success, and satisfaction. It is important to realize that people are actually like magnets. We are pushed away from or pulled toward people and ideas, whether negative or positive. We must make a concerted effort to move away from negative influences and move toward positive concepts such as achieving goals and solutions.

Self-Assessment for Internal Motivation

For students to understand where they stand with regard to self-motivation, they should ask themselves a series of questions, such as:

1. What do I desire most in life?
2. What am I most afraid of?
3. How do my fears affect my life?
4. What emphasis do I place on my desires?
5. Do I see the benefits of success and understand the penalty of failure?

Actions for Self-Motivation

All of us experience times when we just simply do not feel motivated. We have to make a choice. There is a lovely story about a 92-year-old woman who is arriving at a nursing home. She tells the attendant that she loves her new room even though she has not seen it yet. She goes on to explain that happiness is something you decide on ahead of time. She says that whether she likes the room is not based on how it is arranged, but how she arranges her mind. She made the point that she makes a choice every day when she wakes up as to whether she will spend the day in bed recounting the difficulty she has with the parts of her body that no longer work or get out of bed and be thankful for the parts that do. She went on to say that old age is like a bank account—you withdraw from it what you have put in. So her advice was to deposit a lot of happiness in your bank account of memories. What a powerful story! It is important that our students have a reserve of strategic actions they can take to renew their self-motivation, such as the following:

- **Make Positive Choices.** As mentioned in the story being positive is a conscious choice that only each individual can make.
- **Block Negativity.** External forces such as negative thoughts and ideas must be eliminated. It is important to maintain your mental balance and avoid nervousness and depression.
- **List Accomplishments.** Focus on accomplishments you have already achieved. Nothing can make you feel more positive or motivated than identifying all the goals you have already attained.
- **Do What You Enjoy.** Think about giving priority to doing something that you love doing. Perhaps there is a hobby you have always wanted to take up, but never allowed yourself the time. Do it now.

- **Change Your Vocabulary.** Your vocabulary can have a major impact on your attitude. Eliminate negativity. Do not use words like *can't* or *yeah, but*. Replace them with *can* and *that works*. Dwell on things you are going to *do* rather than things you are going to *try*. Make a habit of using positive self-talk regularly.

- **List Your Desires.** Give some thought to at least five things you desire most and create a three-column chart. List the desires and next to them list the payoff or benefit of achieving that desire. In the third column, list the first step you need to take to attain the desire. Once you have taken that first step, your self-motivation will soar.

- **Review Your Successes.** Sit down and make a list of all your accomplishments. If you think you don't have any, start with the beginning of your life. You learned to walk and talk. You learned to read and write and do math. You learned to drive. So, make the list and reflect on how those successes and accomplishments made you feel. Pat yourself on the back and tell yourself that you are terrific!

- **Learn Something New.** Nothing is more motivating than learning. If there is something you always wanted to do or experience, begin to work on it. Seek out individuals who are expert on the subject. Conduct Internet research on the topic or task. Make a project of learning everything you can about people who are successful at it already. Take a course or lessons to generate excitement and then visualize yourself succeeding at your interest.

- **Read Inspirational Books.** Listen to motivational tapes and CDs. Watch motivational movies, such as *Rudy or Pollyanna*. This will help improve your attitude and heal your mind (Figure 18–5). Spend time perusing the self-help section of the local bookstore and read a new book each week or month. Identify at least five ideas you glean from each that will help you achieve your desired success.

- **Concentrate on Success.** When you start a project and take any action toward achieving your desires, give yourself to it 100 percent. Concentrate all your energy and intensity on the achievement of the goal. Reward yourself along the way and celebrate your successes.

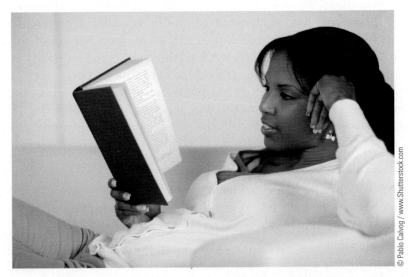

Figure 18–5   Reading inspirational books will improve your attitude and mind.

☑ Expect to Win

CONSIDER AND CONNECT

It stands to reason that if
the idea of self-fulfilling
prophecy works in the
negative, it can also work
in the positive.

pedagogical tool
any tool or aid used in the
art of preparatory training or
instruction.

CONSIDER AND CONNECT

Think of positive self-
expectancy as optimism,
enthusiasm, and hope. When
we fill ourselves with these
positive emotions and
attitudes, there is no room
for fear and anxiety,
which lead to stress.

Winners know that life is a **self-fulfilling prophecy**. We usually get what we actively expect. Twentieth-century sociologist Robert K. Merton is credited with coining the expression "self-fulfilling prophecy." He determined that a false prophetic statement (a prophecy declared as truth when it is not) may sufficiently influence people, either through fear or logical confusion, so that their reactions ultimately fulfill the false prophecy. In his book *Social Theory and Social Structure*, he creates a fictional bank owned by Cartwright Millingville. It is a typical bank, which Millingville has run honestly and properly. As a result, it has liquid assets (cash), but most of its assets are invested in various ventures. One day, a large number of customers come to the bank at once, the exact reason is never made clear. Customers, seeing so many people at the bank, begin to worry. False rumors spread that something is wrong with the bank and more customers rush to the bank to try to get some of their money out while they still can. The number of customers at the bank increases, as does their annoyance and excitement, which in turn fuels the false rumors of the bank's insolvency and upcoming bankruptcy, causing more customers to come and try to withdraw their money. At the beginning of the day, the bank was solvent. But the rumor of insolvency caused a sudden demand of withdrawal of too many customers, which could not be answered, causing the bank to become insolvent and declare bankruptcy.

If we expect to win and see ourselves winning, we may have a greater chance of achieving that success. Further, there is significant research into the effects of the use of self-fulfilling prophecy theories by teachers. It is recommended that teachers read Rosenthal and Jacobson's *Pygmalion in the Classroom* (1968) to learn more about how to use the Pygmalion effect or the self-fulfilling prophecy as a purposeful **pedagogical tool** to convey positive expectations and to avoid conveying negative expectations. As educators, we need to expect our students to succeed and avoid prejudging their performance from a negative perspective. We need to form positive expectations of our students and express clearly what behavior and achievement we expect from them. We need to be consistent in helping our students shape their behavior and achievement into what is expected. If we treat all our students as if they are successful, they will more likely become successful.

We know that stress actually changes the body's production of hormones and antibodies and reduces our resistance to illness and even accidents. On the other hand, if our focus is on harmony and balance, we will be healthier and more energetic. If we expect to win, we naturally develop the ability to attract the cooperation of others in the achievement of our career goals.

Self-Assessment for Expecting to Win

For students to fully grasp the concept of expecting to win, they need to take a close look at their perspective of life. They should ask themselves a series of questions, such as:

1. Am I optimistic (expecting the best possible outcome) or pessimistic (expecting the worst possible outcome)?
2. Am I generally more negative or more positive?
3. Am I healthy or sickly?

4. Do I view challenges as roadblocks or opportunities for growth?
5. Am I a "Gloomy Gus" when things go wrong or do I learn from the mistake and go forward?

Actions for Expecting to Win

After your students have performed their self-assessment, they need to consider actions for improving their expectations for success. For example:

- **Practice Optimism.** Plan on starting your day by saying, "It's a great day to be alive." Choose to be happy. Don't let negativity steal your day. Play upbeat music and sing and dance to it in the shower. Post inspirational quotes on your mirror. Listen to motivational CDs. Surround yourself with optimism and optimistic people.

- **Count Your Blessings.** Elsewhere in this book we have discussed the importance of keeping a grateful journal. We could take a lesson from the little girl in the movie *Pollyanna*, who played the Glad Game. She chose to see the good side of even the worst situations. In one scene all the household staff of her embittered aunt spent a great deal of time outlining the numerous negative aspects of Sundays and then challenged her to find just one positive thing about the dreadful day. After a few moments of thought, she said she was glad it was six whole days until Sunday came around again. The point is, that for every negative thing that happens to us, there is likely at least one positive thing that we can make our focus.

- **Develop and Use Positive Affirmations.** These are statements repeated daily that help manifest a more positive reality in our lives. They must always be stated in the personal and in the present tense with a great deal of enthusiasm. By using positive affirmations, we can harness the power of words and use them to our benefit. They can be as simple as, "I choose joy today," "I am successful," or "I am a happy, healthy, enthusiastic, energetic, and accomplished professional."

- **Define Your Challenges.** Think about any circumstances that may be creating barriers to your success. Write a one-line definition that describes the barrier, such as, "My car is broken down and I have no way to get to work." Then use your creativity to rewrite it as a solution. For example, "I can use public transportation to get to work and actually save money by avoiding the high cost of gasoline."

- **Practice Praising.** Avoid being critical of others. Practice being helpful. All people need to feel needed, appreciated, and important. Practice extending yourself and going the extra mile to make someone feel special. When you make someone else feel good, you feel better yourself. Practice random acts of kindness and become a "day-maker."

- **Associate with Winners.** Your mother probably told you that you would be judged by the people you associate with, and she was correct. If we can be found "guilty by association," we can also be found "successful by association." Surround yourself with successful, winning colleagues and friends. You will learn from them and be viewed by others as one who has achieved their same level of success.

- **Be Well.** Practice all the habits for a healthy life. Get plenty of rest and exercise. Maintain a healthy, balanced diet and avoid the fatty, starchy fast foods that have created an obese society. Avoid recreational drugs and the excessive use of alcohol. Project your health to others in your regular conversation. Apply your positive affirmations in this area by saying things like, "I feel young, vital, and full of energy."

goal management
a powerful technique yielding strong returns and giving one long-term vision and short-term motivation; helps organize resources and helps one focus on the acquisition of knowledge.

✓ Effective Goal Management

Educators who teach students how to effectively set and manage their goals are providing a fundamental life skill critical to their overall success, whatever their chosen career path. Goal management is a powerful technique that can yield strong returns in all areas of our lives. At its most fundamental level, the process of setting goals and targets allows us to choose where we want to go in life. By knowing precisely what we want to achieve, we know what we have to concentrate on and improve. We also recognize what may be a mere distraction to our success. Goal management gives us long-term vision and short-term motivation. It helps us organize our resources and focuses our acquisition of knowledge in the right direction.

By setting clearly defined goals, we can measure the achievement of those goals and take pride in our accomplishments. The measurement process allows us to see what we have done and what we are capable of. The process of achieving goals and seeing their attainment gives us the confidence and self-belief that we need to be able to achieve even higher and more difficult goals. Goal management requires self-discipline, but carrying it through can be relatively simple. See Figure 18–6 for a sample goal-management form.

Through goal setting, we achieve more and perform better. We experience greater motivation and pride in our achievements. Our self-confidence soars and our attitude is more positive.

IT'S WORTH REMEMBERING ✳

Rather than following the conditioned habit of most people to think about the negative, think positively. Expect to get a great parking space at the mall. Expect to be the first in line at checkout. Expect to lose that 10 pounds and see yourself in those new skinny jeans. Expect success in all situations. You will be surprised how often success will be yours.

IT'S WORTH REMEMBERING ✳

Winners who effectively manage their goals experience less stress and anxiety. They display better concentration and job performance and are generally happier than those who don't.

GOAL ANALYSIS

If your students are struggling with the determination of whether a goal is worthwhile, tell them to consider the following questions.

- Do they own it? Is it really their goal or is it someone else's? For example, is it what they want or what their parents want for them?
- Is it moral, legal, and fair? If not, it is definitely a goal that should be discarded.
- Do the short-term goals support the long-range objectives or expected outcomes? For example, if the long-range objective is to own a highly successful salon and spa, have the short-term goals of completing school, obtaining a license, obtaining work experience, and taking business courses been identified?
- Is there an emotional commitment? Has the student totally and unequivocally committed to completing the steps required for goal attainment?
- Can they visualize accomplishment? If students cannot see themselves in the role of successful business owner, for example, it will probably never happen.

GOAL MANAGEMENT ACTION PLAN											List Investments and sacrifices	List Personal Benefits — Identify Intrinsic and Extrinsic Motivation	Identify risks and obstacles	Identify Knowledge Required	Identify Support Group	Deadline for Completion
Goal — List preliminary goals in each category; Indicate Short-term (ST), Intermediate (IN), and Long-term (LT); Indicate Priorities by P1, P2, and P3	Is it mine?	Is it right and legal?	Does it support LT goals?	Can I commit to it?	Can I visualize success?	Is it a performance goal?	Is it attainable & challenging?	Is it clear and positive?	Does it contradict others?						
Professional															
Educational															
Personal															
Community															

Figure 18–6 Goal management form.

FICTION	FACT
Setting goals is not important.	Success will not occur without defined goals. It is not accidental.
Keep goals in your head.	Goals must be written for clarification and objectivity. Writing them reinforces commitment.
Goal setting is complicated and time consuming.	The time invested in planning accelerates the performance. Preparation supports success.
The best time to set goals is the first of the year.	The best time is now. It is about deciding, not timing.
Long-range planning is not required.	The future becomes the present and deserves serious consideration.
A good plan is all it takes.	Success is not passive. Any good plan requires both preparation and action.
Just begin.	The underlying cause of most failure is taking action without planning.
Hard work is all it takes.	Working smart achieves more sooner.
I'm the only one that can achieve my goals.	Success requires the cooperation of the individual's support system.
Annual review of goals is sufficient.	Fast-changing times cause goals to shift and flex and need reshaping. Review should be regular, frequent, and consistent.

IT'S WORTH REMEMBERING ✳

Failure to address the "why" will likely result in failure of the "what."

IT'S WORTH REMEMBERING ✳

Clearly defined, written goals make our purpose achievable.

outcome goals
goals that focus on the end result without focusing on the performance required to get there.

People fail to achieve their goals for many reasons. Whether it is acting without a plan or planning without acting, both can prevent success. We need to plan first, take action next, and perfect the action later. Often, people fail to set realistic time frames and expectations and they don't have the patience for the process. If we don't understand why a goal is important, the commitment to its achievement won't exist. Further, if we spread ourselves too thin trying to attain too many goals at once, the most important ones will suffer. It is important to identify what matters most and make that our central focus. The inability to stay focused is a key deterrent to goal attainment. In addition to all these reasons for failure, fear of failing is probably the biggest cause of all. If we can replace our fears with knowledge and understanding, our performance will improve and our goals will be reached.

Goal management can go awry by setting **outcome goals** instead of **performance goals** or by setting goals too high or too low. If we set the goal unrealistically high, it can be perceived as unreachable and cause us to become discouraged. On the other hand, if we set a goal too low, it can be perceived as unimportant or a waste of time. Additionally, if we are vague or unsystematic in our approach, goals can be forgotten or considered useless. Setting too many goals can lead to overload and cause us to just give up. We must believe our goals are attainable and visualize ourselves achieving them. If we never set them, we will never reach them.

Most goal-management experts describe four categories of goals: **professional goals** (financial, career, fame), **educational goals** (formal, informal, personal development, professional development), **personal goals** (attitude, family, health, home, pleasure, spiritual/ethical), and **community goals** (friends, community service). When defining one's goals, it is important to determine how much time it will take to achieve them.

Generally, goals are considered short term (less than one year), intermediate (one to five years), or long term (more than five years).

SMART goals can be determined using a simple formula, as described in the accompanying box, that ensures they will work.

SMART goals must be *specific*. You have to identify exactly what it is you want to achieve. They must be *measurable*. You must be able to determine that you have achieved them. They must be *attainable*. It is pointless to set a goal of being 5 feet 11 inches tall if you are fully grown and only 5 feet 8 inches tall. They must be *relevant*. The specific goal must be related to your overall objective. They must be *time-based*. A goal without a deadline will likely never be reached.

FORMULA FOR SMART GOALS
S: Specific M: Measurable A: Attainable R: Relevant T: Time-based

Self-Assessment for Goal Management

Questions your students must consider when reviewing the strategy of effective goal management include:

1. What are my five most important life goals?
2. What is the most important goal I want to accomplish within the next 12 months?
3. What is the most important goal I want to achieve five years from now?
4. How do I define success and failure?
5. How much time am I willing to spend each day toward the attainment of my goals?

Actions for Effective Goal Management

After answering the important self-assessment questions, students should identify and consider specific actions they can take toward the development, achievement, and management of their goals. For example:

- **Put Goals in Writing.** Write down short-, intermediate-, and long-term goals and divide them into workable segments.
- **Keep Track.** It is important to set deadlines, keep track of your efforts, record your results, and reward your success. You must celebrate the small wins to increase self-motivation and inspire you to keep trying to attain the next level.
- **Take Action.** Don't wait; begin today. You have heard that procrastination is the thief of time. Consider this: a year from now you will be a year older, whether you have set and worked toward achieving your goals or not. Will you be a year older with accomplishments under your belt or not? The sooner you act, the better. Do it now!

performance goals
goals that focus on specific performances that will ultimately result in the desired outcome goal.

professional goals
goals pertaining to financial, career, notoriety, and so forth.

educational goals
goals pertaining to formal and informal education, personal development and professional development.

personal goals
goals pertaining to attitude, family, health, home, pleasure, spiritual/ethical, and so forth.

community goals
goals pertaining to friends, community service, and so forth.

SMART goals
goals that are specific, measurable, attainable, relevant, and time-based.

- **Take Responsibility.** Enlist the support of your family and close friends. Do not, however, let those who think your goals are silly bring you down. They are the losers. Stay focused and recognize that, ultimately, achievement of the goal is up to you.
- **Prepare for Obstacles.** Don't give up. Learn from mistakes. Mary Pickford said that when you make a mistake, don't look back at it long. Take the reason of the thing into your mind, and then look forward. Mistakes are lessons of wisdom. The past cannot be changed. The future is yet in your power.
- **Take Another Look.** Periodically review and update your goals. What you want may change. As you grow, your ideas and your ideals change. Your goals will need to be updated accordingly.
- **Avoid Perfectionism.** It is a fact that expecting perfection only leads to disappointment and failure.
- **Expect Disappointment.** If you set goals too high or expect too much, you will likely be disappointed. Be realistic when you set what you are aiming for, but recognize that unforeseeable circumstances may interfere with the ultimate attainment of the goal. When that happens, reconsider your goals and move forward.

Develop a Strong Work Ethic

work ethic
a set of values based on the moral virtues of hard work and diligence and includes the belief in the moral benefit of work and its ability to improve one's character.

The **work ethic** is a set of values based on the moral virtues of hard work and diligence and includes the belief in the moral benefit of work and its ability to improve one's character. The work ethic generally includes being reliable and responsible as well as having initiative. When schools across the country were surveyed to learn what qualities and characteristics were desired in the educators they hired, those qualities that make up a strong work ethic were found to be among the most important. Businesses are looking for employees who are dependable, loyal, and committed to the mission of the business. When 150 human resource directors from some of the largest U.S. companies were surveyed, 59 percent ranked work ethic as the number one necessary job skill, aside from the basic occupational skills needed to perform the job.

Other surveys also identified interpersonal skills and a positive attitude toward work as among the most important qualifications for employment. Often, it is believed that the skill set needed to do the job can be learned through training and development. However, the attitudinal skills involved in having a strong work ethic come from within. Our mandate is to provide business and industry with trained workers who possess both strong occupational skills and good work habits.

Research shows that all it takes to be considered in the top 20 percent of your profession is to show up, on time, ready to work. Winners don't stop there—not only do they show up, on time, ready to work, they work while they are there. They give 100 percent to their responsibilities on the job. In fact, winners are willing to go the extra mile and aren't concerned about whether the task is part of their job description, but whether it will contribute to the team's ultimate goals. Winners see the big picture and know that by contributing to the team's success, they will also achieve their own professional goals.

Winners understand and respect the employer–employee relationship and are committed to the need to deliver worthy service for value received. In other words, winners always give a full day of work for a full day of pay. They are totally loyal to their company and their superiors and would never do anything to criticize or bring harm to the organization. Winners take proactive measures to bring about positive change rather than complaining or causing problems.

In 1995, baseball legend Cal Ripken, Jr., broke Lou Gehrig's record of playing in 2,130 consecutive baseball games. He received great accolades for his accomplishment, but he brushed them off and instead offered up praise for the work ethic of America's real working heroes. He referred to Mildred Parsons, who at that time was 82 years of age and had never missed a day of work as a secretary for the Federal Bureau of Investigation (FBI) in 56 years of employment. Ms. Parsons finally retired in March of 2003 after working for 62 years, 9 months, and 2 days, and never once calling in sick. At 88, she was the longest-serving employee in FBI history. Her sick-free record became a matter of pride and legend at the FBI. Just imagine the impact we could have in our schools and salons with that kind of commitment, dedication, and work ethic.

Business and industry leaders have identified 10 work ethic traits that must be taught and practiced in order to develop a viable and effective workforce.

IT'S WORTH REMEMBERING ✳

Winners see themselves as part of the solution, not part of the problem.

TOP 10 WORK ETHIC TRAITS

1. Appearance

2. Attendance

3. Attitude

4. Character

5. Communication

6. Cooperation

7. Organizational skills

8. Productivity

9. Respect

10. Teamwork

Self-Assessment for a Strong Work Ethic

Graduates must ask themselves some key questions to evaluate where they stand with respect to having a strong work ethic:

1. Do I show up every day on time, ready to work, and seek ways to go above and beyond what is expected?
2. Do I plan and organize my day and cooperate with my team?
3. Am I mindful of the goals of my colleagues and employer?
4. Do I always look my best and give a full day of work for a full day of pay?
5. Do I seek creative solutions to daily challenges rather than complaining about them?

Actions for Developing a Strong Work Ethic

After your students or graduates have completed their self-assessment and determined that they need to improve their work ethic, they may want to consider the following actions:

- **Make a Plan.** Create a "to do" list every evening that includes everything you need to accomplish the following day. Plan your day all the way down to what you are going to wear and what you will eat for lunch. If the clothing you want to wear needs pressing, do it the night before. If you can make a sandwich or salad to take to school or work with you, you could even save as much as $100 over the course of a month. If your list includes picking up the dry cleaning or a birthday card for a relative, leave early enough to get it on the way to work or school.

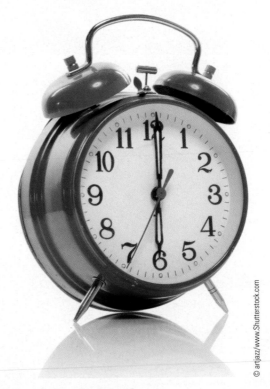

© artjazz/www.Shutterstock.com

Figure 18–7   Set the alarm clock early.

- **Set the Alarm Clock.** Consistent with the plan you made for the following day, plan to go to bed early enough to get the requisite seven to eight hours of sleep and set the alarm clock early enough to accomplish everything you need to do before arriving at work (Figure 18–7). You have heard some people say, "I'm just not a morning person." That is an attitudinal choice you are making. Why not build a bridge and get over it? The morning is a wonderful part of the day that should be enjoyed and appreciated.

- **Build Your Stamina.** Build up your staying power. This relates to getting sufficient sleep as well as adopting a sound exercise regimen that includes at least 20 minutes of exercise no less than three to five times each week. Exercise will improve your stamina and endurance. There are all kinds of little things you can do throughout the day that will help you become more fit. For example, when seeking a parking place at the supermarket, instead of driving around for 20 minutes waiting for a close space to become available, park where you can and take a brisk walk to the building. In the long run, this will save time and improve your health. When visiting or working in a building with multiple floors, take the stairs instead of the elevator if it's not more than six or seven floors. Stand up and pace while on lengthy calls rather than lounging on the sofa or at your desk. Stand up and dance while watching the television (Figure 18–8). All these physical activities will make you more fit while improving your stamina and ability to give a full day of work for a day of pay.

stamina
endurance; the physical or moral strength required to resist or withstand fatigue or hardship.

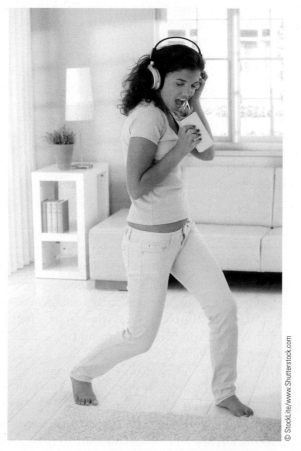

© StockLite/www.Shutterstock.com

Figure 18–8   Dance while watching television to stay fit.

- **Find Role Models.** Build relationships with friends and colleagues who already possess a strong work ethic. Observe them. Ask them how they do it. Mirror their behavior. Before you know it, you will be displaying a strong and valuable work ethic.
- **Meet Deadlines and Persevere.** As we discussed earlier, we need to put our goals in writing (even if it's a daily goal that is part of your "to do" list) and put a timeline on them. Be persistent and stick to your projects even when you undergo challenges or frustrations.
- **Be a Problem Solver.** Practice active listening. Pay attention to details. Use the information you glean to assist you in solving problems. Learn how to consider all the options in a given situation that will result in a "win–win" outcome for all those involved. Once you have facilitated a solution, you will have gained important experience critical to success in the workplace.
- **Be a Risk Taker.** Estimate your chance of success or failure relative to a number of courses of action and be willing to take risks. Without risk, growth and success are hindered.
- **Be Ambitious.** Your dreams are the springboard for your goals, which come in many sizes and shapes. Be ambitious and set your sights high enough that you are challenged to achieve them. Aspire to be the best you can be. It will take a strong work ethic to accomplish this goal.
- **Love What You Do.** It is a whole lot easier to give 100 percent to a job that you enjoy than it is to one that you hate. If you are a teacher who does not love to teach and has compassion for the students, then you should seek another position. If you are a cosmetologist who does not love people and making them feel better about themselves, then you should absolutely look for another avenue to pursue. A motivational speaker once said, "Do what you can't not do!" While grammatically confusing, it really does say it all. When you do what you can't keep yourself from doing, you are probably going to perform well.
- **Take Pride in Your Work.** Consider every task you perform a work of art. Make sure it is good enough to carry your signature.
- **Affirm and Celebrate.** Be a self-promoter. When you do a good job, affirm to yourself and others that you did so. Pat yourself on the back and celebrate your success. Reward yourself with a night out, a walk on the beach, a trip to the ice cream parlor, a movie you want to see, or anything else that is meaningful to you.

> **CONSIDER AND CONNECT**
>
> Positively outstanding customer service should be random and unexpected, creating the element of the unexpected and thereby making it even more pleasurable.

☑ Value the Client

As a teacher in a profession of service, our clients include our students and the clients they serve. In many cases, we are being invited to invade the personal comfort zones of our clients on a daily basis. We must recognize the responsibility that comes with that role. Without our clients, the other success strategies we have talked about will not matter much. Without clients, we cannot enjoy any degree of success.

Service should be out of proportion to the circumstances. We should make ordinary customers feel extraordinary. We want them to feel like a VIP or royalty. As a result, they will never forget us. Outstanding customer service should invite clients to play and be involved. It should create client loyalty by making clients feel so special that they come back again and again. It will create compelling word-of-mouth advertising that has been proven to be the most effective form of promoting a successful business. It is definitely easier to keep one satisfied client than it is to attract five new ones. The happy ones will tell others and your business will grow. The whole process should definitely create a vision of wonder and perfection that revolves around the client.

Self-Assessment for Client Service

Your students need to take inventory of their own abilities in providing outstanding client care. They might ask themselves the following questions:

1. Do I make eye contact immediately, greet my clients warmly with a friendly smile, state my name, and shake their hand?
2. Do I discuss their needs before continuing with their service?
3. Am I a good listener, and do I understand exactly what they want?
4. Do I make my clients feel needed, appreciated, and important?
5. What have I done to make my clients feel like VIPs?

TEN COMMANDMENTS OF SUPERIOR CUSTOMER SERVICE AND RETENTION

- Clients are the most important people in any business.
- Clients are not dependent on us; we are dependent on them.
- Clients are not interruptions of our work. They are the purpose of it.
- Clients do us a favor when they call on us. We are not doing one by serving them.
- Clients are part of our business, not outsiders.
- Clients are human beings, like ourselves, with the same feelings and emotions.
- Clients bring us their needs. It is our job to satisfy those needs.
- Clients are not those to argue or match wits with.
- Clients are deserving of the most courteous and attentive treatment we can give them.
- Clients are the lifeblood of our business and every other business.

Reprinted with permission from *Passion: A Salon Professional's Handbook for Building a Successful Business* by Susie Fields Carder.

Actions for Outstanding Client Care

Your students, while in school and after licensure, should consider the following actions for providing outstanding client service:

- **Check Your Image.** Look in the mirror and consider your appearance as well as your attitude, your punctuality, your interpersonal skills, and your willingness to help others. It is critical that you present the best possible image at all times.
- **Practice Your Handshake.** Your handshake conveys a lot about you. A dry, firm but comfortable, full handshake conveys self-confidence and a genuine interest in the other party (Figure 18–9). A wet handshake is repulsive. A soft handshake demonstrates a lack of confidence, lack of interest, and weakness. The fingertip shake indicates a discomfort

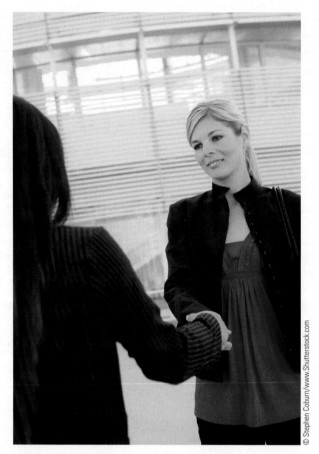

Figure 18–9   A firm handshake conveys self-confidence and genuine interest in your client.

or lack of respect for the whole process. Some men do this with women, either because they are trying to be gentlemanly or because they are trying to intimidate the female. Practice your handshake with fellow students or colleagues until you get it right.

- **Learn Client Names.** There is no sweeter sound than hearing your own name, pronounced correctly and said genuinely. Learning client names is a skill that can be developed. Upon first meeting the client, make a point of repeating his name at least three times in the first few minutes of conversation. Link an adjective to the first letter of the client's name that perhaps describes the client. For example: Amiable Amy, Cool Connor, Kinky Kristie, Laughing Lisha, Petite Patricia, or Terrific Tom.

- **Keep Client Records.** Accurate client records provide a great resource for making clients feel special. In addition to recording important service history and contact information, you might add personal information that you can reference during their next visit. For example, if the client is getting her hair done for little Johnny's piano recital, make a note and ask her if Johnny's performance made her proud. Perhaps the client is getting her hair done for her anniversary and she has told you all about the new dress she is wearing. Make a note of this, and the next time she comes in, ask if her husband liked the peach dress and if they had a wonderful evening.

- **Extend Yourself.** It is important for students to extend themselves when dealing with clients. It simply means saying or doing one extra thing that isn't expected of you. This behavior shows clients that you have noticed them and paid attention to them in some manner.
- **Recognize First-Timers.** Businesses recognize new clients in a variety of ways. It might be a different colored ticket, or a colored dot on the client ticket, or a special ribbon pinned in a visible place that differentiates the client from the others. Whatever method is chosen, acknowledging first-time clients will make them feel special.
- **Provide Refreshments.** Some businesses offer clients herbal teas or even wine to clients. Others have bottled water and cookies available. Whatever refreshments you decide on, having them available will tell the clients you care about them.
- **Give Them a Reason to Return.** Follow the W-I-T (whatever it takes) principle. Network with other professionals to find out what they do to provide outstanding customer service. Ask your clients about the best customer service experience they have ever had and determine if you can adapt it to your business. You can also simply ask clients what types of things they would most enjoy while they visit your school or salon. After all, they are the ones you are trying to please.

Wrapping It Up

As educators, it is critical that we teach our students the valuable soft skills necessary to achieve success in the workplace. Our students must know who they are and what they want in their career. They need to define what success means to them and then create that successful life by envisioning a future and building a plan of action to get there. The students' values and beliefs, their personal motivation, their dreams and goals, their ability to see themselves winning, their commitment to hard work, and their dedication to their clients will all contribute significantly to their overall success. A simple formula that sums up all the strategies is: Dream it, desire it, design it, and do it!

In Retrospect

1. List the six strategies and principles to achieve a winning career.
2. List specific actions students can use to pay value to themselves.
3. List specific actions students can use for self-motivation.
4. List specific actions students can use for expecting to win.
5. List specific strategies students can use to manage their goals.
6. List specific methods students can follow to adopt a strong work ethic.
7. List specific methods students can follow to value their clients.

EDUCATOR SPOTLIGHT

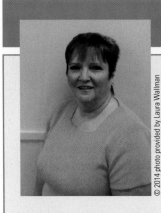

© 2014 photo provided by Laura Wallman

LAURA WALLMAN my philosophy of being an educator is like putting together a jigsaw puzzle: I find an area large enough to work the puzzle. I open the box and start putting the pieces on the table. There are many different sizes, shapes, and colors. I separate the perimeter pieces from the inside pieces. There are several ways to put the puzzle together. Sometimes I arrange the perimeter first and at other times I arrange the inner pieces first. I am a flexible educator and I strive to accurately characterize the learners that I teach so that I can see where they fit into the whole educational picture. When doing a jigsaw puzzle (teaching students) I turn the piece around many times before I am sure it is in the correct place before interlocking it into another piece. I work diligently until every piece fits perfectly. If a student is not "getting it," I use different techniques until the student understands. Many times, just when I start to think that the puzzle is impossible, a light goes off and everything just falls into place.

19 Teams at Work

Objectives (Desired Performance Goals):

After reading and studying this chapter, you should be able to:

- Explain the concept of teamwork.
- List the 10 qualities team members are looking for in their work environment.
- Explain the qualities required of a dynamic leader.
- Identify the six key steps in team building.
- List the 10 elements required in building team essentials.

KEY TERMS

! CRITICAL CONCEPT

Achieving the goal of quality education in any institution cannot be the handiwork of just one educator . . . it takes a village.

The Concept of Teamwork

THE BASIC CONCEPT of teamwork is the key to the success of any business. All of us have had the incredible experience of being part of a team. It is one of life's most rewarding experiences. As adults in the workplace, we sometimes forget the exhilaration we experienced in our youth when we achieved the seemingly impossible by pulling together (in that tug of war, or on the basketball court or track field) and doing what had to be done, not alone as individuals, but as a team. Close your eyes and take an imaginary trip to the summer Olympics and try to picture this powerful image. The event is rowing. Picture a team of eight, rowing through the early morning light, driven by nothing but their faithful steersman and their burning desire to succeed together as a team. That image epitomizes teamwork (Figure 19–1). Each rower has to be in perfect synchronization with his fellow team members to reach the ultimate goal, the goal of winning!

Teams and Teamwork Defined

A **team** is a group of interdependent individuals who have complementary skills and are committed to a shared, meaningful purpose and specific goals. Effective teams display confidence, enthusiasm, and seek continuously to improve their performance. Members have a common, collaborative work approach, clear roles and responsibilities, and hold themselves mutually accountable for the team's performance. **Teamwork**, as defined by *Merriam Webster's Collegiate Dictionary*, tenth edition, is work done by several associates with each doing a part but all subordinating personal prominence to the efficiency of the whole. There is overwhelming evidence that highly successful schools are composed of high-performance teams. Everywhere we look there is confirmation that teams play a key role in enabling strong competitive performance. There is continuing demand to do things better, faster, and at less expense. We have to compete for clients and business today in a way we never have before. The need for responsiveness, service, quality, and sensitivity to customer needs has never been greater.

+ MASTER EDUCATOR

1. Aligns with the overall mission and purpose of the institution.
2. Adapts to needed change to ensure that the institution's mission is achieved.
3. Communicates effectively to ensure collaboration among all members of the institution's team.

---

team a group of interdependent individuals who have complementary skills and are committed to a shared, meaningful purpose and specific goals.

teamwork work done by several associates with each doing a part but all subordinating personal prominence to the efficiency of the whole.

IT'S WORTH ✳ REMEMBERING

Teamwork is the ability to work together toward a common vision. It is the ability to direct individual accomplishment toward organizational objectives. It is the fuel that allows ordinary people to attain extraordinary results.

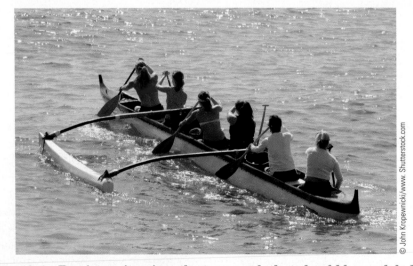

© John Kropewnicki/www.Shutterstock.com

Figure 19–1   Rowing epitomizes the teamwork that should be modeled in every institution.

Team Motivation

Industrial psychologists have determined that human behavior is greatly driven or motivated by the need for sustenance, safety, security, belonging, recognition, and a sense of growth and achievement. Whether the team leader is the business owner or manager, she is responsible for the success or failure of the team. This doesn't mean that a team member's poor performance is the leader's fault; it is, however, her responsibility. Building a team member's self-esteem is a critical part of facilitating self-motivation for each team member. Understanding what team members want and becoming responsive to those interests is a good place to start as a team leader. Research has identified that there are 10 critical desires of team members.

> ☑ **CONSIDER AND CONNECT**
>
> It is a generally accepted principle that people achieve more when they work collaboratively with others than when they work against them.

TOP 10 TEAM MEMBER DESIRES

- Efficient, supportive leadership

- Clear purpose or mission

- Spirit of fellowship and cooperation

- Balanced participation and contribution

- Open communication

- Results

- Challenge

- Responsibility

- Recognition

- Growth

Leadership. Just as a great educator facilitates the circumstances and environment within which students can become self-motivated, a dynamic leader will do the same. Charismatic leaders are highly effective in the short term, but they may not sustain motivation indefinitely. We know that true motivation is intrinsic, coming from within the individual team members. A great leader will be able to help the team members see the best in themselves, which will provide the stimulus for great performance. A strong leader realizes that each team member has needs and that the activities of the team must contribute to meeting those needs for the member's internal motivation to be sustained. The dynamic leader understands all the qualities that team members are looking for and will focus a great deal of time on creating the conditions for each quality to exist.

IT'S WORTH REMEMBERING ✳

It would be a mistake to create an environment where members and leaders depend on each other for their source of motivation.

trust firm reliance on the integrity, ability, and character of a person or thing; confident belief; faith.

Qualities of a dynamic leader include:

- **Being a role model.** A leader will not just give lip service to quality. He will develop energetic, two-way communication with all team members. He will seek input from team members and create an open environment in regular meetings by making them interesting and full of fun surprises.
- **Creating trust.** A true leader will encourage foresight, integrity, and **trust** or firm reliance on the integrity, ability, and character of both sides of the team. She will give direction and then let the team members do their job. She will share her vision and keep the team in the loop on all relevant issues, thereby minimizing rumors and backbiting.
- **Encouraging creativity.** A leader will encourage team members to take risks, which increases creativity. When that risk results in a mistake or something less than the desired result, a true leader will be able to laugh at the mistake. He might even take it as far as Les Wexner, owner of The Limited, a chain of women's clothing stores. He maintains what he calls a "Hall of Shame," where he tells his employees the biggest mistake he made during the week. Then the team members are asked to share their mistakes. The group takes a lesson from Mary Pickford and simply takes the reason for the mistake into discussion and looks at ways they can all benefit from the experience and take measures to prevent its repetition.
- **Being a change master.** Teams must not only respond to change, they must initiate it. Team leaders must acknowledge any perceived danger in the change and then proceed to identify the inherent opportunities with it. This is consistent with the quality of encouraging creativity. The leader can provide the tools that allow team members to innovate. When the team leader models a positive attitude toward change, team members will become more accepting of change.
- **Modeling superior customer service.** A great leader will get team members involved by asking them how the team can exceed their customers' expectations by knowing their needs, emotions, and desires. Team members with a focus on outstanding customer service will naturally be creative and intuitive.
- **Recognizing performance.** Truly dynamic leaders will be able to identify where the team excels as well as team weaknesses. They will reward excellent performance and facilitate open, powerful discussion regarding improvement opportunities. Constant improvement is required for any team to succeed.

☑   **Purpose or Mission.** All teams need a clear sense of direction. Members need to understand how their contribution fits into the objectives or purpose of the school or business. Only then can the team members put aside personal needs for the benefit of the team or company. Team members have to believe in the purpose of the team and hold ownership to sustain the motivation to achieve the desired results. Goals are identified with the business priorities in mind and the ground rules for the team are developed with consideration for both business and individual values. The sad truth is that if team members were asked to write down the mission statement of their organization, research shows that 99 percent of the time, not one person, including the owner or director, can write it down in clear, concise language. For example, every accredited post-secondary institution should publish its mission statement in the school catalog. While most instructors might have a general idea about its intent, none of them is likely able to write it. Therefore, it is appropriate to discuss how to develop a relevant mission statement.

In just one or two sentences, a mission statement should communicate the essence of your organization to your members and the public. It should be a clear, concise statement that says who you are, what you do, for whom you do it, and where you do it. It could even be considered a public relations statement that is easy to remember so that it can be used effectively to promote the organization.

EXAMPLE OF AN ORGANIZATION MISSION STATEMENT

"The mission of Career Success Academy is to ensure the success of our graduates in their chosen career field while providing an energetic environment that facilitates the confidence and skills necessary to attain career success. Our priority is to help our students unlock their creativity and imaginations, improve themselves, and ultimately achieve professional success."

Team leaders might suggest that each institution team develop a team mission and purpose that aligns with that of the business but reflects the individuality of each team. The first thing the work team should do is choose a name and team slogan that will increase awareness of the team's identity and build team spirit. For example, the teachers of the Career Success Academy might call themselves the Career Success Academy Ambassadors and adopt the slogan, "Achieving Excellence in Education."

EXAMPLE OF A DEPARTMENT TEAM MISSION STATEMENT

"The mission of the Career Success Academy Ambassadors is to facilitate energetic, student-centered, discovery-oriented education that inspires, motivates, and supports learner success and excellence."

When a shared purpose is agreed upon by the members, goals and measures can be identified that allow ongoing assessment of progress and allow the team to celebrate periodic successes. Goals and measures for the Career Success Academy Ambassadors' team mission statement might include attendance percentages of students, student grade averages, morale of students, and certification or licensure rates, if applicable. For every week that an instructor gets 100 percent attendance by her students, for example, the class has a brief party or celebration at the end of the last day of the week to celebrate. Students and faculty should feel great about the accomplishment.

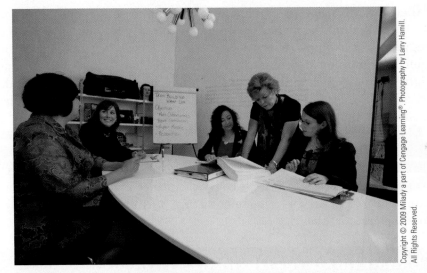

Figure 19–2   Successful teams are comprised of members who like each other and share fellowship.

Students should be recognized for their accomplishment as well. You can also clearly see how the achievement of the *team's* mission will contribute greatly to the achievement of the *institution's* mission.

Spirit of Fellowship. Research shows that highly successful teams are usually composed of members who like each other and feel a sense of fellowship and loyalty with each other (Figure 19–2). They are willing to work harder for the objectives of the team because they don't want to let their fellow team members down or potentially harm their relationship with another member. The result of this type of relationship building is direct and open communication, frequent praising of each team member's contributions, and mutual support of each other's efforts. This behavior is natural when members like each other. However, there are times when members don't particularly like all the other team members. Often, our feelings about other human beings are based on how well we understand them. Adults are a result of many components, including personalities, temperaments, values, beliefs, backgrounds, cultures, ideologies, religions, and so much more. Committed team members will attempt to break down any barriers caused by these differences through education and greater understanding of fellow humans. Teams should not overlook an even simpler solution: design an off-site activity for the team just to play and have fun together and get to know one another better (Figure 19–3). It is a wonderful way to build fellowship and camaraderie.

Diverse thinkers will experience disagreement or differences on occasion. Conflict may occur if those differences are not managed effectively. Misperceptions, ill feelings, and misunderstandings should be dealt with appropriately or they can create tension, stubbornness, and hidden agendas. A good leader will help the team manage the differences by tapping the collective power of the team and maintaining trust. The team should use alignment with purpose, values, and goals to formulate acceptable solutions. Some techniques that have been found effective in helping

fellowship the condition of being together or sharing similar interests or experiences as do members of a profession.

CONSIDER AND CONNECT

Instead of taking the position of, "We are never going to come to agreement on this," master educators will consider "Let's see if we can compromise on this issue and come to a solution where everyone wins."

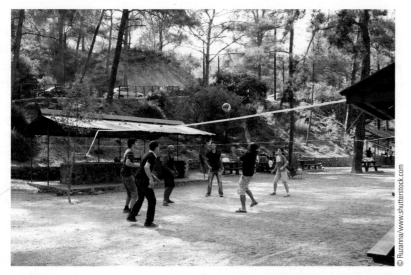

Figure 19–3 Design off-site activities for team play and camaraderie.

teams resolve conflict include affirmations, reframing, and active empathy. Team members use positive affirmation statements before going into a negotiating session to feel more positive. A statement such as, "I am calm and open to options" will allow a team member to shift obstructing patterns of behavior and manage conflict more effectively. In addition, if team members can learn to practice putting themselves in the other person's shoes before responding, differences are less likely to occur in the first place. Finally, team members can reframe their perspective on an issue. **Reframing** is similar to seeing the water glass half-full as opposed to half-empty, or, better yet, seeing a water glass twice as big as what is needed.

Reframing seeing something from a different perspective, or through a different "frame."

Balanced Participation and Contribution. Three factors that dynamic leaders will consider to ensure a balanced contribution from all team members are confidence, inclusion, and empowerment. The more confident a team member feels, the more energy she will exert to achieve the desired end. Leaders will highlight experience, talent, and accomplishments to bolster self-confidence in each team member. Further, the more members feel included as an integral part of the team, the more they contribute. Leaders should solicit input from the members and take steps to keep them informed on every front. Appreciation should be shown for all ideas offered, even those that are not used. Team member empowerment includes involving them in decision making, giving them relevant training, and respecting them for their contributions. When a team member is empowered, she will feel supported and put forth even more effort. Team members should be persuaded to support and praise the contributions of the other members as well.

Open Communication. Communication impacts the energy and effectiveness of the team, whether positive or negative. For a team to achieve optimum results, each member must feel safe in sharing what they think, asking for help when it is needed, offering new and even not-so-popular ideas, and taking risks that may result in mistakes. Effective leaders will provide training in communication skills such as active listening, effective

IT'S WORTH ✳ REMEMBERING

A group becomes a team when all members are sure enough of themselves and their contributions to praise the skill of other members.

responding, rapport building, appropriate business language, negotiating, and consensus building. Open, friendly, positive communication is critical to creating a cohesive, productive team. Team members should be allowed time and encouraged to show caring for fellow team members by asking about their lives outside team responsibilities. Positive communication energizes the entire team.

Challenge. Members of the most dynamic teams will usually say that their most rewarding team experiences resulted after being presented with a stimulating challenge. Driven individuals are highly motivated by challenge. Since such challenges do not necessarily present themselves to a team on a daily basis, a great leader will consider different ways to provide challenges on a more frequent basis. As in goal setting, the level of difficulty of the challenge can cause a team to give up before truly beginning due to the perception that it is impossible. On the other hand, if the challenge is too easy, it may not be viewed as important enough to undertake by the team. A great leader will provide periodic stimulation through a worthy challenge to help maintain team motivation.

Responsibility. Like a good challenge, being given responsibility tends to stimulate a team to action. Responsibility promotes team ownership of the task or project. Dynamic leaders will ensure that teams understand that with responsibility comes authority. Teams must have the authority to make changes, and when they do, they will sustain a higher level of motivation for a longer period of time. An effective leader will know that if the consequences for failure or error are too high, the responsibility can be de-motivating. Teams must view the gift of responsibility as positive, not negative.

Results. Every dedicated team has an internal need to see results. If members don't feel they are getting results, they will lose their motivation. Thus, it is critical to put timelines and benchmarks into the overall objectives. A good leader will provide project wrap-ups when a goal has been met (Figure 19–4). A wrap-up will provide the vital finish to the team's efforts. In a team wrap-up meeting, the leader will answer several key questions, such as:

- What was the original goal?
- What made the goal important or even difficult?
- Who worked on the team?
- What made those team members suitable for the job?
- What were some special aspects of the goal or project?
- How did the team resolve unexpected challenges?
- What performance made the leader proud?

Recognition. All humans share the sophisticated need for recognition, but it happens to be one of the most difficult to get. It is the only need we have that requires complete dependence upon others to obtain. By definition, recognition must come from someone else. You may have wondered why so many recipients of awards or recognition experience the emotional response of tears. It is probably because they finally broke through the "need fulfillment" barrier that they have spent years striving for. They have finally been thanked for their good work. Many years ago a Harris poll asked several thousand workers, "What two or three things do you want most from a job?" The first three most frequent answers were: (1) a good salary, (2) job security, and (3) recognition for a job well done. Recognition is essential to our own

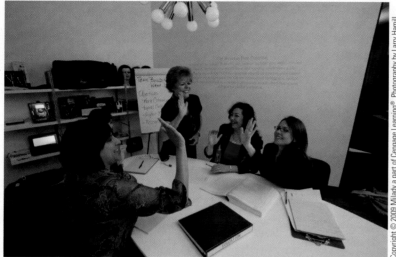

Figure 19–4   Acknowledge the achievement of goals with a project wrap-up meeting.

feeling of self-worth. Recognition sends team members the powerful message that they are important (Figure 19–5). It says that the organization or team leader cares about good performance. Effective leaders will take care to ensure that low performers and high performers are not treated the same way, which would send the message that high performance is not important.

A highly respected leader will not limit the criteria for which a team member can be recognized, and she will open up the recommendations for recognition to all team members because she knows her eyes cannot be everywhere. She will use good judgment and appoint a recognition committee to support this valuable function. A good leader will take the time to make the recognition special rather than expensive and include the recipient's family in the presentation process whenever possible. A highly hands-on team leader might also poll team members to find out exactly what they want from her. A questionnaire, such as the example shown in the accompanying box, might be circulated that allows members to place a mark by the kinds of things they would like the leader to do. She would then make every effort to comply with the most frequent requests.

WHAT WOULD YOU LIKE FROM ME?

_____ Listen to me more often.	_____ Challenge me.
_____ Stop yelling at me.	_____ Involve me in decision making.
_____ Take more interest in my work.	_____ Do not be so negative.
_____ Give me more training.	_____ Show your appreciation.
_____ Give me a pat on the back.	_____ Keep me informed.
_____ Say thank you.	_____ Do not be so demanding.
_____ Consider my suggestions.	_____ Show me more respect.
_____ Laugh more.	_____ Do not talk down to me.
_____ Ask me how I feel.	_____ Give me equal consideration.
_____ Do not be so arrogant.	_____ Be my support system.

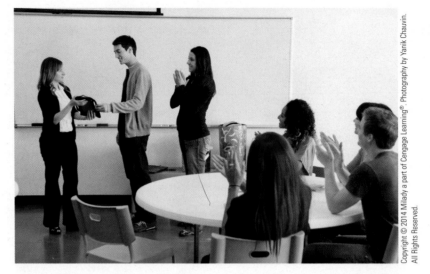

Figure 19–5   Recognition sends team members the message that they are important.

Growth. Just as they need recognition, team members need to experience a sense of growth. A powerful team leader knows the importance of investing in her team members. Personal and team growth are another source for sustained motivation. When team members feel they are moving forward, learning new skills, and stretching their minds, their internal motivation is increased. Regardless of the field, professional development seminars are essential. On-the-job training and peer coaching are other ways to provide opportunities for growth of team members. Field trips and subscriptions to industry journals or memberships in industry organizations are other ways to encourage growth. Growth adds value to the individual team member while also enhancing self-esteem and self-worth. An effective team leader will go directly to the members for feedback on what kind of growth they would like to experience as a result of being on the team.

☑ The Team-Building Process

Effective teamwork is based on clear goals and priorities, which lead to clear roles and responsibilities of team members, which lead to clear procedures and processes for the organization, which lead to good interpersonal relationships and *team success*. The concept of team building has evolved over the past 50 years or so since it was first identified as a foundation of management in the 1960s. It was originally used to emphasize the importance of establishing harmony among employees and building relationships. The focus has expanded to include an emphasis on accomplishing tasks and achieving goals and outcomes. Team building is used to help teams define their purpose and identify the individual roles of the members. It is helpful in formulating business strategies and establishing a vision for the future. In addition, team building can be used to clarify shared values, resolve differences in relationships, and improve job performance. Ultimately, team building can be highly effective in establishing trust and unity among team members.

SIX LEVELS OF EFFECTIVE TEAM BUILDING

1. Determining the need
2. Gaining the team's buy-in
3. Taking the team's temperature
4. Building the team essentials
5. Implementing the plan
6. Evaluating the results

IT'S WORTH REMEMBERING ✳

The age of rugged independent individuals is evolving into the age of the team player.

Determine the Need

Team leaders must watch for key indicators exhibited by the various team members to gain a sense of whether a team-building event is needed. If the team leader sees the following behaviors being exhibited, it is an indication that team building should become a priority.

The team leader needs to determine if the behaviors identified in the "Teams in Trouble" checklist are rampant or limited to the behavior of only one or two team members. Characteristics exhibited in only one team member might be addressed on a one-to-one basis. However, an awareness that team building could help uncover the underlying causes of the behaviors identified is relevant. An effective team-building event could eliminate the high cost of unresolved problems and allow the leader to take full advantage of a prime opportunity.

TEAMS IN TROUBLE

_____	Communication failing	_____	Frequent tardiness
_____	Trust diminishing	_____	Increased conflict
_____	Defensive behavior	_____	Complaints against team members
_____	Playing the blame game	_____	Nonparticipation in meetings
_____	Bad decisions all around	_____	Undermining and backbiting
_____	Apathy	_____	Poor decision making
_____	Overall irritability	_____	Hearing "That's not my job."
_____	Lack of risk taking	_____	Hearing "Nobody tells me anything."
_____	Poor attendance		

Gaining the Team's Buy-in

In education, the *transfer technique* is recognized as a sound way to obtain student involvement and agreement with rules and projects. The same philosophy applies in team building. Before a leader can expect full participation by the team members, she must get their commitment to engage in the team-building process. This can be aided by asking the team member what they think. A simple questionnaire can facilitate the process. The overall purpose and advantages of conducting a team-building exercise should be explained to the team members. The penalties of not addressing the identified issues should also be brought to the table. Ground rules for the event must be established in order to facilitate a feeling of safety and comfort in talking about the issues. Issues should be explained ahead of time to let the team know the leader is sensitive to their needs. The fact that the leadership is interested in obtaining members' buy-in helps gain their support for the team-building process.

WHAT DOES THE TEAM THINK?

Read each of the following statements. Check each statement that you believe applies to your team. Team leaders should analyze the feedback and identify which criteria have *not* been checked. If more than three items have been identified as not applicable to your team, there is a good indication that team building is needed.

_____ 1. Team members have equal input.

_____ 2. All team members can be counted on.

_____ 3. Team members make team meetings a priority.

_____ 4. Team meetings produce excellent outcomes.

_____ 5. Team members are open to new ideas.

_____ 6. Team members respect each other.

_____ 7. Team input is used by management.

_____ 8. Team member roles are clearly defined and accepted by all members.

_____ 9. Team members are kept well-informed.

_____ 10. Team members participate fully in meetings.

_____ 11. Team members routinely help each other out.

_____ 12. Team meetings are upbeat and motivational.

_____ 13. Team members share relevant information with each other.

_____ 14. Team members agree on priorities.

_____ 15. There is a strong feeling of trust among team members.

_____ 16. Team members praise each other's successes.

_____ 17. Open communication exists between all members.

_____ 18. All team members are responsible and accountable.

_____ 19. Team members bring solutions to the table rather than complaints.

_____ 20. Team members share and work toward a common goal.

Taking the Team's Temperature

Team-building data can be gathered from questionnaires, one-on-one interviews, and small-group discussions (Figure 19–6). While the interview may be the most popular, it is also the most time consuming and may not be feasible, especially if an outside consultant has been engaged to facilitate the team-building exercise. Questions that will help the team leader and facilitator assess the team's temperature are divided into three categories: corporate vision, group work dynamic, and general climate.

TEAM TEMPERATURE QUESTIONNAIRE

Answer the following questions to the best of your ability. You may do so anonymously if you choose.

Corporate Vision

What do team members need to do to support the organization's vision and goals?
What can the team do to align its own goals and priorities with those of the overall organization?
How can the team improve the organization's profitability and quality?
What steps can the team take to improve responsiveness and customer satisfaction?
How can the team use technology to operate more efficiently?
How can the team be more flexible in its execution of goal-oriented tasks and procedures?
In what ways can the team be more innovative?
How has the team been effective in delivering excellent client care?
What can the team do to increase client (and student) retention?
In what ways has the team accepted or resisted change within the organization?
If there was one thing you could change about this organization, what would it be and why?

Group Work Dynamic

What types of problems are team members having with each other?
How long have these problems existed?
What is working well with team member interactions?
What needs to change in the way you are working with other team members?
What needs to be done differently among team members?
What can the team leader do differently to improve working relationships?

General Climate

What types of problems are team members experiencing in general?
How long have these problems existed?
What prevents team effectiveness?
What needs to change to improve team effectiveness?
Are there outside factors hindering team effectiveness?
What specific policies or standards are keeping the team from achieving optimum effectiveness?

Building the Team Essentials

Conducting an off-site team-building exercise can be highly motivating to the spirit and morale of the group. Well-designed and properly facilitated team-building events will lead to better understanding of the organization's mission, clearer alignment of the individual and corporate goals,

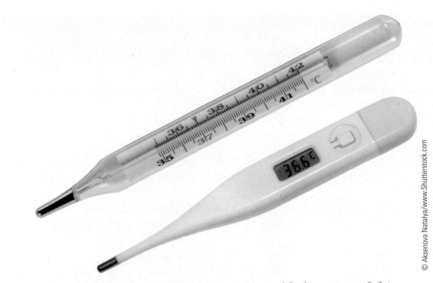

© Aksenova Natalya/www.Shutterstock.com

Figure 19–6   Taking the team's temperature aids in successful team building.

and stronger motivation by the entire team. Several key factors should be considered when conducting a team-building exercise:

1. **Choose an Inspiring Theme.** Just as we encourage our teams to choose a team name and slogan, the same should be done for the team-building event. The event name should be chosen to inspire, motivate, and excite the participants. Instead of "The Fourth-Quarter Team Building Event," why not "Career Commandos Connecting"?

2. **Promote Participation.** It is important to plan the event well enough in advance that it can be properly promoted and team involvement can be established. The interviews and questionnaires that you use to take the team's temperature will help with this step. There should be some type of memo or document circulated at least weekly during the four to six weeks prior to the event. Bulletin boards and staff meetings can also be used to promote the event. You might even consider having employees make a presentation on a topic relevant to the event purpose. Consider after-hours activities. Perhaps your team has talented members who would consider performing for the groups. Get them involved so they will be excited about the process and come with an open mind for growth.

3. **Change the Place.** For optimum results, it is recommended that team-building activities be conducted away from the job. Getting team members away from their regular work environment gives them a physical break and also facilitates a fresh perspective for the issues at hand.

4. **Mix It Up.** Involvement and interest by the participants will be stimulated by scheduling a mixture of activities. There should be ice-breakers during which team members get to know each other and no threats exist. There should be brainstorming about important issues that allow disagreement and even conflict to arise. While little progress takes place during this time, it allows members to get their ideas for consideration. Team-building activities should include brainstorming

and reflecting as well as energizers and team games. Include outdoor activities if weather and space permit. Make sure to sequence the activities throughout the event to vary the stimuli for the participants and maintain a high level of interest. Consider physical activities after meals and always end on a vote of confidence while gaining commitment from all parties.

5. **Reflect, Process, Discuss.** Make sure to allow sufficient time for discussion as well as reflection. Team members need to internalize the information being discussed and give consideration to what it all means and how it will impact their professional lives. Time should be allowed for team members to reach common understanding and respect. It is during this time that teams will reach some consensus, establish rules, and define strategy. They will establish a foundation for cooperation.

6. **Identify the Plan.** Give team members the opportunity to answer a number of questions related to their performance as a team, such as: What do you want to do more of or less of? What do you want to start or stop doing? They should answer these questions as they apply to themselves, another team member, another department, the team leader, the boss, and so forth. For example, they might ask, "What do I want to do more of?" as well as "What do I want my boss to do more of? " During the closing activities of the event, you might consider another series of questions, such as: What am I committed to do more and less of? What am I committed to begin doing or stop doing?

7. **Make History.** Always make plans to take pictures throughout the team-building event. Create a scrapbook that documents the historical event, and give copies to team members. Post the pictures in public areas for all to see. Publish them in the company newsletter or post them on the company website. Make them into a positive reminder of the productive time the team had together (Figure 19–7).

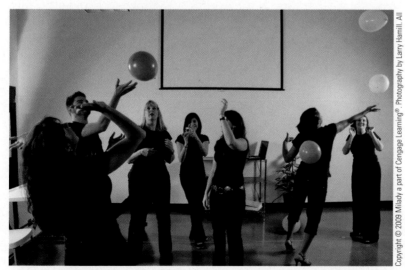

Figure 19–7   Post pictures of your team-building event to remind members of their productivity and commitment to success.

8. **Include Outside Partners.** Depending on your purpose and objectives, you may want to invite participants who are indirectly involved in your organization, such as suppliers, or members of your advisory board. They will often add significant insight and perspective to your program.

9. **Make It Personal.** It is critical to connect the individual actions of the team members to the team at large. Each participant should complete a commitment contract, a personal promise statement, and an action ownership document. The form should help ensure that new behavior will take place. Team members should share their lists with the remainder of the team before departing to gain support and commitment from fellow colleagues.

10. **Recognize the Contributors.** Facilitating an off-site event for an entire group of employees, regardless of how few or how many, is no small feat. The team leader or owner should take care to recognize those efforts with thanks and a token gift at the end of the event in front of the entire team.

Implementing the Plan

A highly motivational and inspirational team-building event will be wasted unless the team leader and facilitator take the necessary steps to ensure effective implementation of the plan. That can be accomplished through documenting the results and distributing the follow-up report to all members within 10 days of the event. The sooner the results are distributed, the less likely momentum will be lost (Figure 19–8). It also sends the message to the team members that their time was valuable and their input important. Leadership should work with team members to manage their commitments. Action items should be prioritized, assigned, and placed in a timetable. Everyone on the team should have specific responsibilities and roles assigned as a result of the team-building exercise. It is at this point that all team members perform. They establish cooperative relationships, focus on the issues,

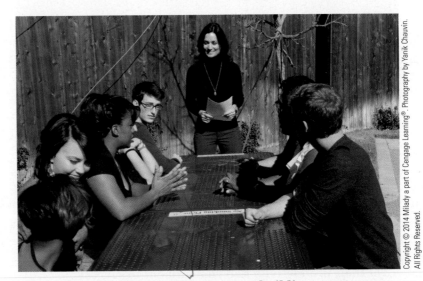

Figure 19–8   Distribute the results of a team-building event as soon as possible.

Chapter 19: Teams at Work

and progress is made. As a result, team pride increases. Finally, leadership should follow up on progress at scheduled increments, not later than 30 days following the exercise. Coaching should be implemented if necessary and encouragement provided where needed.

Evaluating the Results

No plan of action can be effective without proper evaluation and feedback. The very first step will be to obtain feedback from the team members about the quality of the team-building event and whether or not the agreed-upon objectives were met. Participants should be asked to draft their comments on how useful the event was and perhaps list at least three important factors they gained from attending. The team leader, facilitator, and team members should participate in the evaluation process. After the plans have been implemented, the first checkpoint should occur after 30 days. Teams should schedule regular checkpoints after that, ranging from every 30 to 90 days depending on the objectives of the implementation plan. Members should be allowed to bring any challenges or obstacles to the table at any time to ask for input from the rest of the team as to how to overcome them.

Every team member provides input as to how well the team has performed compared to the commitments made as a result of the team-building event. If the team agrees that improvement is not being made to the extent expected, discussions should take place about possible changes to the plan, and then a renewed commitment should be made by the full team. Team members should dig deep into their creative juices to come up with a variety of options for stimulating better performance and working together in a cohesive and harmonious environment.

Think Like Geese

When it comes to teamwork, humans could learn a valuable lesson from geese and wild ducks (Figure 19–9). Consider the following facts and findings about geese and people:

FACT: As each goose flaps its wings, it creates uplift for the birds following. By flying in a "V" formation, the whole flock adds 71% more flying range than if each bird flew alone.

FINDING: People who share a common direction and sense of community can get where they are going more quickly and easily when they are traveling on the trust and strength of one another.

FACT: Whenever a goose falls out of formation, it suddenly feels the drag and resistance of trying to fly alone and quickly gets back into formation to take advantage of the lifting power provided by the birds immediately in front.

FINDING: If we think like geese, we will stay in tandem with those who are headed where we want to go, and we will be willing to accept their help as well as give ours to them.

FACT: When a lead goose gets tired, it rotates back into formation and another goose flies at the point position.

IT'S WORTH REMEMBERING

Evaluation must be a collaborative effort, as it becomes a learning opportunity for all concerned parties.

IT'S WORTH REMEMBERING

E Pluribus Unum—Out of many, one. The motto of one of the greatest countries in the world, the United States, refers to the fact that it was formed as a cohesive single nation as a result of the 13 smaller colonies joining together. What a team!

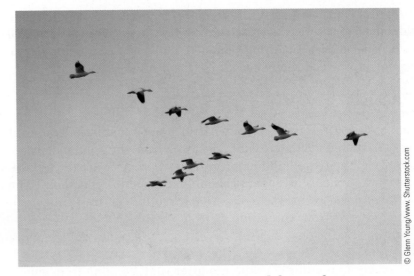

Figure 19–9   **We can learn a valuable teamwork lesson from geese.**

FINDING: It pays to take turns doing the hard tasks and sharing leadership with people interdependent with one another.

FACT: The geese in formation honk from behind to encourage those up front to keep up their speed.

FINDING: We need to make sure our "honking" from behind is encouragement rather than criticism.

FACT: When a goose gets sick, wounded, or shot, two geese drop out of formation and go with their fellow member to help and protect it. They stay with this member of the flock until it is able to fly again or dies. Then they launch out on their own, with another formation, or catch up with their flock.

FINDING: If we think like geese, we will stand by each other in difficult times as well as when we are strong.

Wrapping It Up

Dynamic teams will sustain a high degree of motivation over long periods of time if there is a dynamic leader on board who ensures that all the members are aligned with the overall mission and purpose of the organization and that they feel challenged, respected, and responsible. She will make certain that team members experience a feeling of fellowship and growth as a result of all members providing a relevant contribution. The leader will take the necessary steps to provide appropriate recognition for team members who excel. There will definitely be difficult times. The needs and wants of the individuals as well as the team as a whole will change periodically. As a result, changes to the plan will have to be made accordingly. As long as the lines of communication remain open and the team is open to change and growth through continuous team-building activities, the team and organization will prosper.

In Retrospect

1. Define the concept of teamwork.

2. List the 10 qualities team members are looking for in their work environment.

3. Explain the qualities required of a dynamic leader.

4. Identify the six key steps in team building.

5. List the 10 elements required in building team essentials.

Objectives (Desired Performance Goals):

After reading and studying this chapter, you should be able to:

- Explain the purpose of performance evaluation. List the general standards of performance that may be considered in a formal evaluation.

- Explain the qualities for satisfactory performance within each evaluation area.

- Identify the various sources available for performance assessment and explain the benefits of each.

- List the steps required in preparing a professional development plan.

- Explain the importance of pursuing continuing education as a professional educator.

KEY TERMS

! CRITICAL CONCEPT

One has to first perform well on the job in order to be evaluated and praised for the job performance.

Performance Assessment

EXPERIENCED MASTER EDUCATORS who are successful in producing knowledgeable, skilled, and competent graduates understand the need to remain current with respect to the technology used in the field and the skills taught, as well as the methodologies used to teach that information to learners. They recognize that if they are to continue to meet the challenges presented by their diverse learners, they must engage in constant professional assessment and improvement in personal performance. Generally, the employing institution will have in place an evaluation policy and procedure that provides assessment of the educator's performance on at least an annual basis. Improvement will have a greater impact and will be longer lasting when the educator recognizes the need for improved performance and develops a *professional development plan* to achieve it.

By adopting a positive attitude toward self-improvement and following important self-improvement strategies, educators will inspire and train learners to become highly skilled, competent professionals and, in some cases, the educators of the future. The purpose of evaluation is to improve job performance and promote career development. An evaluation is an appraisal of performance that is based upon expectations. In order to begin the assessment process, educators must first identify the areas of performance that are to be evaluated and the criteria that clarify the performance expectations.

General Standards of Evaluation

In addition to the detailed criteria contained in the educator's defined job duties, general standards of evaluation must also be considered. Depending upon the organization and mission of the institution, those general standards may vary. However, nine areas of performance are usually reviewed:

- **Production**
- **Thoroughness and accuracy**
- **Independent action**
- **Work methods**
- **Problem solving**
- **Interpersonal skills** and professional conduct
- **Work habits**
- **Cost consciousness**
- **Self-motivation**

Each area of performance includes specific criteria that address the expectations that the educator should strive to meet. Examples of performance criteria that might be established for each area are discussed next.

Production

- Meets commitments as assigned and outlined in the job description and duties.
- Goes above and beyond normal production requirements of the job and assumes extra duties when needed.

+ MASTER EDUCATOR

1. Develops and implements an ongoing professional development plan.
2. Obtains quality continuing education in personal and professional development.
3. Does not consider "minimum" standards of performance or education acceptable.

CONSIDER AND CONNECT

Master educators will seek feedback from others in the assessment process, including coworkers and other educators, the students who are being taught, and supervisors and management.

IT'S WORTH REMEMBERING

The primary responsibility for self-improvement lies with the educator.

production one's performance in meeting commitments and producing the expected volume of work or going beyond normal production requirements.

thoroughness and accuracy one's performance in setting high standards, accurately completing assigned tasks, paying close attention to details, and detecting errors and correcting them as applicable.

independent action one's performance in exercising initiative, working independently, solving problems, and maintaining steady performance under pressure.

work methods one's performance in organization skills, meeting deadlines, correcting mistakes, prioritizing and not wasting time.

problem solving one's performance in solving problems, making decision, evaluating outcomes, and striving for a win-win solution.

interpersonal skills one's performance in keeping management informed, working cooperatively with others, communicating clearly, being a role model, never fraternizing with students, and conveying self-confidence.

work habits one's performance in maintaining dependable, regular attendance, arriving promptly, keeping personal time to a minimum.

- Produces the expected volume of work, or more.
- Meets training or other obligations of employment in addition to the regular work schedule.

Thoroughness and Accuracy

- Sets high standards and consistently achieves quality results.
- Accurately completes assigned tasks and job duties.
- Verifies questionable information or procedures.
- Pays close attention to instructions and essential details.
- Provides thorough and accurate written reports when required.
- Detects errors and corrects them or makes appropriate personnel aware of them.

Independent Action

- Exercises initiative in starting and following through on assigned work.
- Works independently, requiring little or no close supervision.
- Initiates action to solve problems whenever possible, without supervisory intervention.
- Maintains steady performance under work pressure.

Work Methods

- Organizes and plans work in advance.
- Sets and meets realistic target dates for project assignments.
- Initiates prompt corrective actions when goals are not met.
- Wastes no time on nonessential work or tasks.
- Organizes priorities and follows through.

Problem Solving

- Solves problems effectively.
- Makes decisions on assigned work without supervisory assistance whenever possible.
- Evaluates all possible outcomes before taking action.
- Strives for a "win, win, win" situation in all solutions.

Interpersonal Skills and Professional Conduct

- Keeps management informed about significant actions or problems.
- Clearly communicates ideas or the essence of a problem or concern.
- Works cooperatively with coworkers, students, clients, and management.
- Maintains a positive, caring attitude at all times.
- Extends courtesy and respect to coworkers, students, and superiors at all times.
- Conducts personal affairs in such a manner that they do not reflect negatively on the school or detract from the normal work day.

- Is a role model for fellow employees and students. Maintains personal hygiene and a professional image at all times according to the institution's dress code.
- Keeps a professional distance and never fraternizes with students. Maintains the relationship of advisor, educator, facilitator, and resource person.
- Refrains from using harsh or loud language and profanity while on the job.
- Develops a positive rapport with area businesses and oversight agencies.
- Develops and conveys self-confidence at all times.
- Practices personal and business ethics (i.e., a system of standards of conduct and moral judgment) at all times.

Work Habits

- Maintains dependable, regular attendance.
- Arrives on time daily (only justifiable reasons cause tardiness).
- Keeps personal time to a minimum (e.g., socializing, personal calls, personal visitors, etc.)
- Doesn't leave scheduled classes or duties to take or make personal calls. Returns calls on breaks.
- Provides a day of work for a day of pay.

Cost Consciousness

- Eliminates nonessential activities.
- Willingly suggests cost-saving measures.
- Does not waste supplies, inventory, or office materials.
- Does not make unnecessary copies on the copy machine.
- Handles monies responsibly and recovers/restores monies lost due to carelessness or mismanagement.
- Observes energy-saving measures whenever possible.
- Respects the property of the institution and takes steps to prevent damage to materials or equipment.

Self-Motivation

- Pursues success and excellence at all times.
- Stretches personal resources for career growth.
- Seeks opportunities to build on strengths.
- Develops an awareness of performance needs and works on deficiencies.
- Sustains a high level of interest and enthusiasm.
- Maintains a minimum of 40 hours of continuing education annually.
- Employs techniques and strategies learned through continuing education.
- Maintains subscriptions to professional trade publications.

Detailed criteria for performance expectations might be found in the job requirements and standards of evaluation sections of the educator's job description, which may vary from institution to institution.

cost consciousness one's performance in eliminating nonessential activities and costs, not wasting supplies, handling monies responsibly, observing energy-saving measures, and respecting the property of the institution.

self-motivation one's performance in pursuing success and excellence at all times, stretching personal resources, seeking opportunities to build on strengths, sustaining a highlevel of interest and enthusiasm, and completing at least 40 hours of continuing education annually.

☑ Educator Position Description

An example of a typical job description for an educator in career education is shown in the accompanying box.

EDUCATOR POSITION DESCRIPTION

Major Goal: To instruct students effectively, which ensures that the institution will achieve its major educational goals, objectives, and continuing purpose.

Summary: To contribute maximum effort through teaching activities toward achievement of the institution's goals and objectives according to the institution's written operating procedures and with the following guidelines in mind:

- To consider first, believe in, and carry out the established policies of the institution.
- To be receptive to competent counsel from colleagues and be guided by such counsel without impairing the dignity and responsibility of the position held.
- To instruct without prejudice and avoid unethical practices.
- To pursue continuing knowledge of the career field and establish practical and current methods of teaching.
- To subscribe to and work for honesty and truth in fulfilling the requirements of the position.
- To respect students, clients, and fellow staff members.
- To counsel and assist fellow educators in the performance of their duties.
- To cooperate with professional organizations and individuals engaged in activities that enhance the development of career education.
- To project a professional image with appropriate grooming and dress at all times.
- To perform all duties and responsibilities as stated in the position requirements and standards of evaluation in a satisfactory manner.
- To maintain a continuing, realistic analysis and appraisal of the needs of students.
- To teach students effectively using proper and current methods for the courses taught.
- To maintain efficiency and consistency in the performance of the administrative tasks of the position.
- To be constantly aware of all work methods, self-improvement, and career development opportunities.

Each job description prepared for a master educator will usually be accompanied by a detailed list of job duties and various abilities and levels of knowledge that are expected of the educator. The list will rarely be conclusive, and most job descriptions will reserve the right to require additional tasks or performance by the educator as deemed necessary by the management. Following is an example of a list of job duties that might apply to an educator in career education.

Job Knowledge and Job Duties

Teaching Responsibilities (90 percent or more of daily scheduled work time)

- Read, understand, and follow the responsibilities and policies outlined in the institution's written operating procedures.
- Gain a working knowledge of the institution's satisfactory academic progress policy, standards of conduct, practical course requirements, grading policies and criteria, and state regulations within 30 days of employment.
- Teach and follow the institution's published curriculum, using all teaching aids and handouts provided unless deviations are approved.
- Learn any new teaching methods introduced during employment and follow them consistently.
- Maintain a thorough knowledge of the school's mission statement and objectives and strive to attain them at all times.
- Greet all students daily with a smile and a positive comment.
- Write an inspirational thought for the day on the board or project on the screen.
- Prepare for and participate in new-student orientation according to school policy. Conduct complete orientation if assigned.
- Prepare a dated class schedule for applicable courses and post in the classroom.
- Organize and prepare for each class presentation. Organize the necessary handouts, teaching aids, and equipment prior to starting the class. Plan which learning reinforcement ideas or activities will be incorporated into the lesson.
- Always begin and end class on time as scheduled without exception.
- Follow and supplement published lesson plans. Present the information without reading from the text or lesson plan.
- Avoid monotone in classroom presentations—project enthusiasm and excitement. Practice proper grammar and pronunciation. Be careful of tone, volume, and clarity of expression.
- Maintain a thorough, accurate, and current knowledge of the subject matter taught.
- Ask open-ended questions; encourage class participation that involves all students, not just a select few.
- Vary the stimuli for learners during presentations. Use body movement and gestures effectively.
- Write practical and/or written assignments on the chalkboard daily.
- Stress which areas of the lesson should be recorded in notes or highlighted in the text for needed emphasis or state board exam preparation.
- Do not embarrass or intimidate students. Never use a condescending tone or manner. Maintain a friendly but businesslike atmosphere.
- Inspire pride in workmanship and a professional attitude in your students toward their training and work responsibilities by your example.
- Be fair and impartial in your dealings with all students.
- Practice active listening skills when interacting with students. Listen carefully to their comments and questions.
- Avoid personal mannerisms or habits that may be distracting to the learning environment.
- Research questions to which you do not know the answer. Stimulate students to think for themselves and research the answers themselves. Use examples for clarification. Use effective review questions and procedures. Ensure tests are graded promptly and give immediate feedback to students whenever possible.

- Control argumentative or disruptive students by getting them involved. Assign them leadership tasks. Praise their accomplishments.
- Grade practical skills according to established grading criteria. Record grades as required by the institution. Explain and clarify grading criteria as needed.
- Conduct practical skills tests as scheduled for all students in accordance with published guidelines, as applicable.
- Ensure that phase I or first-year students complete the required theory and practical skills training and pass the required competency evaluations.
- Complete and conduct progress evaluations and perform academic advisement for students according to the institution's policy. Discuss areas needing improvement as well as areas of accomplishment. Identify a plan of action for improvement as needed. Follow up on plans for improvement during subsequent evaluations.
- Keep equipment needed for classroom or laboratory instruction clean and in good operating order.
- Encourage students to use the extensive reference materials found in the institution's library or resource center.
- Each month, assign different students a bulletin board project with a motivational and educational theme.
- Properly prepare graduating students for the applicable state licensing examinations and strive for a 95 percent annual examination pass rate, if applicable.
- Monitor and fairly enforce the institution's policies, standards of conduct, and oversight regulations.
- Conduct emergency evacuation exercises according to the institution's published policy.
- Never release private information on any student without obtaining written authorization from the student (or parent/guardian if applicable) on the designated form.
- Be readily available for students. Never make them have to search for you when they need a grade or assistance.

Other Duties (never more than 10 percent of scheduled work time)

- Attend staff meetings as scheduled and participate in discussion of all required agenda items.
- Provide employment assistance for graduating students as needed. Document efforts and strive for a rate of 85 percent placement or better. Post job openings found in area newspapers and other publications on a "Career Opportunities" bulletin board.
- Monitor inventory needs according to policy and report needs to campus administration or other appropriate personnel.
- Complete any administrative tasks as assigned in a timely and accurate manner.

Sources of Performance Assessment

As mentioned earlier, the educator can pursue many sources to obtain feedback and assessment of personal performance. Many such sources are readily available within the institution and should be taken advantage of by the educator, as discussed next.

Supervisors

Formal performance evaluations are generally conducted by supervisory personnel on at least an annual basis. Supervisors are responsible for training educators in the proper procedures and expected behaviors as well as providing assistance, coaching, or direction to educators. During that process they will also monitor the educator's performance and progress, much in the same way you monitor your students' progress. They will identify strengths exhibited by the educator and also discuss any weaknesses that need to be improved. Generally, a plan of action for improvement will be identified and agreed upon by both the educator and supervisor. Supervisors may be far more experienced than the educators they oversee and should be considered a source of advice by the educator. A typical evaluation policy and form that could be used by career institutions is shown in the accompanying box.

EXAMPLE OF AN EMPLOYEE EVALUATION POLICY

The performance of staff members is reviewed annually with respect to the tasks specified in the position description and standards of evaluation. Evaluation of employee performance will aid in recognition of excellence and encourage individual improvement when needed.

The ultimate purpose of evaluation is to improve job performance and promote career development. An evaluation is an appraisal of performance that is based upon expectations.

During the employee review, there will be a discussion and summary of job performance and, where appropriate, recommendations for improvement. To determine the overall performance of the employee, the supervisor will consider all evaluation data, including observation of job performance as well as coworker and student surveys conducted in relation to the requirements of the position.

The purpose of the employee review is to help the employee achieve a professional level of conduct and performance. To accomplish this, employees need to clearly understand what is expected and be committed to achieve quality results. Open communication between the employee and the evaluator is needed to conduct a successful review. The employee review should be structured as follows:

1. State the results of the evaluation.
2. Learn the employee's view of his performance.
3. Further investigate, if necessary, to get all the relevant facts.
4. Generate a plan of action.
   a. State what is expected and when.
   b. Determine how these expectations will be measured.
   c. Clearly define next steps if the expected improvement is not achieved.
5. Form a commitment and sign and date the evaluation.

The employee review is utilized in all steps of employee counseling, including regular evaluations, and may result in any of the following:

- Employment promotion
- Employment probation
- Leave of absence (voluntary or involuntary)
- Employment termination

Employee review results are recorded on the employee review report. Performance is evaluated as follows (Figure 20–1):

STRENGTH:	Consistently exceeds requirements
SATISFACTORY:	Consistently meets requirements
DEVELOPMENT OPPORTUNITY:	Room for improvement or needs development
UNSATISFACTORY:	Performance has negative impact on results and improvement *must* occur

EMPLOYEE REVIEW REPORT

NAME _____ POSITION _____

PURPOSE OF REVIEW: _____ Performance Evaluation _____ Employment Counseling

EVALUATOR NAME _____ DATE _____

PERFORMANCE FACTOR	ST.	SAT.	D. O.	UNSAT.	COMMENTS
PRODUCTION					
THOROUGHNESS/ACCURACY					
INDEPENDENT ACTION					
WORK METHODS					
PROBLEM SOLVING					
INTERPERSONAL SKILLS/ PROFESSIONAL CONDUCT					
WORK HABITS					
COST CONSCIOUSNESS					
SELF MOTIVATION					
JOB KNOWLEDGE DUTIES					

STUDENT RETENTION GOAL _____   STUDENT VOLUME GOAL _____

LICENSURE GOAL _____   PLACEMENT GOAL _____

ACTION PLAN _____

_____

_____

_____

_____

EMPLOYEE ACKNOWLEDGMENT	DATE	EVALUATOR SIGNATURE	DATE

Figure 20–1   Employee evaluations should be documented on an employee review report.

Other Educators and Coworkers

Other educators can be extremely helpful in providing you with information in regard to your performance (Figure 20–2). They are in the same profession and work in the same environment. They are familiar with the students you teach. They are very likely familiar with the curriculum or lesson plans you are teaching. It doesn't really matter if they are more or

Educator Classroom Assessment by Peer

Educator Name _____ Class Presented _____ Date _____

Observe the educator for no less than 30 minutes. Rate the educator during a classroom presentation in the following areas. Rate each category from 1 to 4, with 4 considered the best performance. Make constructive suggestions for improvement as applicable.

Educator Image

1.   _____   Hair is styled appropriately.
2.   _____   Makeup is applied appropriately (if applicable).
3.   _____   Clothing/shoes are neat and clean.
4.   _____   Hands/nails are well manicured.

Preparation and Organization

1.   _____   Classroom was organized.
2.   _____   Class began on time.
3.   _____   Visual aid equipment was set up and checked before class.
4.   _____   Demonstration materials were arranged ahead of time (if applicable).

Presentation Skills and Attitude

1.   _____   Projected self-confidence.
2.   _____   Projected positive, professional attitude.
3.   _____   Demonstrated leadership qualities.
4.   _____   Utilized good voice pitch, rate, and intonation.
5.   _____   Utilized visual aids effectively during presentation.
6.   _____   Demonstrated thorough knowledge of subject matter.
7.   _____   Maintained professionalism with all students during presentation.
8.   _____   Maintained good eye contact with learners.
9.   _____   Encouraged participation by all learners.
10. _____   Did not read from the text or lesson plan.
11. _____   Varied the stimuli for the learners.
12. _____   Lesson objectives were met.
13. _____   Learners were attentive, interested, and motivated.
14. _____   Learners actively took notes.
15. _____   Classroom control was maintained.

Testing and Review

1.   _____   Asked open-ended questions during class.
2.   _____   Called upon a variety of learners for participation.
3.   _____   Answered questions accurately.
4.   _____   Involved all learners in the review process.
5.   _____   Questions asked were relevant to the objectives of the lesson.

Demonstration Skills (if applicable to lesson)

1.   _____   Demonstration was seen and heard by all learners.
2.   _____   Demonstration was accurate and used the most current techniques and implements.
3.   _____   Class members participated during demonstration.
4.   _____   Questions were appropriately answered.

Strengths: _____

_____

Suggestions for improvement: _____

_____

Overall Assessment Summary:

_____ Exceeds Standards _____ Meets Standards _____ Development Opportunity _____ Unsatisfactory

Evaluator Name _____ Date _____

Figure 20–2   Peer evaluation is a great source of feedback for educators.

less experienced than you; they can provide you with a nonthreatening, fresh perspective of how you are doing. They may also be able to share techniques with you that they have found effective over the years. Other coworkers who are not educators can also provide relevant feedback, especially when using a standard peer evaluation form. For example, almost anyone could sit in your classroom and observe whether certain criteria or factors are being adequately addressed. Refer to the example of a typical peer evaluation form that could be completed by both fellow educators and other personnel.

Learners

Probably one of the most effective sources of educator assessment is the learners who are actually taught by them. The achievement of learner outcomes may directly relate to the educator's ability and performance. In addition, learners, more so than anyone else, know how the educator performs in the classroom on a regular basis. They can give valuable feedback to the educator regarding the educational methods used, the relationships established with the learners, the use of visual aids, and so much more. An example of an evaluation that can be completed by learners is shown in Figure 20–3.

Graduates and Their Employers

After learners have completed the course of study and entered the workforce, they become another source for feedback regarding the educator's performance. Their achievements on the job and the competitiveness of their entry-level skills may directly or indirectly relate to the educator's ability and performance during the graduate's educational process. Institutions often utilize surveys of both graduates and employers of graduates to obtain feedback about the school's educational programs and support services. Employers of graduates are in a perfect position to assess their skills and abilities, and can therefore provide additional feedback to the educator regarding educational methods and programs. Examples of surveys used for graduates and employers of graduates are shown in Figures 20–4 and 20–5.

You, the Educator

In your quest to become a master educator, you must recognize that absolute perfection is never attained in any career pursuit. However, you must also acknowledge that your abilities as an educator will continue to improve as you learn and grow. Your experiences in the classroom, in the clinic, and during field trips and other educational activities will provide insight into how you can achieve greater outcomes and success with your learners. The growth you experience will be aided by regular self-assessment. Figure 20–6 depicts an educator self-evaluation checklist that can be used to help you personally identify strengths and weaknesses. After completing the checklist, you can use the results to develop your own plan for improvement and set goals for future accomplishments.

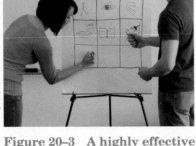

Figure 20–3   A highly effective source of educator assessment is the learners they teach.

Graduate Employer Survey

We are conducting a survey of employers of our graduates in an attempt to determine how they are doing on the job and determine ways to improve our educational programs and methods. If you have received this survey by mail, please take a few minutes to answer a few questions about _____, who is (or has been) an employee in your establishment.

(If this survey is conducted by phone, the school employee must be sure to ask the salon owner or manager if they are busy with a client and if so, determine a convenient time to conduct the survey.)

Graduate's Position: _____ Date Hired: _____

What type of establishment do you operate? ___Full Service ___Nail Salon ___Barber Shop ___Day Spa ___Massage Therapy Clinic ___Esthetics Salon ___Other

Do you agree that a graduate directly out of training will not usually possess the speed and degree of technical skill as a seasoned professional? ___Yes ___No Comment: _____

_____

Do you feel the graduate you employ(ed) was prepared with basic job entry-level skills? ___ Yes ___ No

Comments: _____

_____

_____

Do you have any suggestions that might help us improve education in the previously discussed technical areas?

_____

_____

At our institution we focus a great deal of emphasis during the student's training on the importance of developing people skills, communication skills, goal orientations and professionalism. Please rate the graduate from 1 to 5 (with 5 being the best) in the following areas:
Attitude _____ Self-motivation _____ Personal Desire to Succeed _____
Attendance _____ Promptness _____ Professional Image _____ Cooperation _____

Would you care to serve on our industry advisory council which consults with us on at least an annual basis? _____ Yes _____ No

Would you care to appear as a guest speaker on career related topics for our students? ___ Yes ___ No

Have you taken advantage of our Job Placement Assistance Program in filling open positions in your establishment? _____ Yes _____ No   If not, please feel free to contact us anytime in the future and we will be happy to arrange an interview with any available, qualified graduates.

Thank you for your assistance. Please feel free to call on us if we can be of assistance to you in any way. We feel strongly that all sectors of our industry must unite and work together to achieve success.
Name and telephone number of employer surveyed: _____
Phone survey conducted by: _____ Date: _____

Figure 20–4 Graduate surveys provide valuable feedback on how well the training has prepared the graduate for the workforce.

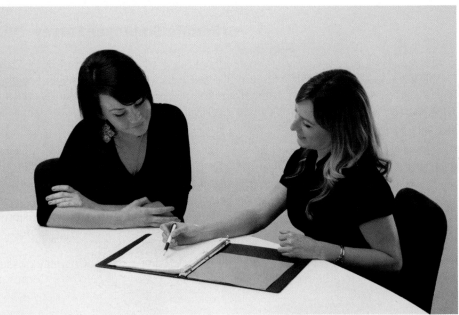

Figure 20–5   Employers of the school's graduates can also provide input on how to improve performance and programs.

The checklist in Figure 20–6 is one example of how an educator can conduct a self-evaluation to determine areas of strength as well as those needing improvement. A similar approach is the use of a climate self-assessment inventory; the example shown in Figure 20–7 is a 34-item chart that is completed using a four-point rating scale.

✓ Professional Development

Master educators will participate in the various forms of assessment previously mentioned and use that valuable feedback to create a professional development plan. The completed evaluations, whether done by peers, students, graduates, or self, will help to identify any problem areas or concerns that need to be strengthened or resolved. The educator can then establish a *long-term goal* for improvement that is supported by measurable *short-term objectives*. Educators should also correlate any *objectives for improved student outcomes* in the development plan. Once the objectives and goals have been identified, the educator can then outline the *strategies or activities* required to achieve the objectives. As with any improvement plan, the master educator will periodically *evaluate the plan* to determine if it is working and if the goals and objectives of the plan are being met.

Sample Professional Development Plan

1. **Problem Area or Concern.** The educator will simply state any concerns that have been identified through the various assessments that have been conducted. The statement should include the source or evidence of the concern. For example:

Educator Self-Evaluation Checklist

Read each standard or performance behavior and check the response that best applies to you.

PERFORMANCE	YES	NO	UNSURE	SOMETIMES
COMMUNICATION SKILLS I maintain a friendly but purposeful atmosphere in class.				
I maintain a direct rapport with the learners.				
I give attention to the entire class.				
I speak loudly and clearly enough to be understood.				
I vary the pitch, volume, and tempo of speech.				
I am clear and precise in my presentation of ideas.				
I use proper grammar and pronunciation.				
I actively listen to all learners.				
I show respect for learners' comments or questions.				
I remain up to date on all curriculum topics.				
I organize course materials properly.				
I properly plan and prepare for each lesson.				
When unsure of answers, I acknowledge my uncertainty.				
I research material and find answers to all questions.				
CLASSROOM ATTITUDES I enjoy teaching.				
I exhibit energy and enthusiasm in the classroom.				
I make every subject seem important to the entire course.				
Teaching stimulates me to increase my own knowledge/skills.				
I foster a professional attitude in students.				
I am fair and impartial with all students at all times.				
I inspire learners to apply their own experiences to learning.				
I stimulate learners to relevant discussion of class material.				
I inspire students to seek further knowledge outside school.				
Most of my students complete their training and attain career success.				
Students appear at ease in my classroom.				

Figure 20–6   (Continued)

PERFORMANCE	YES	NO	UNSURE	SOMETIMES
TEACHING SKILLS AND TECHNIQUES I start every class promptly at the scheduled time.				
I continue class activity until class is scheduled to end.				
I review each lesson before moving to the next one.				
I use concept connectors to tie new material to prior learning.				
I keep learners busy with worthwhile activities and projects.				
I incorporate a variety of teaching methods into every lesson.				
I frequently use a variety of teaching aids.				
I create an interesting and cooperative environment.				
I encourage group synergy, self-expression, and creativity.				
I show the relevance of class work with practice in the field.				
I talk with students in a challenging but unpretentious manner.				
I learn all students' names, talents, abilities, and needs.				
I encourage appropriate relationships among learners.				
My students know I take a personal interest in their learning.				
I use a variety of measures to evaluate learner performance.				
I follow grading criteria fairly and equitably for all learners.				
I confront disruptive learners appropriately and sensitively.				
I hold private conferences with learners when issues mandate.				
I refer learners with special counseling needs to qualified professionals.				

After completing the checklist, think carefully about each strength and weakness that you have identified. For areas of relative strength (yes or sometimes answers), consider the positive effects that those behaviors may have on student learning and on motivation levels of both you and your learners. For areas of weakness (no answers), consider how to improve performance through better planning or additional training. Statements that received an "unsure" response may be unclear because you have not yet considered the effects of those behaviors on student learning. Review all questions and answers carefully and incorporate them into the planning and evaluation phases of your teaching. It is recommended that you conduct this self-evaluation on a quarterly basis and retain in your personnel file.

Figure 20–6   Your professional growth will be aided by regular self-assessment.

Climate Self-Assessment Inventory

Rate yourself on each of these items, using the following codes:

1 = Almost never   2 = Occasionally   3 = Frequently   4 = Almost always

I. Relationships with Learners

_____ 1. I treat learners fairly. I don't play favorites or punish the entire class for the actions of a few.

_____ 2. I operate on the assumption that the learners want to do the right thing.

_____ 3. I make ample use of rewards and praise and show appreciation for all learners.

_____ 4. I am perceived by my learners as a sincere person.

_____ 5. I treat learners as valuable human beings.

_____ 6. I respect learners regardless of their ability levels.

_____ 7. Learners believe that I care about them and that I am there to help them.

_____ 8. Learners can count on me to listen to their side of the story and take appropriate action.

_____ 9. Learners easily approach me for advice and assistance.

_____ 10. I set a positive example for students to follow.

_____ 11. I listen carefully when students voice their opinions and needs.

_____ 12. I emphasize success and potential with learners rather than focus on behaviors that result in failures and shortcomings.

II. Structuring and Managing the Classroom

_____ 1. I attempt to recognize and identify problems concerning students before they develop.

_____ 2. I monitor and enforce the rules in my classroom in a fair and equitable manner.

_____ 3. I discipline the learner's behavior rather than the learner.

_____ 4. I show respect for my students in spite of what they do.

III. Instruction Techniques

_____ 1. I establish realistic and attainable standards for my learners in their behavior and their work.

_____ 2. I vary my instructional techniques so that students with varying learning styles can benefit.

_____ 3. Assignments I give are perceived as useful and meaningful by my students.

_____ 4. I utilize learning activities that require active participation by all learners.

_____ 5. I incorporate greater learner–educator interactions to achieve better outcomes and results for all learners.

_____ 6. During class discussions and reviews I call on individual learners by name rather than asking for responses from volunteers only.

_____ 7. I ask questions that are challenging but allow the learner reasonable opportunity for success.

_____ 8. I utilize questions that encourage productive, divergent thinking abilities in my learners.

_____ 9. I encourage student-to-student discussion as a learning activity.

_____ 10. I provide as much praise to low achievers as I do to high achievers.

IV. Expectations

_____ 1. I instill the importance of high learning and behavioral standards in all my learners.

_____ 2. The expectations that I set for my learners include clear goals for achievement.

_____ 3. My students are instructed in such a manner that supports an atmosphere of confidence so that they can and will succeed.

_____ 4. My instructional effectiveness determines learner achievement levels far more than family background or ethnicity.

V. Physical Environment

_____ 1. My classroom or laboratory is neat, bright, cheerful, and attractive.

_____ 2. The materials, equipment, and facilities I utilize are in good condition and well cared for.

_____ 3. The materials and visual aids on display are interesting and stimulating.

_____ 4. My classroom or laboratory arrangement is conducive to orderly behavior and the delivery of instruction.

_____ **TOTAL SCORE**

Figure 20–7 **Use the results of self-assessment to develop a plan for improvement.**

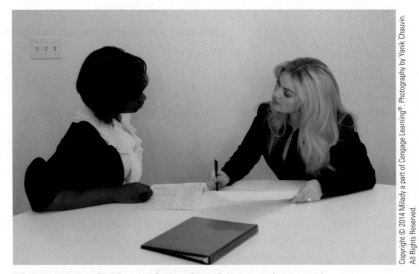

**Figure 20–8   Seek employer involvement in creating a
professional development plan.**

*A few learners in the class appear inattentive, disinterested, and lack
motivation, as evidenced by both peer and student evaluations and my
own observations. Their lack of interest can be defeating and discouraging to the remainder of the class.*

2. **Long-Term Goal for Improvement.** In this step, the educator will
   briefly identify one or two long-term goals for improved performance or
   behavior. For example:

   - *To establish a learning environment in which all students are moti-
     vated, interested, attentive, and actively participate.*
   - *To improve my skills in creating an exciting, energetic environment
     and my ability to bring learners into active participation in the
     class.*

3. **Short-Term Objectives.** Here the educator will list specific objectives
   that are measurable and may include timelines for achievement. These
   objectives will tie directly to the educator's performance and abilities.
   For example:

   - *To prepare more thoroughly for each class presentation.*
   - *To review specific teaching methods and techniques known to improve
     learner attention, interest, and motivation.*
   - *To incorporate those teaching methods and techniques into each les-
     son presentation or class project.*
   - *To reconsider the classroom arrangement to ensure that maximum
     participation by all learners can be achieved.*

4. **Expected Learner Outcomes.** In this step, the educator will list
   behavioral or performance changes that can be expected of the learners
   with the use and implementation of the educator's objectives and strategies. For example:

   - *Increased learner attention and participation.*
   - *Improved learner outcomes with respect to grades and skills abilities.*
   - *Improved attitudes of all learners due to the more enthusiastic
     environment.*

5. Strategies and Activities. Here the educator will identify specific actions that should result in the achievement of the stated objectives. For example:

- *To incorporate dynamic openings into every class in order to gain the attention of all learners.*
- *To utilize concept connectors at the opening of each lesson to ensure that all learners are interested in the day's lesson.*
- *To employ small-group activities in which group leaders are rotated so that all learners become involved, regardless of interest level.*
- *To reward learners for volunteering and participation so that less participatory learners will be motivated to get involved with the lesson.*
- *To incorporate activities that require working in pairs and match less motivated learners with those who are more active and involved.*
- *To conduct more stretch breaks and energizers for a change of pace and to bring life and enthusiasm into the lesson.*
- *To involve the less interested learners by giving them responsibilities such as being the "handout control officer" or the designated scribe during flip-chart activities.*
- *To vary my speech tone, pitch, volume, and pace to increase interest.*
- *To vary the stimuli for learners as often as possible in each lesson to retain learner attention.*
- *To employ the use of circle, half-circle, or crescent rounds in the classroom arrangement to facilitate better eye contact and participation among all learners.*

6. Evaluation of Professional Development Plan. After the educator has developed and implemented the strategies for improvement, the final step is to evaluate the effectiveness of the plan. It must be determined which strategies or activities were effective and which were not, if any. That information will determine if any changes need to be made in the plan. The educator can conduct the evaluation through the use of repeated peer and student evaluations, checklists, notations of personal observations, self-evaluations, student outcomes, and more. For example:

- *Completion of my climate self-assessment inventory indicated that I had made significant improvements in the categories stated in Instruction Techniques.*
- *Learner assessments of educator surveys indicated improved ratings by nearly all learners in criteria 12, 14, 17, and 25.*
- *Educator classroom assessment by peer conducted by Ms. Rogers indicated improvement in criteria 3, 4, 5, 8, 9, 11, 13, and 14 of the Presentation Skills and Attitude category.*

7. Supervisor Assessment of Professional Development Plan. Having supervisory feedback is recommended in order for the educator to obtain the support of a professional who has a vested interest in the educator's success. Because they are normally more experienced, their ability to interpret the feedback and recommend actions for improvement can be highly beneficial. For example:

> *My supervisor observed at least two of my classes during the past month. She observed increased enthusiasm and participation on the part of the learners. That improvement was noted in my annual performance evaluation conducted recently. She encourages the continued implementation of the strategies and activities identified in the plan. She suggested that I might also incorporate more use of team contests, especially when teaching the more difficult subjects.*

☑ Resources for Professional Development

A sure step toward the attainment and maintenance of your master educator status is to constantly further your education. We have stressed throughout this text that educators must stay abreast of changes in technology, products, and tools in order to remain effective in the classroom. Continuing education is the measure that should be taken by all educators to help ensure that performance evaluations from learners, peers, and supervisors result in the best possible ratings. Sources of continuing education and professional development vary. As stated in Chapter 1, "The Career Education Instructor," it is recommended that a master educator obtain at least 40 hours per year of professional development training, regardless of whether the hours are required for license renewal.

Resources for obtaining continuing education include state school associations, online learning modules from Cengage Learning, state regulatory boards, national accrediting agency seminars, national trade association workshops and seminars, annual conventions, and more. All such continuing education events promote serious opportunities for networking with educators of varied backgrounds, interests, and experience. This informal interaction among educators allows you to share ideas, experiences, solutions to problems, and any other concerns or issues relevant to the professional of teaching.

☑ Wrapping It Up

We have focused on the importance of assessment and evaluation of the educator's performance in achieving the status of master educator. We outlined several strategies and formats of evaluation to aid you in your quest of becoming a master educator. We have described steps to develop and implement a professional development plan. Emphasis has again been placed on the importance of remaining abreast of industry trends, technologies, tools, and techniques. We have also identified several resources for obtaining quality training in personal and professional development. As a reminder, when surveying institutions across the nation to determine the qualities and characteristics sought in educators, one of the first and foremost requirements was that the educator independently pursued professional continuing education and went above and beyond the "minimum" required. Master educators will avail themselves of every opportunity for continued growth and professional development and will not consider "minimum" standards of performance or education acceptable.

In Retrospect

1. Explain the purpose of performance evaluation.

2. List the general standards of performance that may be considered in a formal evaluation.

3. Explain the qualities for satisfactory performance within each evaluation area.

4. Identify the various sources available for performance assessment.

5. List the steps required in preparing a professional development plan.

6. Explain the importance of pursuing continuing education as a professional educator.

Glossary

Academic advisement: the process of advising a student regarding his academic performance, including written grades, practical skills, and attendance, and developing a plan for improvement, if needed.

Accommodation plan: an accommodation plan provides the necessary information for the learner regarding the steps the school is able to reasonably take to accommodate the individual learner's needs.

Achiever: achiever communicators score high in self-control and resist impulses to reveal much about their inner selves; they are very sensitive and express their expectations clearly.

Active listening: active listening means being with the speaker, concentrating on what is being said; not interrupting; repeating what the speaker has said and paraphrasing it to make certain you have understood; establishing that what you repeated was what was meant.

ADA: The Americans with Disabilities Act signed into law in 1990.

ADHD: attention deficit hyperactivity disorder, a chronic neurological dysfunction within the central nervous system that is not related to gender, level of intelligence, or cultural environment.

Advisory council: a committee composed of school owners and directors, educators, and employers within the applicable field of study; graduates of the institution; representatives from local or state professional trade organizations; and even, perhaps, representatives from the regulatory oversight agencies. The focus of the council should be curriculum, facilities, equipment, and institutional outcomes, at a minimum.

Affective domain: in the affective domain, the desired performance objective includes the demonstration of feelings, attitudes, or sensitivities toward other people, ideas, or things.

Amphitheater arrangement: an arrangement that is highly effective for lecture, demonstration, slide or video projection, and role-playing; facilitator has high degree of control; provides poor opportunity for participation and interaction.

Analogy: similarity in some respects between things that are otherwise dissimilar.

Anecdote: a short account of some interesting or humorous incident.

Anticipatory set: a process that begins before students enter the classroom and continues during the activity that occurs when learners are arriving physically and then mentally adapting to what is about to occur in the classroom. Essentially, it is the process of getting students ready to learn.

Articulation: the act or process of pronouncing distinctly and carefully; enunciation.

Assertiveness: the degree of boldness or confidence one has in dealing with others.

Authority: an individual cited or appealed to as an expert; the power to influence or command thought, opinion, or behavior.

Boardroom arrangement: an arrangement suitable for roundtable-type discussions or meetings; not often used in career education classroom; facilitator has medium control.

Bodily/kinesthetic intelligence: the ability to use the physical body skillfully to solve problems, create products, or present ideas and emotions as well as take in knowledge through bodily sensation such as coordination or working with the hands.

Character role-playing: the learner plays the part of a specific person and acts as that person would in the given situation.

Characterizations: characterizations are used in the classroom by the educator to allow the learners to translate the content of the lesson into personage.

Checklist: a variation of the rating scale that contains fewer rating categories; generally, a specific performance is rated as *adequate* or *inadequate* or *satisfactory* or *unsatisfactory*.

Chevron-style arrangement: an arrangement also known as the V-shape; can be used for lecture, demonstration, discussion, role-playing, and case studies; suitable for small and large groups; facilitator has medium control.

Chronic barrier: a chronic barrier to learning occurs when a learner behaves in a difficult manner consistently and creates a barrier to learning for other students.

Circle arrangement: an arrangement for small classes up to 15; effective for lectures, discussion, role-playing, and completing case studies; facilitator has high control.

Classroom arrangement: an arrangement commonly used in traditional education; can be used for lecture, demonstration, discussion, or panel discussions; facilitator has high control; provides poor opportunity for participation and interaction.

Cognitive domain: the cognitive domain includes those performances that require knowledge of specific information, such as principles, concepts, and generalizations necessary for problem solving.

Combative: in this closed/forward mode, the listener presents resistance.

Communication: the act of transmitting information so that it is satisfactorily understood.

Community goals: goals pertaining to friends, community service, and so forth.

Compassion: the deep feeling of sharing or feeling the pain or suffering of another; sympathy.

Competent: In some rubrics, "competent" indicates that the student displays detailed and consistent evidence of competency; task is completed alone; performance includes rare errors.

Confidential student profile: a document containing personal student information and other relevant information, including copies of successful projects, thoughts on what motivates the student, goals and interests of the student, and any learning obstacles that affect the student.

Conflict management: conflict management involves implementing strategies to limit and manage negative aspects of conflict and to enhance learning and group effectiveness or performance in an educational setting.

Conscious (humor) competence: the educator understands or knows how to interject humor into the educational process. He possesses both a sense of humor and sensitivity to humor. However, demonstrating the humor requires a great deal of effort and concentration.

Conscious (humor) incompetence: the educator neither understands how to interject humor in the educational process nor recognizes the deficit, or doesn't have a desire to address it. At this stage, individuals don't appear to have a sense of humor, and the humor they do display is negative and demeaning.

Constructive criticism: a well-meant critique intended to help someone improve.

Consumption supplies: those supplies used in the daily operation of the institution.

Cost consciousness: one's performance in eliminating nonessential activities and costs, not wasting supplies, handling monies responsibly, observing energy-saving measures, and respecting the property of the institution.

Culture: the school's culture defines how students are trained, developed, and nurtured into professionals; the traits or distinguishing characteristics or qualities that make up the institution; the institution's personality.

Curriculum: a set of courses constituting an area of specialization.

Customer service: the set of behaviors that a business or institution undertakes during its interactions with its clients and/or students.

Decode: interpreting the message.

Deductive reasoning: This process allows learners to reach a probable conclusion by employing logical reasoning.

Demographics: The characteristics of human populations such as size, growth, density, distribution, and vital statistics.

Desire: a wish, longing, or craving; something longed for.

Destructive tactics: tactics used to take away and/or harm an individual's creation, prestige, or self-esteem.

Development opportunity: in some rubrics, "development opportunity" indicates that the student displays little or no evidence of competency; assistance is needed; performance includes multiple errors.

Distance learning: any mode of instruction in which there is a separation, in time or place, between the instructor and the student.

Downtime: salon time during which the student or professional is not serving a client; when used effectively, downtime becomes productive.

Dyslexia: a neurologically based, specific learning disability that hinders the learning of literacy or reading skills and creates a problem with managing verbal codes in memory.

Educational aids: aids that boost student success in the classroom and reinforce what a teacher says while helping to ensure that main points are understood. Educational teaching aids highlight important information, engage students' other senses in the learning process, and allow for different learning styles.

Educational goals: goals pertaining to formal and informal education, personal development and professional development.

Educational objective: a clear goal indicating what the student should be able to know or do as a result of the training.

Empathetic: characterized by an understanding so intimate that the feelings, thoughts, and motives of one individual are readily comprehended and understood by another.

Encode: packing information so that it is understood to achieve the desired results.

Ethics: the moral principles by which we live and work.

Facilitate: make easier, aid, assist.

Failure behaviors: any behavior that prevents a student from completing course requirements, achieving educational objectives, and preventing the student from attaining success.

Fear: a feeling of alarm or disquiet caused by the expectation of danger, pain, disaster, or the like; terror; dread; apprehension.

Fellowship: the condition of being together or sharing similar interests or experiences as do members of a profession.

Forward/back body posture: indicates that the listener is actively accepting the message.

Fugitive: the closed/back mode suggests the listener is trying to escape, either physically or mentally.

Fundamentals: in some rubrics, "fundamentals" indicates that the student displays beginning evidence of competency; task is completed alone; performance includes a few errors.

Gelotology: the formal name for the physiological study of humor and laughter and their effects on the human body.

Goal management: a powerful technique yielding strong returns and giving one long-term vision and short-term motivation; helps organize resources and helps one focus on the acquisition of knowledge.

Grading: the process of evaluating a student's performance or knowledge and assigning a letter or number that shows the student's level of achievement.

Half-rounds arrangement: an arrangement also called cabaret; most popular for learner-centered education; used for lecture, demonstration, discussion, slide or video projection, role-playing, group projects and activities; facilitator has lower degree of control, but this arrangement provides for high degree of eye contact, participation, and interaction.

Hitchhiking: taking an idea or information from another and hitchhiking or piggybacking off of it.

Human relations: the study of how people relate to each other in group situations, especially at work, and how communication skills and sensitivity to other people's feelings can be improved.

Idea: a formulated thought or opinion.

Incongruity theory: laughter occurs when the outcome is different from what is expected.

Independent action: one's performance in exercising initiative, working independently, solving problems, and maintaining steady performance under pressure.

Initiative: the power, ability, or instinct to begin and/or follow through with a plan or task.

Input: one of four stages of information processing used in learning; the information perceived through the senses, such as visual and auditory perception.

Integrate: one of four stages of information processing used in learning; in this stage perceived input is interpreted, categorized, placed in a sequence, or related to previous learning.

Interpersonal intelligence: the ability to relate to others, noticing their moods, motivations, and feelings.

Interpersonal skills: one's performance in keeping management informed, working cooperatively with others, communicating clearly, being a role model, never fraternizing with students, and conveying self-confidence.

Intrapersonal intelligence: the ability to understand one's own behavior and feelings.

Laughter: (1) the sound of laughing; (2) the cause of merriment, and *laugh* as "1) to show mirth, joy . . . with a smile; 2) to find amusement or pleasure in something."

Learning: to acquire knowledge, understanding, skills, or behavioral tendency by study, instruction, or experience.

Learning disability: a group of disorders that affect a broad range of academic and functional skills, including the ability to read, speak, listen, spell, reason, and organize information; it does not necessarily indicate low intelligence.

Likert scale: a measurement that uses a five-point rating scale ranging from "strongly agree" to "strongly disagree" or from "poor" to "excellent."

Liquid crystal display (LCD): an LCD projector is a device that is used to display video images or data. Light from a halogen lamp passes through glass panels and produces an image that can be projected onto any flat surface.

Logical/mathematical intelligence: the ability to understand logical reasoning and problem solving in areas such as math, science, sequences, and patterns.

Major life activities: human functions including caring for self, performing manual tasks, walking, seeing, hearing, speaking, breathing, learning, and working.

Mind mapping: creates a free-flowing, graphic organizing system to outline material or information.

Mission statement: describes the identity of the institution; it says what the school is, what it does, what it hopes to accomplish or what it is trying to change, who it services, and where it provides its services.

Mnemonics: any aid that is used to assist the learner's memory.

Multiple-category grading: an evaluation chart that incorporates scoring of more than one area of learner assessment.

Multipurpose board: a white magnetic marker board that functions in much the same way as a chalkboard but with many more uses.

Musical/rhythmic intelligence: the ability to comprehend and/or create meaningful musical sounds. This intelligence indicates an understanding and appreciation of music and ability to keep rhythm.

Mutuality: the act of having the same relationship each to the other; being directed and receiving direction in the same amount; each party having the same commitment to the relationship.

Naturalist intelligence: the ability to make consequential distinctions in the natural world and to use this ability productively such as in farming or biological science.

New-student orientation program: a briefing designed to acquaint students with the institution's educational programs and objectives, administrative policies and procedures, and student support services.

Objectives: something that one's efforts or actions are intended to attain or accomplish; purpose; goal.

Orientation program: a program or class that occurs on or before the first day of class that provides information about the educational program. It should cover the detailed program course outline and all its elements, school policies and procedures, and any other general information pertinent to the student's success in the program.

Outcome evaluation: grading that determines what the student knows after having been taught certain material or skills.

Outcome goal: a goal that focuses on the end result without focusing on the performance required to get there.

Output: one of four stages of information processing used in learning; in this stage information comes out of the brain either through words (language output) or muscle activity (gesturing, writing, or drawing).

Pedagogical tool: any tool or aid used in the art of preparatory training or instruction.

Peer coaching: a method that provides for one-on-one, personalized instruction that can increase learning results by allowing learners to set their own pace and receive individualized feedback on a regular basis.

Performance checklist: a factual and objective form of grading that uses specific performance criteria that help to remove educator bias from the rating process, resulting in more consistency.

Performance goal: a goal that focuses on specific performances that will ultimately result in the desired outcome goal.

Personal goals: goals pertaining to attitude, family, health, home, pleasure, spiritual/ethical, and so forth.

Point grading: grading that assigns specific weights or points to each criterion or task, which allows the educator to place emphasis on the more important tasks during evaluation.

Portfolio: a folder or binder used to sell services or obtain employment that includes key items such as a resumé, certificates, awards, before-and-after pictures of services, pictures from photo shoots, and so forth.

Position role-playing: the learner plays the part of a particular position (such as a technician, manager, or educator), rather than the part of a specific individual.

Praise: an expression of warm approval or admiration; strong commendation.

Private conference: a private meeting between the educator and learner that gives both the opportunity to discuss concerns (whether performance or behavioral) and potential solutions.

Problem solving: one's performance in solving problems, making decision, evaluating outcomes, and striving for a win–win solution.

Procrastination: to put off doing something until a future time; to postpone or delay needlessly.

Production: one's performance in meeting commitments and producing the expected volume of work or going beyond normal production requirements.

Professional goals: goals pertaining to finance, career, notoriety, and so forth.

Psychomotor domain: Objectives in the psychomotor domain relate to skill performance, which requires tools, objects, supplies, and equipment.

Rating scale: a grading chart similar to Likert scales but usually containing fewer rating categories; it can be used to compare a student's performance or behavior with specific standards established for a designated learning category.

Rebook: refers to a client booking a future appointment before leaving the student salon or professional service facility.

Referral: a client obtained from another client who has recommended that client to the student or professional for a service.

Reflective: the open/back mode indicates the listener is interested and receptive, but not actively accepting the information.

Reframing: seeing something from a different perspective, or through a different "frame."

Relater: relater communicators are warm and friendly and less concerned about themselves than others; they can ask questions of a personal nature.

Relationship: refers to the state of affairs existing between those who have an aspect or quality that connects them as being or belonging or working together.

Relief theory: laughter that occurs after a long period of tension, stress, suspension, or danger. This aspect of laughter is used in films quite effectively.

Repeat service: a service completed for a regular client such as a haircut scheduled every four to six weeks.

Responsive: the open/forward mode indicates the listener is actively accepting the message.

Responsiveness: the degree to which a person is open in interactions with others.

Retail supplies: those supplies sold to clients.

Retention plan: begins when a student walks in the door for the first time and continues until he or she graduates; it involves all institution personnel, regardless of position, and includes key elements such as establishing a vision and mission, sound ethical administrative policies, defining the school's culture, sound admissions procedures, a detailed new-student orientation program, instilling student ownership of the institution, developing and following a creative curriculum, employing energized educators, developing outstanding customer service, investing in the institution's educators, employing a praise policy.

Role-reversal role-playing: Learners assume the roles of other persons with whom they interact on a regular basis. For example, the student might play an educator or a client.

Rubric: a clearly developed scoring document used to differentiate between levels of development in a specific skill performance or behavior; it may also be used as a self-assessment tool.

Self-esteem: pride in oneself; the deep-down feeling you have in your own soul about your own value or self-worth.

Self-fulfilling prophecy: refers to the philosophy that we usually get what we actively expect. In education it is believed that conveying positive expectations, students have a greater chance to succeed.

Self-motivation: motivation fueled by one's dreams, ideals, and visions for the future.

Self-motivation: one's performance in pursuing success and excellence at all times, stretching personal resources, seeking opportunities to build on strengths, sustaining a high level of interest and enthusiasm, and completing at least 40 hours of continuing education annually.

Seller: seller communicators are "people" persons; they are touchy, feely, warm, and outgoing with others and assertive.

Semi-circle arrangement: an arrangement effective for small classes up to about 10 learners; effective for informal discussion; facilitator has high degree of control.

Situational barrier: a situational barrier to learning occurs when a learner temporarily exhibits difficult behavior that is different than the personality or behavior usually exhibited.

SMART goals: goals that are specific, measurable, attainable, relevant, and time-based.

Spontaneity theory: laughter that occurs as a result of an unplanned, momentary impulse.

Stamina: endurance; the physical or moral strength required to resist or withstand fatigue or hardship.

Stimuli: anything causing or regarded as causing a response; something that incites or rouses to action.

Storage: one of four stages of information processing used in learning.

Strength: in some rubrics, "strength" indicates that the student displays detailed evidence of highly creative, inventive, mature presence of competency.

Stress: a physical, chemical, or emotional factor that causes bodily or mental tension and may be an aspect in the cause of disease; the inability to cope with a threat, real or imagined, to our well-being that results in a series of responses and adaptations by our minds and bodies.

Study group: a group of like-minded students who get together to share notes, questioning, discussions, and so forth to prepare for each class or scheduled tests.

Summative evaluation: the process of assigning grades after testing has occurred.

Superiority theory: laughter that, albeit inappropriate, occurs at the expense of someone else's mistake or misfortune causing us to feel superior.

TASK: Technical Assessment of Skills and Knowledge; a practical and written test performed at various levels of training to determine the student's level of competence.

Team: a group of interdependent individuals who have complementary skills and are committed to a shared, meaningful purpose and specific goals.

Teamwork: a cooperative effort by a group of individuals working together to achieve a common goal.

Teamwork: work done by several associates with each doing a part but all subordinating personal prominence to the efficiency of the whole.

Telecommunications courses: courses offered principally through the use of one or more technologies to deliver instruction to students who are separated from the instructor and to support regular and substantive interaction between students and the instructors. These technologies include television, audio, or computer transmission through open broadcast, closed circuit, cable, microwave, or satellite, and audio and computer conferencing.

Test plan: consists of an outline of the content that will be covered by each test, applying weights to particular test questions based on lesson objectives.

Theater arrangement: an arrangement suitable for lecture, slide use, and video projection; can be used for small or very large groups; facilitator has high control; provides for poor opportunity for participation and interaction.

Thinker: thinker communicators are guarded in interactions with other thinkers; they are not outgoing; self-control is important to them.

Thoroughness and accuracy: one's performance in setting high standards, accurately completing assigned tasks, paying close attention to details, and detecting errors and correcting them as applicable.

Ticket upgrade: refers to the technician "adding on" additional services to what was previously booked for the client.

Time: a continuum that is measured in terms of events that succeed one another from past through present to the future.

Time Utilization Log: a document used to help you track how you spend your time, which is the first step in changing your ways and using your time more efficiently.

Transfer technique: a process that involves learners in decision making, establishing rules, and designing projects and contests, which ultimately results in the students taking ownership of the project or policy.

Transferable skills: the skills mastered at other jobs that can be put to use in a new position.

Trust: firm reliance on the integrity, ability, and character of a person or thing; confident belief; faith.

Unconscious (humor) competence: the educator has had so much practice with using humor in the classroom that it becomes "second nature" and can be performed easily (often without concentrating too deeply). The educator's humor is spontaneous, warm, and appropriate.

Unconscious (humor) incompetence: the educator neither understands how to interject humor in the educational process nor recognizes the deficit, or doesn't have a desire to address it. At this stage, individuals don't appear to have a sense of humor, and the humor they do display is negative and demeaning.

Unconscious incompetence: Abraham Maslow's theory states that *unconscious incompetence* means that "we don't know that we don't know."

U-shaped arrangement: an arrangement for small classes up to 15; effective for lecture, demonstration, and discussion; facilitator has high control.

Values: principles, standards, or qualities considered worthwhile or desirable.

Verbal/linguistic intelligence: the ability to communicate through language, which includes listening, reading, writing, and speaking.

Vision statement: outlines where the institution wants to be and concentrates on the future; it should be a source of inspiration and will provide clear decision-making criteria.

Visual aids: an instructional tool, such as a video, poster, model, chart, graph, or slide, that presents information visually.

Visual/spatial intelligence: the ability to understand spatial relationships and comprehend and create images.

Visualization: the process by which the mind translates the content of a lesson into visual imagery.

Weighting: the process of determining the importance of each content area that has been selected to test.

Window paning: window paning is the process of transferring key elements, points, or steps in a lesson to visual images that are then hand-sketched into the squares or "panes" of a matrix.

Work ethic: a set of values based on the moral virtues of hard work and diligence and includes the belief in the moral benefit of work and its ability to improve one's character.

Work ethic: taking pride in your work and committing yourself to consistently doing a good job for your students, clients, employer, and school team.

Work habits: one's performance in maintaining dependable, regular attendance, arriving promptly, keeping personal time to a minimum.

Work methods: one's performance in organization skills, meeting deadlines, correcting mistakes, prioritizing and not wasting time.

Zone teaching: a method of student salon supervision that considers three elements—student and client safety, client comfort, and practical teaching.

Biblography

Frost, R. (1920). *The road not taken*. New York: Henry Holt and Company.

Larson, C. (1912). *Your forces and how to use them: The optimist's creed*. Los Angeles: The New Literature Pub. Co.

McCarthy, B. (2013). *What is 4MAT? About Learning*. Official Site of Bernice McCarthy's 4MAT System. Retrieved from http://www.aboutlearning.com/what-is-4mat

Index